Seven Countries

This volume is published as part of a long-standing cooperative program between Harvard University Press and the Commonwealth Fund, a philanthropic foundation, to encourage the publication of significant scholarly books in medicine and health.

SEVEN COUNTRIES
Ancel Keys

A Multivariate Analysis of Death and Coronary Heart Disease

with
Christ Aravanis
Henry Blackburn
Ratko Buzina
B. S. Djordjević
A. S. Dontas
Flaminio Fidanza
Martti J. Karvonen
Noboru Kimura
Alessandro Menotti
Ivan Mohaček
S. Nedeljković
Vittorio Puddu
Sven Punsar
Henry L. Taylor
F. S. P. van Buchem

A Commonwealth Fund Book

Harvard University Press
Cambridge, Massachusetts
and London, England
1980

Copyright © 1980 by the President
and Fellows of Harvard College
All rights reserved
Printed in the United States of America

Library of Congress Cataloging in Publication Data
Keys, Ancel Benjamin, 1904–
Seven countries: a multivariate analysis of
death and coronary heart disease.

"A Commonwealth Fund book."
Includes bibliographical references and index.
1. Coronary heart disease—Europe—Statistics.
2. Coronary heart disease—United States—
Statistics.   3. Coronary heart disease—Japan—
Statistics.   4. Coronary heart disease—Etiology.
I. Title.   [DNLM: 1. Coronary disease—
Occurrence.   2. Coronary disease—Etiology.
WG300.3 K44s]
RC685.C6K42   616.1'23'071   79-9163
ISBN 0-674-80237-3

Foreword

Ancel Keys's *Seven Countries* is a monumental study, awesome in its dimensions, of a major biomedical problem. It is a meticulously planned and executed ten-year investigation of the epidemiology of coronary disease in six Western countries and Japan. Sixteen groups comprising 12,763 men, aged 40–59 at the outset, were followed in the seven countries: Yugoslavia, Finland, Italy, the Netherlands, Greece, the United States, and Japan.

Introductory comment is difficult because there is no prototype with which to compare Keys's opus. There have been other epidemiologic approaches to the problem of degenerative vascular diseases in the past, and all the significant ones are quoted in *Seven Countries*. They are, however, minuscule by comparison. Dr. Keys's book, although nominally covering a ten-year span, actually represents the coherent and concerted effort of a long professional career. It began in 1947, long before the vague and deceptive term *risk factor* had been coined. At that early date Keys and his colleagues recognized that the causes, and thus the possibilities for prevention, of coronary disease were not to be identified by clinical studies in hospital or by laboratory experimentation, however sophisticated. Such efforts might offer clues, as some indeed did; but they could do no more than that. What was required was the systematic observation of groups likely to be at risk, over relatively long spans of time and under conditions that could be defined but very deliberately left as uncontrolled as possible. This, a special application of the epidemiologic method, was not easy to apply convincingly and effectively even in the United States; to do so under so many different cultural conditions was a formidable undertaking, to say the least.

Yet, with the help and understanding of foreign colleagues, the work got done. Through the sixties and early seventies, Dr. Keys's perception and great energy kept the efforts in the seven countries moving, and some interim results were published as they became available. The present work surveys and summarizes the whole.

The chief effect of Dr. Keys's work is to provide critical new insights into the relationships between cultural conditions and the operation of certain of the usually accepted risk factors. No less important, the study tends to deflate the evangelical hysteria of those who would have us believe that if a person eliminates all suspected risk factors, freedom from coronary disease and a life span of a century or more are guaranteed. For example, in Finland the incidence of clinically significant coronary disease rose as the level of serum cholesterol rose, but in other populations this relationship was of negligible significance. As for cigarette smoking, it was "less predictive of heart attacks and premature death in southern Europe and Japan than in the United States and northern Europe." Nor do the studies (and the survey of the literature) bear out standard dogma, so important until very recently to American life insurance companies, concerning the relation between the incidence of obesity and the incidence of clinically significant coronary disease. Of even greater interest to Americans, in view of the great resurgence of interest in regular and vigorous physical exercise, is the conclusion that there is no "indication that the proportion of sedentary men in the population makes any difference to the average risk of developing coronary heart disease in that population." Even more startling was the finding that moderately active Finns were more susceptible to attacks of clinically significant coronary disease than those who were sedentary.

From these findings one can, depending on one's preconceptions, leap to the conclusion that such attractive vices as cigarette smoking and indolent living habits may safely be discounted as threats to health, at least insofar as coronary disease is concerned. But to draw such conclusions is clearly ill-advised.

Seven Countries is not to be read in a hurry, since the approach and treatment of data are of necessity highly sophisticated. Tentative conclusions, as often as not, are offered as questions or statements that do no more than emphasize the differences, startling in some instances, between population groups. They also serve as strong suggestions for further investigations by future workers. But they cannot safely be lifted out of context. Of the traditional risk factors, only two seemed to be positively related to the incidence of coronary disease in all the populations studied: arterial blood pressure and dietary intake of saturated fatty acids and cholesterol. This is not to say that other risk factors, such as heavy cigarette smoking, may safely be ignored for all populations and social conditions. Age is yet another risk factor usually taken as too obvious to require mention; quantitative expression of its effect is, however, difficult because it is usually expressed as a range, such as 10–20 years, 20–40 years, and so forth.

The Seven Countries Study is a massive and supremely important beginning, a classic-to-be that is already playing a role in influencing the design of research plans and, for that matter, the shape of research careers. How, apart from the use of the epidemiologic method as Keys has applied it, can one explain the high incidence of coronary deaths among the eastern Finns and Americans, as compared with the extremely low incidence in certain Greek and Japanese populations? And investigators who enter the field must reckon with the fact, deducible from the nature of the problem and of the research method, that their commitment is for decades, not months or years.

The genesis of coronary disease and its prevention are far more complex matters than was thought to be the case when Dr. Keys and his colleagues began their investigations soon after World War II. *Seven Countries* in an important sense represents the end of intellectual innocence. The study and its successors may one day permit Greeks, Japanese, Finns, and other nationals, including Americans, to discover the full extent of the evils of omission and commission we still inflict upon ourselves.

Carleton B. Chapman, M.D.

Acknowledgments

The many sources of financial support that carried the Seven Countries Study through the entry examinations and the first five years of follow-up have been acknowledged in previous publications (Keys et al. 1967; Keys 1970; Keys et al. 1972a, 1972b, 1972c; Hartog et al. 1968; Taylor et al. 1966; Menotti et al. 1977). The support needed to complete the ten-year follow-up came, for the most part, from the same sources, but with crucial additional grants from the U.S. Public Health Service (HE 3088, HE 4672, HE 4697, HE 4774, HE 4854, HE 5471), the American Heart Association, the Finnish Heart Association, the Japanese Ministry of Education, the Chiyoda Mutual Life Subsidiary Fund, the Institute of Public Health of Croatia, the Finnish State Science Board, the Sigrid Juselius Fund, the Yrjö Jahnsson Foundation, the Netherlands Nutrition Council, the Organization for Food and Nutrition Research, the Royal Institute for Research of Greece, Elais Oil Company, the Serbian Ministry for Health, the Serbian Council for Research, the International Cardiology Foundation, the International Olive Oil Council, U.S. Counterpart Funds for Yugoslavia, and private individuals and anonymous donors.

Publication of this book has been aided by a grant from the U.S. National Heart, Lung, and Blood Institute and by the Commonwealth Fund.

Persons who aided in the research through the first five years of follow-up have been cited in the publications referred to above. We do not forget their essential help, but it is proper here to emphasize our indebtedness to those who provided assistance after the five-year re-examinations, notably in the ten-year re-examinations, in the check on interim mortality, and in data processing.

Most of the data processing was done at the Laboratory of Physiological Hygiene of the University of Minnesota in Minneapolis, mainly by Rosemarie Hilk, David R. Jacobs, Norris Schulz, John Vilandré, and Allan Womelsdorf. Additional computer work was done at the Laboratory of Epidemiology and Biostatistics of the Istituto Superiore di Sanità, Rome, Italy, and at the Department of Community Health and Preventive Medicine of Northwestern University Medical School, Chicago, Illinois. At Rome, computer analysis was done by Gino Farchi, Arduino Verdecchia, Riccardo Capocaccia, Sergio Mariotti, Susanna Conti, and Piero Corradini. At Chicago, computer analyses were made by Dan Garside. We are grateful to all of these persons. Readers of this book will appreciate the central importance of the data processing and computer analyses.

The experience of the American railroad men after the five-year follow-up was learned from the records of the Railroad Retirement Board, Chicago, and the death certificates of the states in which the men died. It is a pleasure to acknowledge the help of H. Benjamin and J. Klein of the retirement board.

The research team in Finland included Drs. Matti Arstila, Martti Helin, Veikko Kallio, Martti J. Karvonen, Heikki Peltola, and Sven Punsar, nurse Laila Tolppanen, Mrs. Pirkko Saarelainen, and Mrs. Kaija Nygård. Dr. Alessandro Menotti contributed his experience and helped in the study. The following persons performed various tasks and did much work in the study: the late health-nurse Impi Lavikainen, nurse Pirjetta Hirvisalo, Mrs. Ester Ehnberg, Miss Sirpa Kontkanen, school teacher Reetta Rintala, nurse Aino Toivonen, Mrs. Aila Mikkola, Mrs. Anja Rantasalo, Miss Ulla Tammi, and Mrs. Kirsti Haapanen. The local physicians, Dr. Tauno Koistinen in the East and Dr. Pentti Vaittinen in the West, were helpful in many ways. Professor Leo Noro, then director of the Institute of Occupational Health, placed members and facilities of the institute at the disposal of the study.

In rural Italy, the ten-year re-examinations were aided by Drs. Paolo Dini, Giuseppe Messina, and Paolo Signoretti (all of Rome), Gÿorgÿ Lamm (then of Budapest, Hungary, now of Copenhagen, Denmark), and Josef Pokorny (of Prague, Czechoslovakia). Special help was given at Crevalcore by Antonio Pedretti and Alfonso Barbieri and at Montegiorgio by Egidio Marziali and Giuseppe Allessandrini. The ten-year work with the Italian railroad men involved the help of Drs. Francesco Ceccherini, Giuseppe Lobefaro, and Paolo Signoretti (all of Rome). We are also grateful to Aldo Bellini, Cesare Coluzzi, and Antonio DeBartolomeo of the Ministry of Transportation, Rome.

The physicians who aided the ten-year re-examintions in Serbia were Drs. Vladan Josipović, Ljubica Božinović, Dusan G. Stojanović (who died in

1978), Vladimir Slavković, Gradomir Stojanović, Srboljub Sekulić, Borica Balog, Natalija Simin, Dejan Bošković, and Miodrag Ostojić. We are also grateful to nurse Desa Lovrić. Petar Vulicević at Velika Krsna and Danilo Babić at Zrenjanin gave much help, as did Milica Dodić, secretary at the University of Belgrade.

The responsibility for the work in Japan, under the direction of Noboru Kimura, was shared by Hironori Toshima, Yukki Nakayama, and Hiromi Tashiro (all of Kurume), Ichiro Furukawa (Fukuoka), Fuminobu Mori (Shimonoseki), Shunichi Kodama (Beppu), and Syoji Nishimoto (Kitakyushu). The professional staff on the team at Tanushimaru and at Ushibuka in the ten-year follow-up study comprised Drs. K. Takayama, T. Fukami, T. Mizuguchi, M. Yoshinaga, K. Abe, T. Arima, F. Katayama, Y. Yokata, T. Tanioka, S. Nanbu, E. Minagawa, K. Yamada, S. Shimada, R. Tanaka, T. Akiyoshi, F. Ohshima, K. Soejima, K. Tanaka, A. Mizunoe, K. Akasu, H. Ikeda, K. Nakamura, T. Niizaki, E. Nishi, M. Ageta, T. Inoue, T. Nakagawa, Y. Miike, M. Takagi and Y. Inaba. The local physicians, Drs. Y. Egami, R. Harada, T. Nakano, K. Nakano, M. Kimura, and T. Onizuka in Tanushimaru, and Drs. A. Kukumoto, Y. Hamasaki, H. Hatta, M. Kawano, M. Nishimura, T. Sato, T. Takahira, and T. Tateshi in Ushibuka, provided information about previous illnesses of the subjects. Special thanks are due to Major T. Inoue and Major A. Urata for local help in Tanushimaru and Ushibuka, respectively.

Important help in the ten-year followup at Zutphen was provided by Drs. F. S. P. van Buchem, E. B. Bosschieter, and Th. F. S. M. van Schaik and by A. H. Thomassen-Gijsbers, J. Brands-Thomassen, and N. H. Meures-Blom.

The work of the ten-year follow-up in Croatia was greatly aided by Drs. Ivan Mohaček, Miljenko Marinković, Djordje Vukadinović, Ante Smetiško, and Zdenko Radošević, all of Zagreb, by Dr. M. Marinović, pharmacist M. Barbieri, and I. Kosović of Makarska, and by Drs. C. Vugrinčić, B. Miljuš, and I. Vlahović of Osijek.

In the ten-year follow-up in Greece, the assistance of George Arnoukatis and Dr. E. Staphylakis in Crete was valuable. Direct help was also given by Dr. Adrian Corcondilas, by Drs. L. Anthopolous, C. Vasilikos, and D. Lekos in the field clinical examinations and by Maria Tzelisi, M. Papadatou, E. Sdrin, and the members of the diet group in the field laboratory. Dr. D. Galanos, Professor F. Fidanza, and Professor J. T. Anderson were helpful in performing the chemical analyses.

Contents

1 Introduction *1*
2 Methods *17*
3 Prevalence of Cardiovascular Disease at Entry *34*
4 Ten-Year Deaths *64*
5 Ten-Year Incidence of Coronary Heart Disease *85*
6 Age *96*
7 Blood Pressure *103*
8 Serum Cholesterol *121*
9 Smoking Habits *136*
10 Overweight and Obesity *161*
11 Physical Activity *196*
12 Resting Pulse Rate *218*
13 Respiratory Function *235*
14 Diet *248*
15 Multivariate Analyses *263*
16 Change at the Ten-Year Follow-up *296*
17 Some Conclusions *315*
Appendix *345*
References *362*
Index *373*

Seven Countries

1 | Introduction

The prospective research program known as the Seven Countries Study was a logical outgrowth of explorations on the epidemiology of coronary heart disease (CHD) that began early in 1952 in Italy and Spain (Keys 1952, 1953a). Those international studies, in turn, had their inspiration in a prospective study on Minnesota business and professional men that started in 1947. The aim of this study was to find individual characteristics in apparently healthy middle-aged men related to future tendency to develop CHD, an aim based on the conviction that "the physico-chemical characteristics of the individual should have predictive value" (Keys 1949). It was believed that the discovery of predictive variables—what we now call *risk factors*—should point the way to preventive efforts (Keys 1953b).

The results of the early work in Italy and Spain stimulated an international group to join in larger surveys in Italy in 1954 (Keys 1956; White 1956). The findings in Naples, Cagliari, and Bologna, compared with similar hospital surveys in the United States, confirmed the belief in marked differences among populations in the frequency of CHD. The feasibility of organizing international teams of clinicians and medical scientists to produce comparable measurements and diagnoses in different populations was further demonstrated in South Africa in 1955 (Bronte-Stewart, Keys, and Brock 1955) and in Japan and Finland in 1956 (Keys 1957a; Keys et al. 1958; Roine et al. 1958; Keys, Karvonen, and Fidanza 1958). Those studies also indicated that populations differing in the fats in the diet also differ in the concentration of cholesterol in the blood serum, and these two features are associated with contrasts in the frequency of CHD. By that time, too, follow-up studies in Framingham, Massachusetts, Albany, and Los Angeles were clearly pointing to the importance of arterial blood pressure and serum cholesterol as risk factors (Chapman et al. 1957; Dawber, Moore, and Mann 1957; Doyle et al. 1957).

Clearly it would be important to extend to samples of populations in other countries similar examination and follow-up studies, assuring comparability with international teams using a common protocol, standardized methods and criteria, and exchanging professional personnel between the countries concerned. Further to assure comparability, it seemed essential to concentrate at a single center the evaluation of electrocardiograms, measurement of cholesterol in blood serum, review of diagnoses, and all data processing. The Laboratory of Physiological Hygiene at the University of Minnesota was designated as the central headquarters.

Aims

One aim of such a collaborative international study was to discover to what extent the incidence rates of the various cohorts could be predicted from the experience of earlier follow-up studies in the United States, taking into account the characteristics of the cohorts in regard to the risk factors stressed in the American studies. A high degree of consistency in the experience of major prospective studies in the United States had become evident from the Pooling Project analysis of data from Albany, Chicago, Framingham, Los Angeles, Minnesota, and Tecumseh, Michigan, but that fact was not known until recently. Moreover, the samples of men in the Pooling Project analysis did not differ enough in regard to socioeconomic, ethnic, cultural, and genetic characteristics to allow universal conclusions for other populations.

A broader aim was to attempt to relate differences in incidence among cohorts to the average or general characteristics of the men in the cohorts, including their living habits. Does the incidence of CHD and of death in the various cohorts differ from that in the United States? Does the incidence vary among the cohorts? Are the differences, if any, from experience in the United States explained by the risk factors as weighted according to the experience of studies in the United States? To what extent can differences in incidence among the cohorts be explained by a multivariate analysis of characteristics of the makeup of those cohorts as indicated by the variables recorded for the subjects?

Some of the populations sampled differed markedly in the average diet, so dietary characteristics could be treated as a variable in comparisons between cohorts. Another aim of this study was to see whether consideration of dietary variables could help explain differences among the cohorts in their disease experience.

Definition of the Cohorts

For practical reasons the study is confined to men aged 40 through 59 at the entry examination. Women or younger men would yield relatively low incidence rates and therefore would require much larger numbers. Moreover, younger men are generally less stable in residence and therefore more difficult to follow. Men over 60 at entry would yield higher incidence rates, but a large proportion of them would have excluding prevalence conditions at entry. Also, considering possible future preventive efforts, relationships that might be found in old age seemed likely to be less relevant to younger ages when, presumably, the prospects for prevention would be better. Similar considerations have dictated the selection of middle-aged men as the subjects in most other prospective studies.

We wished to keep self-selection of the subjects to a minimum and to strive for near-zero loss to follow-up. Both goals were achieved by concentrating on rural areas. Rural men aged 40 or more are less likely than urban and younger men to change occupation, habits, or residence. Community spirit and cohesiveness tend to be inversely related to the size of the community, thus assuring good response in small communities if we had the cooperation of local leaders. It was decided to invite all men aged 40–59 in the selected areas to participate because an attempt to sample within an age class might be divisive.

Elsewhere we have reported details of the selection of the areas for study, the organization of the study teams, and the general characteristics of the cohorts at the entry examinations (Keys et al. 1967; Keys 1970), and only brief notes are given here. For each cohort a roster was compiled of men eligible because of age and geographical location of residence. At the entry examinations, some men not on these rosters presented themselves for examination, and in some cases they were examined. However, they were not enrolled in the cohort unless the original omission of their names had been in error.

Rural men. Of the sixteen cohorts, eleven were strictly rural; they lived and worked in areas of low population density where agriculture, forestry, and fishing are the only industries. Forestry is an important activity only in the two areas of east and west Finland, and only for the Japanese men of Ushibuka, Japan, is fishery the major activity, though a few of the men in Dalmatia were fishermen.

The rosters of men eligible for the study in the eleven rural areas included all men then 40–59 permanently residing in geographically defined regions. The lists were compiled from local registers and tax and voting lists and were checked against church, police, and other records. In Japan and the European countries, all adults have identity documents that are locally registered. For five cohorts the geographical areas consisted of single large villages: in Italy, Crevalcore in the Po Valley and Montegiorgio in the Region of Marche near the Adriatic Coast; in Japan, Tanushimaru and Ushibuka on the big southern island of Kyushu; in Serbia, Velika Krsna south of Belgrade, Yugoslavia. For each of the other six rural areas the geographical definition embraced a number of villages clustered in a limited area. Dalmatia refers to a series of villages strung along 60 kilometers on the Dalmatian coast of Yugoslavia, with Makarska the nearest town. Slavonia comprises Dalj and nearby small villages near the Danube River and the Hungarian frontier, with Ossiek the nearest town of any size. East Finland was represented by villages in north Karelia near the Russian border centering on the town of Joensuu. West Finland comprises villages of similar character not far from Turku; Crete, eleven villages southeast of Heraklion on the Greek island of Crete; Corfu, seven villages in the northeast part of the island of Corfu, Greece.

Railroad men. In the United States it was not considered feasible to establish rural cohorts comparable to those organized in Europe and Japan because of the geographic and occupational mobility characteristic of many men in the United States. However, men employed by the railroad industry are relatively stable in these respects and are very rarely lost to follow-up, because the pensions, death, and disability benefits of the Railroad Retirement Board provide powerful incentives to maintain contact with the board. Accordingly, with the cooperation of the board and the railroad unions and management, a statistical sample was drawn of men employed in specified occupations by the major American railroad companies in the northwest sector of the country, roughly defined by the quadrangle of Green Bay, Wisconsin, Saint Louis, San Francisco, and Seattle. Sampling took account of the size of the community and the geographic region and attempted to provide subsamples defined by occupation so as to afford contrasts between sedentary and more physically active men. Sedentary railroad men were represented by executives, dispatchers, and sedentary clerks (not all clerks in the lists of railroad employees are sedentary in their work). Physically active men were represented by switchmen.

Details of sampling the American railroad men and a discussion of the question of self-selection have been published by Taylor et al. (1966). Self-selection is particularly important for the American railroad men because their rate of response to participate in the study was lower than in the other cohorts. Of those invited, only 75 percent came in for examination (the 68 percent figure given in Taylor et al., p. I-22, refers to the least responsive group, the switchmen). Apparently, some switchmen refused examination because they feared that revealing a disability would mean transfer to a less active job with lower pay. However, detailed analysis of the data on the railroad men failed to indicate any significant difference between the occupational classes in either risk factors or subsequent incidence of disease. Accordingly, in the present report the railroad occupations have been pooled in most of the analyses.

To provide a European sample to compare with the American railroad men, all men aged 40–59 in specified occupations employed by the Italian State Railroad in the Rome division were invited to join the study. The Rome division extends 318 kilometers along the west coast of Italy. As in the United States, railroad men in Italy are stable in their occupations, and their status is easy to follow because of the provisions for disability, retirement, and death benefits. Although the response of the Italian railroad men to the invitation to participate was better than that of their American counterparts, it did not approach the nearly perfect response of the rural Italians. Not all men who failed to present themselves for examination actually selected themselves out of the study of Italian railroad men. Unlike the relatively convenient arrangements for the other cohorts, the examinations of the Italian railroad men were made at the main Rome railroad station, and for many of the men it was difficult to adjust work schedules for a long trip to and from Rome.

Lack of funds prevented ten-year examinations for the American railroad men. However, with the help of the Railroad Retirement Board, a careful check was made of mortality in the ten years after the entry examinations. For the Italian railroad cohort it was not possible to examine all survivors at precisely ten years after the entry examination; men were examined over a span of about ten to eleven years after entry, some examinations being made in their homes.

Zutphen, the Netherlands. In the Netherlands the Dutch investigators selected the small commercial market town of Zutphen in the eastern part of the country because it offered practical advantages of local hospitals and physicians and had been the site of earlier health surveys. Because Zutphen had more men aged 40–59 than could be covered with the resources available, a statistical sample was drawn of four out of nine men of the eligible age. That roster took so long to prepare that when the examinations were made only one man remained in the age 40 category; men listed as that age in the roster had graduated to the age 41 class.

At Zutphen only 84.3 percent of the invited men presented themselves for examination. This response, much lower than in the rural areas, bears out the rule that cohesiveness diminishes as the size of the community increases. However, a check on the subsequent disease and mortality experience of the no-shows with the local physicians and hospitals failed to show that they were, in this respect, different from the men who formed the active cohort. It does not seem, therefore, that self-selection at Zutphen created a bias in regard to future disease in the cohort actually enrolled for examination and follow-up.

Serbia: Zrenjanin and the Belgrade University faculty. Zrenjanin, in Serbia north of Belgrade, is an agricultural town with a little light industry. A cohort of men 40–59 for the Seven Countries Study was organized in a large cooperative in Zrenjanin that operates farms, a slaughterhouse, processing plants for foods, and other agricultural products, and a small packaging factory for chemicals and cosmetics. Of the men aged 40–59 associated with the cooperative, 98 percent agreed to form the Zrenjanin cohort.

Of the sixteen cohorts for which ten-year results are reported here, the last to be formed comprised members of the faculty of the University of Belgrade who were 40 through 59 years old in 1964. Because of some questions about which men in the employ of the university should be classed as faculty, there is some uncertainty about the precise percentage response to invitation, but it was at least 80 percent. Although university professors are not representative of the general population, the relationships between their entry characteristics and subsequent disease experience was examined.

Selection of the Areas

Opportunity and practicability determined the selection of the several areas for inclusion in the Seven Countries Study. The decision to work in Italy reflected personal contacts made in our first explorations in that country. In the absence of any detailed information about the incidence of disease, the diet, and the characteristics of the men of Crevalcore and Montegiorgio, it was enough to have the assurance of our colleague Flaminio Fidanza that we would have good cooperation in those rural areas and that the cost of the work would be within our resources. It was suggested that the two areas might differ much in the diet, but this was not borne out by the dietary surveys.

Friendship with our colleague Ratko Buzina led to selection of areas of Dalmatia and Slavonia where he had friends to help and where, again, we could expect low cost and high cooperation. Although the two areas were expected to offer a dietary contrast, almost nothing was known about the incidence of CHD and other disease.

Japan was a natural selection because, of all countries with anything like credible vital statistics, it seemed to be the lowest in CHD. The compelling practical reason was that Noboru Kimura, who had once worked with us in Minnesota, offered enthusiastic help at little cost. The farming village of Tanushimaru and the fishing village of Ushibuka were selected because local physicians in those areas offered to help.

Similarly, collaboration with Martti J. Karvonen, initiated during work on committees of the World Health Organization and the Food and Agriculture Organization of the United Nations, led to the choice of Finland, which had the appeal of the world's highest CHD mortality according to vital statistics, very competent clinical help, and a cooperative population.

In Greece, friends A. S. Dontas and Christ Aravanis led us to Crete where the diet was said to be remarkably high in olive oil but where there were no reliable data on the incidence of CHD. The island of Corfu was selected because the Greeks consider it to be far more "European" than Crete.

Personal contacts with M. J. L. Dols of The Hague, developed during joint work on United Nations committees, resulted in the presence of a Dutch observer at the international trials of protocol and methods for the Seven Countries Study. As a result, the Dutch government proposed that the Netherlands be represented in the study.

B. S. Djordjevic, then president of the Jugoslav Society of Cardiology, was an observer at the entry examinations at Corfu in 1961. He returned to Belgrade determined to organize Serbian cohorts to be included in the study. Because little was known of the frequency of CHD or the character of the diet, these variables were not involved in the selection of the areas in Serbia. As elsewhere, the determining factors were proffered aid, little expense, and assurance of cooperation.

The foregoing information about the selection of the areas for the Seven Countries Study is offered to counter unfounded suggestions that the cohorts were chosen on the basis of prior knowledge that promised to support a hypothesis of a causal link between diet and incidence of CHD.

Entry Examinations

In 1957 full-dress trials of the protocol, methods, and organization proposed for the present study were carried out in the village of Nicotera near Reggio Calabria on the Italian boot and in a number of villages on the island of Crete in Greece. Physicians and medical scientists from England, Finland, France, Japan, the Netherlands, the United States, and Yugoslavia joined the Italian and Greek teams. Most of the key persons in the later long-term study took part in the preliminary work in Italy and Greece.

After refinements of protocol, methods, and organization, the present long-term study was started in 1958 with the establishment of rosters and entry examinations for two areas of Croatia, Yugoslavia, the farming village of Tanushimaru, in the northern part of the island of Kyushu in Japan, and railroad workers in the northwestern part of the United States. As indicated in table 1.1, over the next six years the program was extended to cover a total of 12,763 men aged 40 through 59 at the time of their examinations. There were sixteen cohorts in seven countries enrolled by 1964. The next year the program was extended to Hungary with the leadership of George Lamm, then on the faculty of the medical school of the University of Budapest, now in the European office in Copenhagen of the World Health Organization. Three rural areas of southern Hungary near Szeged were represented by 1,041 men examined in 1965 and 1966. In 1976 ten-year reexaminations were begun in those areas with Dr. Ivan Gyarfas in charge, but a full report on the ten-year experience must await receipt and analysis of the data.

Table 1.1 shows that, in general, a high proportion of the men eligible to participate responded to the invitation for the entry examinations. For all sixteen cohorts combined, 90.4 percent of men invited appeared for examination. We have already discussed the relatively low response rates of the railroad men, the men on the faculty of the University of Belgrade, and the men of Zutphen. Except in the case of the United States railroad men, there is no reason to suggest that self-selection in regard to response might have biased the rates of prevalence of CHD and of cardiovascular disease (CVD) including CHD indicated by the entry examinations. The present report focuses on the incidence of disease and death among men found to be CHD- and CVD-free at entry. In view of the high response rate in the present study, it seems unreasonable to suggest that the men found to be CHD- and CVD-free might not be representative of all men similarly free of these diseases in the eligible sample. In any case the findings on incidence of disease and death among sizable groups of men in ethnically diverse cultures are of independent interest, regardless of whether these findings can be generalized to the entire population of the countries concerned.

Ten-year Follow-up

Of the 1,512 deaths in the ten years following the entry examinations, 413 were attributed to coronary heart disease, or a total mortality of 11.85 percent, and a CHD mortality of 3.23 percent. In the fourteen cohorts fully covered by ten-year reexaminations (9,424 men at entry), 435 men suffered hard CHD, that is, either dying from CHD or having a definite nonfatal infarction, making a ten-year incidence of 4.62 percent.

Table 1.1 indicates the magnitude of the data available for the present

Table 1.1. Definition of the sixteen cohorts (CHD-free = number free of coronary heart disease; CVD-free = number free of cardiovascular disease; N = number of men, aged 40–59, examined).

Entry year	Cohort	Response rate (%)	N (men examined)	CHD-free	CVD-free
1958–60	U.S. railroad	75.0	2,571	2,454	2,315
1958	Dalmatia, Yugoslavia (Croatia)	98.0	671	670	662
1958	Slavonia, Yugoslavia (Croatia)	91.0	696	692	681
1958	Tanushimaru, Japan	100.0	508	506	504
1959	East Finland	99.3	817	775	728
1959	West Finland	97.0	860	845	806
1960	Ushibuka, Japan	99.6	502	498	496
1960	Crevalcore, Italy	98.5	993	982	956
1960	Montegiorgio, Italy	99.0	719	713	708
1960	Zutphen, Netherlands	84.3	878	864	845
1960	Crete, Greece	97.6	686	682	655
1961	Corfu, Greece	95.3	529	526	525
1962	Rome railroad	80.6[a]	768	758	736
1962	Velika Krsna, Yugoslavia (Serbia)	96.7	511	504	487
1963	Zrenjanin, Yugoslavia (Serbia)	98.0	516	508	476
1964	Belgrade, Yugoslavia (Serbia)	80.0	538	532	516
	Total	90.4	12,763	12,509	12,096

a. Only about half of the men missed were refusals; work schedules prevented many men from keeping appointments.

report. Crude incidence rates can be calculated from the figures in table 1.2, but in the detailed analyses to follow all rates are age-standardized, as explained in chapter 2.

Other Prospective Studies

Prospective studies covering substantial numbers of middle-aged men began in 1948. Table 1.3 lists sixteen major studies with the common purpose of attempting to identify and measure characteristics that predispose to or hinder the development of the disease. The study of longshoremen was

Table 1.2. The Seven Countries Study: Ten-Year Incidence (hard CHD = CHD death or definite myocardial infarction).

Cohort	N	All-causes deaths	CHD deaths	Hard CHD
U.S. railroad[a]	2,571	294	146	—
Dalmatia	671	61	7	14
Slavonia	696	124	15	22
Tanushimaru	508	58	5	9
East Finland	817	147	78	115
West Finland	860	127	30	61
Ushibuka	502	70	4	13
Crevalcore	993	136	24	51
Montegiorgio	719	74	10	27
Zutphen	878	109	38	59
Crete	686	42	1	4
Corfu	529	43	8	19
Rome railroad[b]	768	77	22	31
Velika Krsna	511	63	4	8
Zrenjanin	516	60	8	14
Belgrade	538	27	13	19
Total	12,763	1,512	413	466

a. No 10-year examinations.
b. Ten-year examinations incomplete.

primarily an analysis of death records of men for whom employment and some examination data were recorded in 1951, but in the other studies the methodology was essentially the same as in the present work: selection of a target sample or population, examination with standardized methods of as many of the eligible men as were willing, reexamination at set intervals of follow-up, and diligent search for information about the status of all men who could not be reexamined with the prescribed protocol.

In these studies, as in the present work, questions arise about the relevance of the findings to groups or populations other than the men actually studied. In most of the studies the target sample was preselected according to employment. Are men in particular occupations representative of men of like age in the area and in general? Because men whose activities are limited by disease are underrepresented in samples of full-time regular employees, prevalence data on such men have limited applicability. Another limitation concerns all studies in which a substantial number of men in the target sample failed to appear for examination. The effect of nonresponse to the

Table 1.3. Follow-up studies on men aged 40–59 (except where noted).

Study	Year of entry	N	Response rate (%)
1. Minnesota business, professional men 45–55 (Keys et al. 1963)	1948	300	92
2. Framingham residents, 40–60+ (Dawber, Kannel, and Lyell 1963)[a]	1948–50	1,379	66
3. Los Angeles civil servants (Chapman and Massey 1964)[b]	1950–51	1,092	75
4. San Francisco longshoremen, 35–64 (Borhani, Hechter, and Breslow 1963)	1951	3,263	67
5. Albany, N.Y., civil servants (Doyle et al. 1957)	1953–54	1,829	89
6. Chicago Western Electric Co. employees (Paul et al. 1963)	1957	2,080	67
7. Chicago Peoples Gas Co. employees (Stamler 1973; Stamler et al. 1968)[c]	1958	1,465	92
8. Tecumseh, Michigan, residents (Johnson, Epstein, and Kjelsberg 1965)[d]	1959–60	798	88
9. California corporation employees, 39–59 (Rosenman et al. 1975)	1960	3,524	66
10. Oslo, Norway, employees, 40–49 (Westlund and Nicolaysen 1972)	1960	3,751	?
11. Evans County, Georgia, residents, 45–64 (McDonough et al. 1965)[e]	1960–62	646	92
12. Gothenburg, Sweden, men born 1913, aged 50 (Tiblin, Wilhelmsen, and Werko 1975)	1963	855	88
13. Israel civil servants (Medallie et al. 1968)	1963	7,666	86
14. Two areas of Yugoslavia, residents, 35–62 (Kozarevič et al. 1976)	1964–68	11,121	93
15. Puerto Rico residents, 45–59 (Gordon et al. 1974)	1965–68	6,954	81
16. Japanese in Honolulu, residents, 45–59 (Gordon et al. 1974)	1965–68	6,217	81

a. About 15 percent of the 1,379 men were volunteers not on the original invited list.
b. One-fourth of the 1,092 men were alternates to replace men who refused examination.
c. Reported on 667 men in the gas company whose medical records started in 1954.
d. A response rate of 88 percent was reported for the total of both sexes and all ages 15 and over at Tecumseh.
e. Combining sexes and ages, 92 percent response rate.

invitation for examination is considered further in chapter 3. A major bias could result from men who refuse examination because they know or suspect they are abnormal or diseased. The converse situation, men who refuse examination because they believe they are perfectly healthy and do not need examination, is of less concern because the true prevalence of detectable serious disease is low in samples, such as in these studies, and it is unlikely to be higher among men who feel particularly healthy.

The studies listed in table 1.3 were concerned with incidence, and the real question concerns the relationship between entry characteristics and the future appearance of disease. Whether the men in the follow-up study are representative of some larger population in regard to particular characteristics at entry is not the issue. We are interested in relationships. The mean blood pressure in the sample may differ from that of all men of the same age in the community, but that does not necessarily mean that a relationship between blood pressure and the frequency of later CHD found in the sample is irrelevant to the men in the community or in some other community. So we conclude that the significance of relationships emerging from the studies listed in table 1.3, and those found in the present study, is not limited to the particular studies, provided, of course, that other things are equal or at least comparable. Multivariate analysis is a powerful method in the attempt to satisfy this last stipulation.

The studies listed in table 1.3 cover something like half a million man-years of follow-up of men middle-aged at the start. Unfortunately, it is not possible to pool that great mass of data for a giant analysis extending to six countries and the United States. Data from eight of the American studies have been pooled to some extent (Pooling Project Research Group 1978). Those studies are numbers 1, 2, 3, 5, 6, 7, and 8 in table 1.3; some data from the United States railroad men in the Seven Countries Study were also included in the Pooling Project. It should be noted that the numbers of men in table 1.3 for the studies in the Pooling Project are somewhat larger than the numbers actually included in the analyses in the project because men with coronary heart disease at the entry examinations were excluded from the analyses.

Although useful, the results from the Pooling Project present many problems. In general, the methods and criteria in the several studies were similar but not identical because the studies were independently planned and operated; pooling was attempted long after the work was finished. Furthermore, with the exception of the Framingham and Tecumseh studies, the men in the Pooling Project are not samples of ordinary populations; they are somewhat self-selected samples of particular work forces. That limitation also applies to the studies on the San Francisco longshoremen, the California corporation employees, the Oslo employees, and the Israeli civil servants.

Because the studies focused on the incidence of coronary heart disease and not total mortality, comparison of death rates and of the ratio of coronary to other deaths is not possible from the published reports. Another point of interest is the fact that a substantial number of eligible, invited men did not participate in the studies. An average of 82 percent of the men invited for examination responded. In the Seven Countries Study the average response rate to the invitation to participate was 90.4 percent; excluding the United States railroad men, the response rate was 93 percent. However, as will be shown in chapter 3, even that high level of response does not guarantee a good estimate of the prevalence of disease in the target population. Unless the response rate is extremely poor, there is little danger of an overestimation of prevalence, but unless substantially 100 percent response is obtained an important underestimation of prevalence is possible.

Accordingly, we do not emphasize comparisons among samples or populations in regard to prevalence. Moreover, all men given a diagnosis of coronary heart disease at the entry examination were excluded from all analyses of incidence. However, the subsequent experience of men found to have coronary heart disease at entry is of interest in regard to prognosis (see chapter 3).

Any attempt to compare incidence rates among these studies must raise serious questions about diagnostic comparability. Recognition of that difficulty led the collaborators in the Pooling Project to confine the analyses to myocardial infarction and death as manifestations of coronary heart disease. In this book we also concentrate on the incidence of myocardial infarction and death from coronary heart disease, that is, hard CHD. As will be seen, the incidence of angina pectoris and other soft diagnoses is much less closely related to the risk factors than diagnoses of coronary heart disease that involve electrocardiographic criteria. Furthermore, the experience of this study is that, although uncomplicated angina pectoris carries the risk of future more serious manifestations, the prognosis is much less ominous than that of myocardial infarction, even when the infarct survivor has no clinical signs of disability after the acute episode.

In many reports on the epidemiology of coronary heart disease, the various manifestations of the disease are combined. This is understandable in view of the desire to offer a significant number of cases, but it also means that reported incidence rates are often of uncertain comparability. Another reason why it is generally difficult to compare incidence rates of different studies is the common practice of reporting incidence by ten-year or even twenty-year age groups. As will be emphasized in chapter 6, age is the most important of the risk factors, and incidence rates for ten-year age groups are not comparable unless the age distributions are essentially identical. Even though the age distributions of the men in the sixteen cohorts of the Seven Countries Study are closely similar, we have used age-standardized rates in all cohort comparisons. Furthermore, because some important characteristics, notably blood pressure, respiratory function, and smoking habits, are related to age, age must be allowed for in evaluating risk factors; here, also, age groupings may confound age and the risk factors of concern.

Death from coronary heart disease generally raises fewer questions about comparability than diagnoses of angina pectoris, coronary insufficiency, and many cases of previous infarction. Thus it might seem reasonable to compare coronary death rates in various studies. However, for the studies listed in table 1.3, death rates standardized by single years of age are not available.

Summary

Prospective studies on the epidemiology of coronary heart disease began in the late 1940s in the belief that, if clinically healthy persons were examined, queried, and followed over the years, it would be possible to identify characteristics associated with the development of clinical coronary heart disease. It was hoped that such knowledge would provide a basis for preventive measures. These programs started in the United States because the coronary problem seemed most serious there, but it was soon realized that comparisons with other populations would be instructive. Are there, as rumored, large differences among populations in the frequency of the disease? If so, what are the characteristics of the populations, including their mode of life, associated with differing rates of incidence of the disease? The cholesterol hypothesis, then being revived, needed test of the idea, derived from animal experiments but rejected by leaders of clinical medicine in the 1930s, that the diet of a population would be reflected in the level of cholesterol in the blood which, in turn, would affect susceptibility to coronary heart disease. Finally, questions were asked about the natural history of the disease. Are there population differences in the manifestations or in the force of what, years later, would be called risk factors?

In 1952 explorations in Italy and Spain showed marked differences in the average blood cholesterol level of men subsisting on the contrasting diets of working men in Naples and Madrid, (Keys 1953a; Keys 1956). Local physicians insisted that coronary heart disease was very rare in the working class of Naples and Madrid. Still greater contrasts were found when the explorations were extended to South Africa, Hawaii, Japan, California, and Finland. Obviously, a systematic international prospective study, with common protocol and fixed criteria, was needed.

In 1957, full-scale trials were made in Italy and Greece to test methods and work out the organization of international teams and a common center for all data and analyses. Medical scientists participating in that work in 1957 came from England and France and the seven countries—Finland, Greece, Italy, Japan, the Netherlands, the United States, and Yugoslavia—in which the long-time collaborative study was organized. The prospective program began in 1958 with the establishment of rosters and entry examinations of men 40–59 years old in the two rural areas of Croatia, Yugoslavia, a farming center in Japan, and the start of examinations of men employed by railroad companies in the northwestern sector of the United States. The last entrants into the study, members of the faculty of the University of Belgrade, were examined in 1964.

The study concerns sixteen cohorts of men in areas suggested as affording a wide range of contrasts in the mode of life. All men aged 40–59 in the specified areas, or in the designated samples, were invited to participate. The phrase *designated samples* refers to men in certain railroad occupations in specific regions in the United States and Italy and a randomly selected 44.4 percent sample of all men 40–59 in the small town of Zutphen, the Netherlands. All men 40–59 on the faculty of the University of Belgrade and in a big cooperative at Zrenjanin, a Serbian agricultural center, were invited to make up two cohorts. The other eleven cohorts comprised the responders to invitations to participate in geographically defined rural areas in Croatia, Finland, Italy, Japan, Greece, and Serbia. A total of 12,763 men, over 90 percent of those invited, are covered by this study. Deaths and major illnesses were checked annually. Reexaminations were made yearly at Zutphen and at the five- and ten-year anniversaries of the other cohorts except for the American railroad men who were reexamined at five years; at ten years finances permitted only a thorough review of mortality.

All examination records, medical histories, electrocardiograms, and copies of death certificates were sent to the University of Minnesota for central processing and diagnostic review. Measured samples of blood serum, dried, were analyzed at the University of Minnesota, as were the lyophylized samples of the diets. Professional personnel were exchanged among the areas, and representatives of the area teams worked from time to time at the University of Minnesota center so as to assure standardization of methods and criteria.

The present book reports characteristics of the men in the sixteen cohorts at entry, intercorrelations among the several entry variables, and the differences among the cohorts. The major focus of the book is the ten-year experience of death and the incidence of coronary heart disease and the relationships of the incidence rates to the characteristics recorded at entry. During the ten years, 1,512 men died, 413 from coronary heart disease. Most of the analyses concern the 12,095 men who showed no evidence of cardiovascular disease at the entry examinations.

2 | Methods

The examination and analytical methods used in the Seven Countries Study have been described elsewhere in some detail (Keys et al. 1967, 1972a; Keys 1970), but some important items will be spelled out here. In the preparation of the protocol and in the conduct of the examination, great efforts were made to assure comparability of the data obtained in the various areas. Evaluation and coding of the electrocardiograms (ECGs) and the serum cholesterol analyses were done at the University of Minnesota, as was all statistical work.

Blood Pressure

In spite of standardization of instructions and equipment for measuring blood pressure, it became obvious in the entry examinations that the recordings were not always strictly comparable, even in the same examination period in a given area. The standard arrangements included avoidance of smoking, eating, and vigorous exercise for at least a half hour before measurement in a room at a temperature that would not provoke sweating or shivering in seminude subjects. Two physicians took alternate subjects for the physical examinations, including the measurement of blood pressure. The standard instructions were: Allow at least five minutes of supine rest after the examination. Then make two successive readings in the right arm, allowing the mercury to return to zero between readings. Read to the nearest 2-mm mark and record the fourth and fifth phase diastolic.

We have reported in some detail the evidence leading to the conclusion that in some areas the two examining physicians produced different distributions of blood pressure from what should have been random samples from the same population (Keys et al. 1967, pp. 28–41). Differences of up to 10 mm in the mean systolic and diastolic pressures of such parallel samples were fairly common. Accordingly, caution is advised in comparing the prevalence of hypertension based on the frequency of readings above a given fixed point. We have no evidence of bias among areas in the recording of blood pressure, but in considering blood pressure as a risk factor it would seem wise to emphasize the relative blood pressure of men within each cohort.

Diagnosis and Disease Classification

From the first planning sessions, it was agreed that every effort should be made to assure comparability of diagnoses. With the exception of Zutphen, in each area at least one member of the local medical team had worked as a postdoctoral fellow or research associate at the Laboratory of Physiological Hygiene at the University of Minnesota. Diagnoses of disease at entry and follow-up examinations were made by experienced internists using standard medical history and physical examination forms (Keys 1970, pp. I-205–211). Relative uniformity of diagnostic criteria and interpretation was further promoted by the participation in the examinations in the several areas by members of the central staff of the study and by representatives of other local area teams. Because funduscopic examination was not made in all cohorts, comparison of the frequency of hypertensive vascular disease is not warranted. Several internists were consulted and concurred in all diagnoses of cardiovascular disease and other serious disorders. For deaths, final attribution of cause was made by members of the central staff of the study, Henry Blackburn and Alessandro Menotti after reexamination of the records.

The diagnostic criteria and the codes for categories of cardiovascular disease are as follows:

Code Criteria
00   ECG corresponding to Minnesota code 1.1 (major Q waves; old infarction)
01   ECG corresponding to Minnesota codes 1.2 and 5.1 or 1.2 and 5.2 (lesser Q waves plus major T wave findings; old infarction)
03   clinical judgment of heart disease (definite or possible) *and* etiology specified as myocardial infarct (by history) and any of the following Minnesota codes: 1.2, 1.3, 5.1, 5.2, 6.1, 6.2, 7.1, 7.2, 7.4, or 8.3 (clinical infarction with abnormal but nonspecific ECG findings)
04   clinical judgment of definite heart disease and etiology specified as myocardial infarct by history (clinical infarction without ECG confirmation = possible myocardial infarction)
08   clinical judgment of definite heart disease and etiology specified as coronary insufficiency (equivalent to angina pectoris by history); definite angina pectoris

09   clinical judgment of definite heart disease and etiology specified as chronic heart disease of probable coronary origin (chronic heart disease manifested as arrhythmias and failures without obvious etiology)
10   clinical judgment of definite heart disease and etiology other than those specified above
11   ECG corresponding to any of the following Minnesota codes: 1.2, 1.3, 4.1, 4.2, 4.3, 4.4, 5.1, 5.2, 6.1, 6.2, 7.1, 7.2, 7.4, or 8.3 (nonspecific resting ECG abnormalities)
20   clinical judgment of hypertensive vascular disease and finding of hypertensive fundi (hypertensive vascular disease)
21   clinical judgment of peripheral arteriosclerotic disease and medical history of claudication (peripheral vascular disease)
22   clinical judgment of cerebral arteriosclerotic disease and medical history of stroke (cerebrovascular disease)

The history taking was structured on the London School of Hygiene Cardiovascular Questionnaire (Rose 1962; Rose and Blackburn 1968).

The prevalence codes are hierarchical, that is, they are mutually exclusive with priority given to the smallest code number that can be assigned. A man who warrants the diagnosis of old myocardial infarction who also suffers from angina pectoris and has a diagnosis of definite stroke is given only the infarct code for identification in this system. A man with angina and evidence of definite hypertensive vascular disease is coded only 08.

In the analysis of incidence in the ten years after the entry examination, the information about prevalence is used in defining three kinds of cohorts: (1) all men, (2) CHD-free men (excluding all men with codes 00 through 09), and (3) CVD-free men (excluding all men with codes 00–09, 10, 20–22). The greatest emphasis is placed on the CVD-free cohort in the search for and evaluation of risk factors. The subsequent medical experience of the men excluded from the CVD-free cohort provides data for the study of prognosis, a subject to be examined in later reports.

Criteria for the diagnosis and classification of nonfatal incidence of coronary heart disease, with identifying codes used in data processing at the Laboratory for Physiological Hygiene (LPH) are as follows:

LPH code	Definition
30	same as prevalence code 00 (major Q waves)
31	same as prevalence code 01 (lesser Q waves plus major T wave findings) when no such Q or T waves at entry
32	same as prevalence code 03 except that clinical judgment of

	definite heart disease is required (clinical infarction with abnormal but nonspecific ECG findings)
34	same as prevalence code 04 (clinical infarction without ECG confirmation)
35	follow-up examination judgment of possible heart disease and etiology specified as myocardial infarct (by history and Minnesota codes 1.2, 1.3, 5.1, 5.2, 6.1, 6.2, 7.1, 7.2, 7.4, or 8.3 at the follow-up examination)
36	Minnesota ECG code 1.2 at the follow-up but not at the entry examination
37	Minnesota ECG codes 1.3 and 5.1 or 1.3 and 5.2 at the follow-up but not at the entry examination
38	same as prevalence code 08 (definite angina pectoris)
39	same as prevalence code 09 (chronic heart disease manifested as arrythmias and failure without obvious etiology)

The incidence criteria are almost identical with those of the prevalence criteria except for the requirement of changes from the entry ECG in codes 31, 36, and 37. For analytical purposes codes 30–32 are taken to be hard CHD; any of codes 30–39 qualify for diagnosis of incidence of any CHD. Codes 34–37 and 39 are labeled possible coronary heart disease. As in the prevalence codes, the arrangement is hierarchical in order of presumed importance or severity, that is, in order from smallest to largest number.

Codes 00–09 were interpreted as coronary heart disease, but only codes 00, 01, and 03 were considered hard criteria indicating definite old myocardial infarction. A medical history indicative of old infarction but without confirmatory signs in the ECG, code 04, was considered to be softer evidence and was labeled as possible myocardial infarction. Cardiovascular disease was taken to be present when a subject had any of the codes except 11. The ECG abnormalities in code 11 are not, by themselves, diagnostic of cardiovascular disease, but follow-up may reveal prognostic significance. A diagnosis of definite angina pectoris was made from a history of classical chest pain of brief duration, commonly provoked by exercise.

Definitions and codes for causes of death used in this report are given below. ICDA code refers to the International Classification of Diseases adapted for use in the United States based on the eighth revision of the *International Classification of Diseases*.

LPH code	Definition
71	myocardial infarction with death (ICDA codes 410 and 412 and their subdivisions)
72	angina pectoris with death (ICDA codes 411 and 413 and their

	subdivisions), sudden death of probable coronary origin (similar to ICDA code 795 but with the requirement of reason to judge probable coronary origin), deaths from heart disease excluding hypertension, and known heart disease other than coronary heart disease (ICDA codes 427.2 and 427.6)
73	death from congestive heart failure or arrhythmia or both without hypertension or other known causes (ICDA codes 427.0 and 427.9)
74	death from other heart diseases (ICDA codes 390–398, 400–404, 420–426, 427.3–427.5, 429)
75	all other deaths
750	death from infectious diseases
751	death from malignant neoplasm of trachea, bronchus, and lung (ICDA codes 162.0 and 162.1)
752	death from other neoplasms (ICDA codes 140–161 and 163–239)
753	death from cerebrovascular diseases (ICDA codes 430–438)
754	death from other arterial diseases (ICDA codes 440–448)
755	death from accidents, poisonings, violence (ICDA codes E 800–E 999)
759	death from all other causes not covered by the preceding codes

For the purpose of this book, death from CHD (codes 71–73) and definite nonfatal myocardial infarction (codes 30–31) are taken to be incidence of hard CHD. Causes of death other than those listed are, of course, in the mortality records, but no detailed analysis of these is attempted here.

The diagnosis of nonfatal incidence was based on the medical history, findings in the physical examinations, and the electrocardiographic data obtained by our own examining teams in the field; no search was made for preexisting medical records. The decision to make this restriction was dictated by realization that the areas involved in the study differ in the extent, reliability, and availability of medical records and in the frequency of medical consultation and hospitalization. More complete medical histories and data useful for retrospective (interim) diagnoses could be obtained by a search for other medical records, but certainly the results would not be comparable among the several cohorts. Even within cohorts bias could arise because of socioeconomic variations in the use and quality of medical services.

Although this restriction to the same sources of information contributes to the comparability of the incidence data from the several areas, it also means that some diagnoses might be missed. We have previously reported an attempt to estimate the effect of using our restricted sources of information as contrasted with using those findings plus a full search for other medical information on the same subjects (Keys, 1970, p. I-14). Full search yielded 16 percent more cases of definite myocardial infarction among United States railroad men in five years, but there was no difference in the estimated number of cases of the incidence of angina pectoris. Full search also resulted in a slight decrease in the number of cases classified as possible infarction. Accordingly, it is believed that the system adopted for the Seven Countries Study makes a slight underestimation of the incidence of any CHD and a more significant underestimation of definite infarction.

Attribution of cause of death involved not only inspection of death certificates but also information from local physicians, families, and friends of the deceased. The records of previous examinations of the deceased in this study were also useful in the assignment of probable cause of death.

A final point in regard to deaths was the effort to ascertain whether men not known to be dead were actually alive at the end of the ten-year period. Insistence in every case on the facts of life as well as of death discovered a few deaths that had been missed in the early years of this study. The extra efforts on this score delayed closing the books on the ten-year experience and hence the preparation of this book.

Age Distribution and Standardization

Rates of prevalence and of incidence were age standardized by single years of age to the age distribution of all men 40 through 59 at the entry examinations. The formula is: $R = r_{40}(p_{40}) + r_{41}(p_{41}) \ldots r_{59}(p_{59})$, where R is the age-standardized rate; r_{40}, the observed rate for the men aged 40 at entry in the cohort of interest; and p_{40}, the proportion of all men 40–59 in the Seven Countries Study represented by men aged 40. Table 2.1 shows the age distribution of the men at entry in the Seven Countries Study and the corresponding distribution for all white men in the United States reported by the U.S. Vital Statistics for 1965.

At the time of the entry examinations some of the men examined were found to be outside the specified range of 40 through 59 years. The data on those men have not been used in the present analysis.

In table 2.1 the unduly small proportion of men aged 40 at entry reflects the fact that in some cohorts considerable time elapsed between the establishment of the rosters of eligible men and the actual examinations. At the time of the examinations, there were no men still aged 40 at Crevalcore and Montegiorgio, and at Zutphen only one man was 40; the 40-year-old men listed in the rosters were now 41.

Besides the deficit at age 40, the age distribution in the Seven Countries

Table 2.1. Age distribution, percentages of men 40–59, at entry, all cohorts combined, and for white men in U.S. Vital Statistics for 1965.

Age	Cohorts	U.S. white	Age	Cohorts	U.S. white
40	2.45	5.33	50	5.67	5.04
41	4.97	5.31	51	5.18	5.00
42	5.25	5.29	52	5.32	4.94
43	5.00	5.27	53	5.57	4.89
44	5.57	5.25	54	5.61	4.83
45	4.67	5.22	55	4.89	4.76
46	4.71	5.19	56	5.41	4.69
47	4.83	5.16	57	5.13	4.61
48	4.94	5.13	58	5.07	4.53
49	5.11	5.09	59	4.65	4.45
40–49	47.50	52.24	50–59	52.50	47.76
			40–59	100.00	100.00

Study shows greater proportions at the older ages than were reported in the range 40–59 for United States white men in 1965. There are two reasons for this difference. First, the excess mortality in World War II was much greater in Europe and Japan than in the United States, and that mortality was particularly excessive in younger men. Over three-fourths of the non-American men in this study were first examined in the years 1958–1961, fifteen to eighteen years after the middle of the war. Thus men in their forties at entry would have been in their twenties or early thirties and at greater risk of being killed than their older compatriots. A rural-urban population shift after the war also contributed to a relative deficit of the younger men. The younger men tended to seek jobs in the cities; the older men were more tied to their homes and had less wish or opportunity to move away. Of the men in this study, 70 percent were rural in residence.

It is useful to compare age-standardized rates using the age distribution of the Seven Countries Study as base a and that of United States white men as base b. Base a seems more appropriate for comparisons among the cohorts of the study, but for comparisons with the general population of the United States perhaps base b would be preferred. Practically, however, the conclusions from such comparisons would be very similar with both bases. Because the rates of death and the incidence of coronary heart disease increase with age, standardization with base a will give slightly higher rates than will base b because the men in this study were, on the average, slightly older than white men 40–59 in the general population of the United States.

The effects of using the two bases for age standardization may be illustrated by comparing the Dalmatia cohort, in which only 14.6 percent of the men were 40–44 at entry, with the east Finland cohort, in which 25.7 percent were in the 40–44 year class. Standardized to the seven countries age distribution, the ten-year all-causes death rates per 10,000 men were 801 (SE = 105) for Dalmatia and 1,864 (SE = 136) for east Finland. Standardized to the United States white male age distribution, the corresponding rates were 681 (SE = 97) and 1,812 (SE = 135), respectively. With either base the conclusion about mortality in east Finland compared with that in Dalmatia is similar. Using the seven countries age distribution, the ratio of mortality rates is 1,864/801 = 2.33; with United States white men as the base, the ratio is 1,812/681 = 2.66.

Parenthetically, it may be noted that east Finland did not follow the general rule of a relative deficit of younger men. One reason is that in east Finland almost all men of all ages fought the Russian invaders. The older men were equally exposed and because of their age were less able to withstand the rigors of the winter war. Another reason for the relatively high proportion of younger men in east Finland is that in the resettlement of the Finnish refugees from the land seized by the Russians the younger men were encouraged to remain in eastern Finland to rebuild after the devastation of the war.

The need for age standardization is shown when the death rates are compared for two populations of men aged 40–59 but with different distributions of age within that range. For all-causes ten-year deaths of all men 40–59 at entry, the crude rates per 10,000 were 10,000(61)/671 = 909.1 for Dalmatia and 10,000(63)/511 = 1,232.9 for Velika Krsna. This indicates a nonsignificant difference in mortality rates, $\Delta = 323.8$, SE $\Delta = 179.9$, $t = 1.79$, and $p = 0.074$. However, the age-standardized rates are 800.7 and 1,188.9, respectively, with $\Delta = 388.2$, SE $= \Delta = 173.6$, $t = 2.23$, $p = 0.026$, indicating that the observed difference in favor of Dalmatia would arise by chance fewer than 3 times in 100.

In the tables in this book rates per 10,000, and their standard errors, are generally given without decimals. However, in the computations the rates were not rounded, so SE, t, and p values may not correspond exactly with those that would be computed from the values for rates in the tables.

Incidence Rates

Emphasis is placed on the ten-year age-standardized incidence rate per 10,000 men standardized by single years of age, as described in the preceding section.

The proportion, p, of the number of men at risk, N, who become incidence cases is $p = C/N$, where C is the number of incidence cases. We have calculated the standard error of the proportion, SE_p, as $(SE_p)^2 = p(1-p)/N$, when both pN and $(1-p)N$ exceed the value of 5. Per 10,000 men, the incidence rate, R, and its standard error, SER, are $10,000p$ and $10,000SE_p$, respectively. Here, where N is generally of the order of several hundred or more, approximately 95 percent and 99 percent confidence limits for the rate are $R \pm 1.96\ SER$ and $R \pm 2.58\ SER$, respectively.

For comparing incidence rates R_a and R_b of cohorts a and b we have calculated the standard error of the difference between the rates at 10,000 times the standard error of the difference, Δp, between the proportions of incidence cases to men at risk in the two cohorts: $(SE\Delta_p)^2 = p(1-p)/N_a + p(1-p)/N_b$, where p is the mean proportion of cases in the two cohorts combined, $p = (C_a + C_b)/(N_a + N_b)$. The ratio $Z = \Delta R/SE\Delta R$ follows approximately the normal distribution (Brownlee 1965). The probability that ΔR is not equal to zero may be estimated from the usual normal or t table. Z^2 is equal to the usual chi-square calculated from a 2-x-2 contingency table without Yates's correction for continuity.

Our decision to omit Yates's continuity correction in the use of the chi-square test was explained in the report in the five-year experience in the seven countries study (Keys 1970, p. I-11.). The usual chi-square test (or the equivalent Z test) has been restricted to cases in which the smallest expected frequency in any cell of the 2-x-2 table is 5 or greater. In a few cases where a comparable test seemed desirable but the expected smallest frequencies did not meet this requirement, we have used Fisher's exact test to evaluate the significance.

Multivariate Analysis

It is commonly agreed that the development of CHD may be promoted by a number of variables, some of which at least are interrelated. Thus it is obviously desirable to explore the use of multivariate methods in which a number of independent variables are considered simultaneously in regard to relationship to the dependent variable, CHD.

It is sometimes useful to look at the results of summation of 2-x-2 tables in which subsamples have been matched in one or more variables to reduce their possible confounding effect on the independent variable of interest. For those analyses we have used the method of Mantel and Haenszel (1959) in which summary chi-square with only one degree of freedom is calculated from the sums of the observed and the expected cases and the variances in the matched subsamples. The calculation does not depend on the assumptions about the distributions and linearity involved in both multiple regression and multiple logistic analyses.

The most common multivariate methods so far applied to the analysis of data from prospective studies on the incidence of CHD are those of the multiple linear and the multiple logistic equations. Both depend on the proposition that the contributions to the development or clinical expression of CHD of the several independent variables are additive. The multiple linear regression model is: $y = a + b_1 x_1 + b_2 x_2 \ldots b_k x_k$, where $x_1 \ldots x_k$ are the variables such as age and blood pressure proposed as possibly useful in the estimation or prediction of the dependent variable y. With observed values for $y, x_1 \ldots x_k$, it is possible to solve the general equation so as to find the values of $a, b_1 \ldots b_k x_k$, that give the best estimate of y, where best is defined as the result in which the sum of the squares of the deviations of predicted y from observed y is least (least-squares criterion). In the case where the dependent variable is the incidence of CHD, y is a categorical variable and the solution is an attempt to discriminate between the persons who become CHD cases from those who do not. The solution of the equation y may be set as 0 for noncases and 1 for cases. When the results of the solution of the equation, the best values of $a, b_1 \ldots b_k$, are applied to an individual's values for the independent variables, $x_1 \ldots x_k$, the result can be thought of as an estimate of the relative degree of CHD in that individual.

The multiple logistic regression equation has the property that the resulting solution for y is an estimate of probability which has the limits of 0, or zero probability of CHD, and 1, or certain CHD; the distribution is S-shaped. The equation is: $y = 1/(1 + e^z)$ where e is the base of natural logarithms (2.718 . . .) and the exponent $z = -(\alpha + \beta_1 + \beta_2 x_2 \ldots \beta_k x_k)$ in which α is a constant and $\beta_1, \beta_2 \ldots \beta_k$ are coefficients of multiplication to be applied to the variables $x_1, x_2, \ldots x_k$ as in the case of the multiple linear regression equation. Here again y is a categorical variable taking the value 0 for noncases and 1 for cases.

Truett, Cornfield, and Kannel (1967) developed a method of solving the multiple logistic regression equation on the assumption that the variables $x_1 \ldots x_k$ are multivariate normal in distribution with equal variances and covariances. In spite of the fact that these assumptions are commonly far from being warranted, their method of solving the equation has generally proved to be useful (Keys et al. 1972b).

Walker and Duncan (1967) developed an iterative method of solving the multiple logistic regression equation without the assumptions made by Truett and colleagues. Their method, although theoretically superior, is much more costly in computer time. Data from the Seven Countries Study have been used in many parallel analyses with the multiple linear regression and with both methods of solving the multiple logistic regression equation. In practical results all three have been remarkably similar in success in discriminating between cases and noncases and in classifying persons according to degree of risk.

The effectiveness of the solutions of the multiple logistic or linear regression equation can be evaluated by estimating the value of y (the probability of developing CHD in the logistic solution) for each individual and comparing the estimates with the observed outcome. It is convenient to place the individuals in an array from lowest to highest values of estimated values of risk probability, p, and then to group them into decile or 5-percentile classes of the distribution of p. The distribution of the observed cases of CHD among those groupings of estimated or predicted cases indicates the effectiveness of the solution for discrimination or, when tested with data from another population, for prediction. The computer programs that solve the multiple linear or multiple logistic regression equations also provide estimates of the standard errors of the coefficients, $b_1 \ldots b_k$ or $\beta_1 \ldots \beta_k$. The coefficients divided by their standard errors are approximate t values which can be used to estimate confidence limits of the coefficients and the probability that they are not zero. Those t values are also useful indicators of the relative discriminating power of the several independent variables, but it must be emphasized that they do not necessarily have any significance in regard to etiology or causation.

In the evaluation of the discriminating power of solutions of the multiple logistic equation, Truett, Cornfield, and Kannel (1967) used the coefficients found in the solution to calculate the risk, or probability, of the event in question for each of the individuals in the study so as to classify them into deciles of estimated risk and then noted the number of events observed in each of those risk decile classes. Comparisons of the deciles in terms of the number of cases or events observed in them illustrate the discriminating power of the solution but do not summarize the picture over the whole series of decile classes. A simple plot of the number of cases observed in each decile against the number expected from the application of the multiple logistic solution to each of the individuals in the decile class provides an excellent display, but there are problems of numerical evaluation.

The correlation coefficient is readily calculated from the ten pairs of observed and expected values. Some critics object that the unwary reader may be thereby misled, not realizing that the correlation refers only to that between the numbers of the decile classes, not to individuals. A more serious limitation to the use of the coefficient of correlation to evaluate the discriminatory power of the solution is the fact that with only ten pairs of values the confidence limits of the coefficient are very wide. For example, with $N = 10$ and $r = 0.8$, the 95 percent confidence limits are approximately $r = 0.56$ and $r = 1.0$. The difficulty is that N is necessarily small. With a material providing many incidence cases, 5-percentile instead of decile classes can be examined. But even with $N = 20$ the 5 percent confidence limits are wide; if $r = 0.8$, the limits are approximately $r = 0.64$ and $r = .96$. Clearly, comparison of correlation coefficients between observed and expected numbers in the decile classes has very limited value in evaluating the performance of the model or of different variables used in it.

For these latter purposes, Menotti et al. (1977), with data from the seven countries' five-year experience, have used the likelihood ratio statistic (LRS) and what they term the first and second moments, M1 and M2, of the distribution of the observed cases in the decile classes of estimated probability. M1 is the sum of the products of the decile class numbers times the number of cases, C, observed within the respective decile, the whole being divided by the total of all cases observed:

$$M1 = \sum_{i=1}^{10} C_i \cdot i \bigg/ \sum_{i=1}^{10} C_i$$

M2, the second moment, is similarly calculated, using the squares of the decile class numbers as multipliers, the sum then being divided by 10 times N, where N is the total number of cases observed:

$$M2 = \sum_{i=10}^{10} C_i \cdot i^2 \bigg/ 10 \sum_{i=10}^{10} C_i$$

The upper limit of M1 is obviously 10, the value that would result if all the incidence cases were concentrated in the top or tenth decile. The lower limit is, on the average, $M1 = 5$, the case where the logistic solution has no discriminatory power at all, so the cases are randomly distributed among the ten decile classes. The upper limit of M2 is also 10 and the average lower limit is 3.85, the situation where discrimination is zero and the incidence cases are randomly distributed among the decile classes. Whereas M1 is an indicator of overall performance, M2 stresses discrimination at the upper end of the scale of risk.

Although M1 and M2 are useful indicators of performance, their interpretation is limited by the absence of a way to estimate their standard errors or confidence limits. The same is true of the maximum likelihood statistics (MLS), which have a further disadvantage in attempts to compare discrimination where there is a difference in the number at risk or of cases, for

MLS depends on these numbers as well as on agreement between observations and expectations.

Expected deaths. A common reference point is useful for comparisons of death rates. For the Seven Countries Study we have used as the reference the mortality experience of white men as reported in the *Vital Statistics of the United States,* volume 2, *Mortality,* part A. For all-causes deaths the life tables for single years of age were used, taking the tables for 1962 for the first five years of follow-up, because that year corresponds best to the midpoint of the first five years for the generality of the cohorts and the 1967 life tables for the succeeding five years. The composite 1962, 1967 rates for ten years per 10,000 men, given in table 2.2 were used for calculating the expected all-causes deaths for each of the cohorts.

The same volume of the U.S. Vital Statistics reports the numbers of deaths of white men, in five-year age classes, from all causes and from specified causes. From 1962 to 1967 the basis of classification for specified causes was the seventh revision of the *International Classification of Diseases* (ICD) in which we considered that rubrics 420 and 422 represent deaths from coronary heart disease. An adaptation of the eighth revision of the ICD has been used in the United States mortality statistics since 1968. In the newer classification rubrics 410 through 413 seem to correspond fairly well with 420, 422 in the former classification, though there may be some question

Table 2.2. Expected deaths (ten-year deaths per 10,000 white men calculated from U.S. Vital Statistics for 1962, first five years, and 1967, second five years).

Entry age	All-causes deaths	CHD deaths (%)	Entry age	All-causes deaths	CHD deaths (%)
40	534	35.0	50	1,377	41.5
41	590	36.1	51	1,494	41.7
42	650	37.0	52	1,617	41.9
43	717	37.9	53	1,747	42.1
44	790	38.7	54	1,885	42.2
45	870	39.3	55	2,032	42.3
46	962	39.9	56	2,190	42.3
47	1,057	40.4	57	2,357	42.4
48	1,158	40.9	58	2,534	42.4
49	1,265	41.2	59	2,719	42.4

about 411.0 ("other . . . forms of ischemic heart disease" with several kinds of "hypertensive disease"), which is commonly included in statistics in the United States on coronary heart disease.

From the U.S. Vital Statistics for 1962 and 1967 the proportion of all deaths represented by CHD was plotted against the mid-age for each age group, 45–49 through 65–69. A smooth line connecting those points allowed interpolation to the percentage of CHD deaths for single years of age given in table 2.1. The percentages proved to be closely similar for the 1962 and 1967 Vital Statistics but, as in the calculation of all-causes deaths, we used 1962 data for the first five years and 1967 data for the second five years of follow-up. The composite for the whole ten years of follow-up is shown in table 2.2.

Expected ten-year all-causes deaths were calculated for each cohort, multiplying the number of men at risk at entry for each single year of entry age by the rate of table 2.2 for the corresponding age divided by 10,000. The sum of those 20 sets of expected deaths is the number expected for the men in each of the single years of age 40–59. Expected CHD deaths were calculated by applying the percentage figures in table 2.2 to the expected all-causes deaths.

Measures of variation and significance. The calculation of rates, their standard errors, and the standard errors of differences in rates, was described earlier. The standard errors of means have been calculated in the usual way, that is, as the standard deviation divided by the square root of the number of cases from which the mean was calculated. The standard error of a difference between means, SE *diff*, has been computed taking into account the numbers on which the two means are based and the standard errors of those means: $(SE\ diff)^2 = [(N_1-1)SE_1^2 + (N_2-1)SE_2^2]/(N_1+N_2-2)$.

Some readers may prefer confidence limits instead of standard errors for comparing means or rates, and we have given confidence limits rather than standard errors in some tables. Confidence limits are, of course, readily calculated from standard errors. The 95 and 99 percent confidence intervals are, respectively, 1.96 SE and 2.58 SE, so the confidence limits are the mean ± 1.96 SE and ± 2.58 SE. This calculation was used, for example, to provide the confidence limits shown in table 4.1.

For many purposes in this study it is desirable to report the statistics on each of the separate cohorts, and either standard errors or confidence limits are suitable to indicate the variation around the central tendency. However, it is often desirable to combine cohorts. For example, Crevalcore and Montegiorgio may be combined as rural Italy, Crete and Corfu as rural Greece, and so on. In such cases the standard errors are used to calculate the standard error of the combined cohorts, and that standard error, in turn, is used to calculate the confidence limits. In case the confidence limits but not the standard errors are at hand, the standard errors are readily computed from the confidence limits. For example, given the 95 percent confidence limits x_1 and x_2, $SE = (x_2 - x_1)/2(1.96)$. When two means or rates are being compared, the significance of the difference between them may be judged by inspection of the two sets of confidence limits or from the difference divided by the standard error of that difference. This last is the 5 value, and the probability that the difference is not zero will be indicated by reference to a table of t values.

It has been customary to consider a difference as *statistically significant* if it would not be expected to occur by chance in 20 trials. *Highly significant* is the popular term for a difference that would not be expected to occur by chance in 100 trials. These arbitrary definitions correspond to the probabilities $p = 0.05$ and $p = 0.01$ commonly given as headings in tables of t values. Lately, however, new, small calculators, widely available, make it possible to calculate probability without limitation to the probability classes of t tables, so in this book actual probabilities are generally given instead of classes of significance.

The choice of emphasizing confidence limits or probabilities depends on the end in view. If it is simply desired to give quantitative descriptions of sets of data, confidence limits may be desirable. If testing of hypotheses is the concern, it would seem to be better to show the actual probability that an observed difference would be expected to occur by chance.

Decile classes. In earlier publications we have described how the men in each cohort were grouped into five-year age classes and how the complete distribution of values for a number of variables measured at entry were obtained for each age- and cohort- specific group (Keys et al. 1967, pp. 48, 49; Keys 1970, p. I-10). The decile cutting points describe the distributions without the assumptions involved in the usual mean and standard deviation and are therefore appropriate for data that are either normally or otherwise distributed.

An advantage of the classification into age- and cohort-specific deciles is the ease and propriety of combining age classes or cohorts or both so as to examine, with increased numbers, the characteristics and subsequent disease experience of men who, in respect to a given variable, are relatively high or low in comparison with other men of like age in their own community. Another advantage of the decile classification is in the examination of the character of a relationship between one characteristic and another or between a characteristic and subsequent events. By definition, on the null hypothesis one-tenth of all cases is the expectation for each decile class of each variable. A simple plot of the number of cases per decile class reveals at a glance the tendency, if any, for the condition to be related to the variable. Moreover, such a plot suggests the kind of relationship, rectilinear or curvilinear. The scatter of the observed number of cases in the decile classes about the expected number in those classes is, of course, a measure of the departure from chance expectation.

Cutting points for the age- and cohort-specific classes have been published (Keys et al. 1967, pp. 365–382) for all cohorts except Zrenjanin and Belgrade and separately for the latter two cohorts (Keys 1970, pp. I-125, I-126). Tables of all these cutting points are given, in slightly condensed form, in the appendix.

Summary

Smoking, eating, and vigorous exercise were not allowed for at least 30 minutes before the physical examination. The examining teams, except at Belgrade, Zutphen, and at the entry examinations in Japan, included representatives of the central staff and of other areas of the study. Standard medical history, physical examination, and death record forms were supplied from central headquarters where all original data processing was done. Blood serum and lyophilized food samples were analyzed at central headquarters in Minnesota, some independent analyses being made also in Italy, Greece, and Japan.

Cardiovascular events were recorded only from the evidence of the medical history, physical examination, and 12-lead electrocardiograms recorded before and after exercise, positive diagnoses being verified by two internists of the study teams. The decision to avoid secondhand reports was made to assure comparability of diagnoses in regions varying in amount and sophistication of local medical services. The electrocardiograms were coded according to the Minnesota code, and positive findings were verified by an independent coder. Diagnostic criteria, specified in detail, identified (1) four categories of old myocardial infarction, (2) three categories of changes in the ECG from the entry record suggesting possible interim infarction with nonspecific residue, (3) classical uncomplicated angina pectoris, (4) unexplained arrhythmias associated with heart failure. For subsequent analyses, diagnoses of coronary death and of myocardial infarction were grouped as hard CHD, and those of angina pectoris only and of nonspecific changes from the entry ECG were grouped as soft CHD. Deaths were ascertained yearly in each area, and a member of the area team interviewed relatives and friends in addition to obtaining copies of death certificates and other relevant documents. The attribution of cause of death proposed by the local teams was reviewed at central headquarters.

From the entry data all men were arrayed into decile classes, specific for the cohort and five-year age class, in height, relative body weight, systolic and diastolic blood pressures, skinfold thickness, and serum cholesterol. This facilitated grouping of cohorts for analyses of incidence rates according to the relative position of the men in the distribution of the entry measurements of interest.

Incidence rates were standardized by single years of age to the age distribution of the men in all sixteen cohorts combined. Standard errors and confidence limits were calculated for all rates. Chi-square tests were made in many analyses; Fisher's exact method for the 2-x-2 table was used when indicated.

Multivariate methods were applied in the evaluation of the significance of the characteristics recorded at entry. In some cases a summary chi-square with only one degree of freedom was calculated according to Mantel and Haenszel; however, Walker and Duncan's solution of the multiple logistic equation was the standard method. The analyses concentrated on the men with no evidence of cardiovascular disease at entry.

The observed numbers of deaths from all causes and from coronary heart disease in each cohort were compared with the number expected to match the experience of white men of the same age reported in the U.S. Vital Statistics for the corresponding period of years.

3 | Prevalence of Cardiovascular Disease at Entry

Table 3.1 summarizes the findings on prevalence of cardiovascular disease at the entry examinations of the men aged 40 through 59 at the time. Of 12,763 men, 252, or 2.0 percent, were given a diagnosis of coronary heart disease; of these, 183 were specified as old myocardial infarction. But there were marked differences among the population samples. While CHD was recorded for 4.6 percent of the Americans and 3.6 percent of the Finns, the prevalence of CHD was only 0.9 percent or less in nine of the other cohorts. The prevalence of all cardiovascular disease (CVD) showed less striking but still very large contrasts. For the Americans and the Finns the CVD prevalence rates were 9.9 percent and 8.5 percent respectively; the corresponding rates for the rural Italians, the Greeks, and the Japanese were 2.9 percent, 2.8 percent, and 0.9 percent respectively.

Because the various diagnostic categories are arranged in a mutually exclusive hierarchy, each man is counted only once. The category angina pectoris does not include men who had angina and a diagnosis of myocardial infarction; such men were counted only in the infarct category. Although the totals for CHD and CVD are correct in this system, the frequencies of hypertensive vascular, peripheral vascular, and cerebrovascular disease indicate only those men with no other disease higher in the hierarchy. A man with clear evidence of cerebrovascular disease is not listed in that category if he also was diagnosed as having CHD or other heart disease, or hypertensive or peripheral vascular disease. The analysis of prevalence as well as incidence of conditions other than death or incidence of CHD is not attempted here.

Crude rates without age standardization are given in table 3.1. Table 3.2 shows the age-standardized rates and their 95 percent confidence limits for

Table 3.1. Prevalence of cardiovascular disease at entry (Rate = the crude rate per 10,000 men at risk; infarct code 04 = old infarction by history but no ECG confirmation; CHD code 09 = probable CHD; all men 40–59 at entry).

Item	U.S. RR	Finland	Croatia	Italy	Greece	Zutphen	Serbia	Japan	Total
Men at risk	2,571	1,677	1,367	2,480	1,215	878	1,565	1,010	12,763
Definite old infarction									
Cases	61	20	4	18	4	9	9	5	130
Rate	237	119	29	73	32	103	58	50	102
Infarct code 04									
Cases	29	15	0	4	1	2	2	0	53
Rate	113	89	0	16	8	23	13	0	41
Angina pectoris									
Cases	25	22	1	5	2	3	5	0	63
Rate	97	131	7	20	16	34	32	0	49
CHD code 09									
Cases	2	0	1	0	0	0	4	0	7
Rate	8	0	7	0	0	0	26	0	5
Other heart disease									
Cases	58	44	16	44	17	16	28	4	227
Rate	226	262	117	177	140	182	179	40	178
Hypertensive vascular disease									
Cases	67	27	2	1	12	0	18	0	127
Rate	261	161	15	4	99	0	116	0	100
Peripheral vascular disease									
Cases	9	13	0	4	0	3	15	0	44
Rate	35	78	0	16	0	34	96	0	34
Cerebrovascular disease									
Cases	5	4	1	3	0	0	1	0	14
Rate	19	24	7	12	0	0	6	0	11

Table 3.2. Coronary heart disease at entry (age-standardized prevalence per 10,000).

Region	N	Rate	95% confidence limits	
U.S. railroad	2,571	459	379	539
Finland	1,677	339	253	425
Croatia	1,367	43	8	78
Italy	2,480	109	68	150
Greece	1,215	56	15	97
Zutphen	878	56	7	74
Serbia	1,565	129	72	186
Japan	1,010	30	0	50
Total	12,763	196	172	220

the prevalence of CHD. Clearly the prevalence among the Americans and Finns is much higher than in the other cohorts, and the difference is highly significant; however, there is no significant difference between the Americans and the Finns. Another point of interest in table 3.2 is that the Japanese seem to have a significantly lower prevalence rate than the Italians and Serbs; the issue is in doubt in comparing the Japanese with the Croatians and the Dutch. But it is necessary to consider the possible effect of the response rate before drawing conclusions.

The response rate of the men in the sixteen cohorts varied from 75 to 100 percent (table 1.1); in thirteen other major studies the rate varied from 66 to 93 percent (table 1.3). If the men who failed to appear for examination were a random sample of those invited there would be no problem, but it seems unlikely that nonresponse is determined simply by chance or by factors totally unrelated to the presence of disease. Men who knew or suspected that they had heart disease may have been especially eager, or reluctant, to have the facts come out in examination. Such self-selection could have been different in the various cohorts.

We have already mentioned that some of the American railroad men seemed to have declined examination because they had heart disease and feared disclosure might affect their job security—in spite of repeated assurances that examination findings would not be made available to their employers. Such self-selection would mean that prevalence among the American men is underestimated in tables 3.1 and 3.2. It is possible that similar self-selection operated to produce some underestimation of prevalence for the other groups of men whose eligibility depended on their employment—the Italian railroad men and the Belgrade professors—but there is no evidence to that effect. On the other hand, in the rural areas it was often evident that the men who had, or feared they might have, heart disease were the first to accept the invitation for examination. This suggests that the prevalence figures for the rural men might be overestimations for the populations invited. Any such overestimation would necessarily be slight because few of the rural men invited failed to respond. Among 8,213 rural men invited, 8,008 were examined; the average response rate was 97.5 percent.

It is useful to examine the general situation in which it is desired to estimate the prevalence of a disease in a population from a sample in which not all persons can be examined. Consider the prevalence rate for all men invited, R_0, in comparison with that observed in the men examined, R_1, when R_1 differs from the rate, R_2, in the men not examined. If the number of men invited is N_0 and the number actually examined is N_1, the proportion of all men examined is N_1/N_0. Let $P = R_2/R_1 = (N_1/N_0) + P(1 - N_1/N_0)$. Figure 3.1 shows values for R_0/R_1 for various values of P and of N_1/N_0.

For all cohorts combined, a total of 9.6 percent of the men invited did not appear for examination. If the prevalence of the disease in the nonresponders were double that in the men examined, the recorded prevalence rate would be underestimated by 9 percent. In the case of the United States railroad employees, where the response was only 75 percent, a twofold prevalence among the nonresponders would mean a 25 percent underestimate for the invited sample. Doubts about underestimation of the preva-

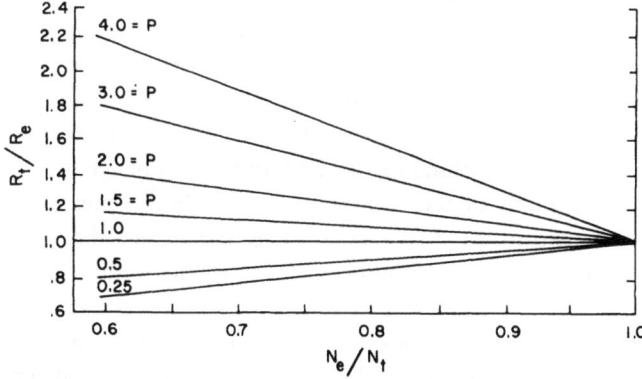

Figure 3.1. Relation of the true prevalence rate in a population (R_t) to the rate observed in an examined sample (R_e) as a function of the rate (R_m) in the persons not examined, the numbers examined (N_e), and the numbers not examined, N_m: $R_t = R_e(N_e/N_t) + R_m(N_m/N_t)$. $P = R_m/R_e$. N_e/N_t = number seen / number in population. R_t/R_e = population rate/rate for men seen.

lence in the other cohorts are smaller, particularly in the rural cohorts. If the prevalence of CHD in the nonexamined rural men were double that observed in the 8,008 men actually examined, the true rural population rate would be only 2.5 percent higher than that recorded at the examinations. Except for Finland, it appears that the prevalence of CHD in all the rural areas could not be more than about one-fourth that in the United States railroad men.

Although CHD is far too common a disease in many populations, in no population does more than a small fraction of the middle-aged men show clinical evidence of the disease. This means that the prevalence rate is calculated from a numerator that is much smaller than the denominator. Accordingly, as can be seen from figure 3.1, when a fairly large proportion of the target population is actually examined, overestimation of prevalence in the population is less of a problem than is underestimation. For the extreme case in the present study, if the American railroad men not examined had a CHD prevalence half that of the examined men, the result would be an overestimate of only 12.5 percent. And, to repeat, it seems that, if anything, the prevalence of CHD in the population was somewhat overestimated from the findings on the men examined.

Other Studies

Comparison with prevalence reported from other studies is difficult not only because of possible bias from nonresponders but also because of varied, often imprecisely stated criteria and the common practice of including both definite and suspect cases in a single category of CHD. Another obstacle to valid comparisons among populations and samples is the fact that rates are commonly only reported for a range of ages—40–49 or even 40–60 or 35–63—without age standardization or specification of cases and numbers at risk for single years or even five-year age classes. Since the incidence rate of CHD increases by something like 10 percent per year of age in mid-life, and the age distributions in the various studies are by no means uniform, it follows that comparisons of rates in broad age classes are subject to the possibility of serious error unless the distributions by age within the age classes are similar.

At the entrance examinations in the Framingham study of 941 men aged 45–62, a diagnosis of myocardial infarction was made for fifteen men, of angina pectoris for another eighteen men, and of possible myocardial infarction from ECG evidence only for ten men (Dawber, Moore, and Mann 1957). Including the cases of possible infarction, this means a prevalence of 3.4 percent compared with the finding of 4.6 percent among the American railroad men. The difference is not statistically significant ($t = 1.85$).

It is interesting that angina pectoris accounted for 41 percent of the CHD prevalence at Framingham, whereas the figure for the railroad men was only 22 percent. This yields chi-square = 5.9 for the comparison of diagnostic categories, and p is less than 0.02, from which it appears that there is a real difference. However, it is not possible to decide whether the difference reflects a difference between the populations or in the diagnostic criteria. The age distributions of the Framingham men 40–59 is similar to that of the railroad men, and the 73 older Framingham men who contributed five of the CHD prevalence cases could scarcely account for the difference in the kind of manifestation reported.

The prevalence of CHD among civil servants in Los Angeles indicated in the report by Chapman et al. (1957) cannot be so readily compared because only coronary disease and coronary and hypertensive disease are tabulated for men under 40, 40–54, and 55–70. Among 692 Los Angeles men aged 40–54, 6 were labeled only coronary and 4 coronary and hypertensive, making a combined prevalence of only 1.4 percent. Of 1,875 American railroad men 40–54, there were 49 men with myocardial infarction diagnoses and 21 labeled angina pectoris, giving a combined prevalence of 3.7 percent. The difference is highly significant with p less than 0.005 (chi-square = 8.46), but again it is not possible to decide whether this reflects differences in populations or diagnostic criteria.

The report on prevalence among civil servants at Albany, New York, is more detailed (Doyle et al. 1957). Of 1,821 men 40–59, 69 were judged to have CHD at entry, giving a prevalence of 3.8 percent, almost identical with that for the railroad men in the same age range and of almost identical average age. The percentage of CHD accounted for by angina pectoris at Albany was 26 percent, closely similar to the finding in the railroad men.

For men aged 40–59 in Chicago industry, a prevalence of 2.1 percent CHD, apparently based on hard criteria, was reported (Paul et al. 1963). For men aged 50–59 employed in another Chicago industry the CHD prevalence was said to be 7.1 percent—3.4 times higher (Stamler et al. 1960). Some of the discrepancy can be ascribed to an average age difference of some five years, but an important factor seems to be a difference in criteria. For the group 50–59 years old the label CHD included suspect cases with only bundle branch block and nonspecific T and S-T peculiarities in the electrocardiogram.

For white men 40–59 in Evans County, Georgia, the reported prevalence of 5.4 percent CHD included twelve cases labeled only as possible among the total of 31 men listed as prevalence cases (McDonough et al. 1965). Without the possible cases the rate for these white men is only 3.3 percent. For 283 black men 40–59 in Evans County the reported prevalence of 2.5

percent was based on one definite, two probable, and four possible cases. Considering only definite and probable cases, the rate for the blacks is 1.1 percent, which is not significantly different from that for the corresponding white men. Obviously the numbers are too few for conclusions.

In Gothenburg, Sweden, a prevalence of 2.4 percent CHD was recorded for 855 men, then aged 50, in 1963; in 1971–1972 a prevalence of 4.0 percent was recorded for 5,361 men aged 51–55 by the same team in the same city (Wilhelmsen, Wedel, and Tibblin 1973). In neither series was the response to invitation for the examination perfect (88 percent in 1963, 76 percent in the later series), but there is no reason to suggest a difference in any bias caused by the nonresponders. It is tempting to propose that the frequency of the disease in Gothenburg increased substantially in just under ten years; the difference in prevalence rates is statistically significant ($p = 0.04$). In the later survey the men averaged a little over three years older than those in the earlier Gothenburg survey. That fact alone would be expected to be associated with a somewhat greater prevalence, perhaps as much as 20 percent. Allowing for the age differential, it could be suggested that men aged 51–55 in Gothenburg in 1963 should have had a prevalence of perhaps 2.8 to 2.9 percent. So the data still suggest an increasing frequency of CHD among middle-aged men at Gothenburg. Such findings are a reminder that changes in true frequency over time among men of the same age may cause confusion in comparisons of studies.

Comparisons of populations in respect to the prevalence and incidence of CHD are most acceptable, of course, when the methods and criteria have been carefully standardized beforehand and the clinical judgments centrally reviewed, as in the present study. The parallel epidemiological studies in Puerto Rico and on men of Japanese ancestry in Hawaii conform to these specifications (Gordon et al. 1974). The findings from both studies offer convincing evidence that at the entry examinations the prevalence of old myocardial infarction was of the order of only half that found at Framingham for men of the same age. The lower frequency of CHD in both areas was confirmed by the incidence findings in seven years of follow-up.

As indicated above, it is more difficult to compare the reports from different studies of angina pectoris than of myocardial infarction. Often the two conditions coexist, of course, and frequently one or the other or both together are used to define CHD. A large study in Israel on civil servants (Medallie et al. 1968) reported that the prevalence of definite angina pectoris was 3.1 percent and that of verified previous myocardial infarction was 1.8 percent. It was also stated that 2.5 percent of the men had angina and a "verified history of a previous heart attack." This seems to suggest that angina pectoris as the only indication of CHD was much less common than evidence of previous infarction. This would be similar to the findings in the present study.

The foregoing brief review of prevalence data from leading studies illustrates the difficulty of drawing valid conclusions about prevalence from comparisons of reports from independent studies involving different protocols and investigators. An extreme example is in a recent report from a survey of a "random sample" of men aged 50–54 in Czechoslovakia (Geizerova, Hejl, and Santucek 1975). Eleven percent of the men were judged to be suffering from angina pectoris, and among the men with "low physical activity" the prevalence rose to 17 percent!

Some Characteristics of Prevalence Men

It is interesting to compare characteristics of men given a diagnosis of coronary heart disease with their fellows not so judged, but conclusions about cause and effect are not warranted from such data. Many of the characteristics of interest are so interrelated that in single-variable analysis it would be easy to mistake secondary for primary associations. This is a problem in the analysis of incidence data, but in prevalence data there is also the possibility that observed peculiarities of the prevalence men may be a product of the disease rather than a factor in etiology.

Smoking habits. Table 3.3 summarizes smoking habits of men who were given a diagnosis at the entry examination of either old myocardial infarction or angina pectoris and compares them with the men in their own cohorts who were judged to be free of disease. In all populations most of the men were or had been cigarette smokers, but there were differences in detail among the several cohorts. The percentages of men who had never regularly smoked ranged from a low of 7.6 percent in Zutphen to a high of 34 percent in Serbia. The percentages of the men who, at the time of the entry examinations, were smoking twenty or more cigarettes daily ranged from a low of 19 percent in Italy to the high of 41 percent in Japan. In Zutphen the figure of only 10.7 percent heavy cigarette smokers, twenty or more daily, is deceptive because many of these men, like their countrymen in general, are mixed smokers, smoking pipes, cigars, or both, as well as cigarettes, and many smoke only pipes or cigars.

Perhaps the most significant point in table 3.3 is the fact that the percentage of men who had never smoked was much lower among those with coronary heart disease than those without the disease. Among the American railroad men, 115 had coronary heart disease at entry, and only 13 of them had never smoked. Had they been like the other railroad men without the disease, the expectation would be 22 never-smokers (chi-square = 4.52,

Table 3.3. Smoking status of men with and without coronary heart disease at entry (numbers of men and percentage of all men in the coronary class).

Cohort	Entry status	N (%)	Never smoked (%)	Stopped (%)	Cigarettes per day		
					<10 (%)	10–19 (%)	≥20 (%)
U.S. railroad	OK	2,568	494	560	154	734	627
		(100)	(19)	(22)	(6)	(29)	(24)
	CHD	115	13	46	10	18	28
		(100)	(11)	(40)	(9)	(16)	(24)
Finland	OK	1,615	317	306	204	462	383
		(100)	(19)	(48)	(12)	(28)	(23)
	CHD	57	7	13	5	18	14
		(100)	(12)	(23)	(9)	(32)	(25)
Croatia	OK	1,364	382	170	113	415	284
		(100)	(28)	(13)	(8)	(30)	(21)
	CHD	6	3	0	0	2	1
		(100)	(50)	0	0	(33)	(17)
Italy	OK	2,472	577	355	564	602	470
		(100)	(23)	(14)	(19)	(24)	(19)
	CHD	26	5	5	5	5	6
		(100)	(19)	(19)	(19)	(19)	(23)
Greece	OK	1,207	293	193	141	268	319
		(100)	(24)	(16)	(12)	(22)	(26)
	CHD	7	0	4	1	1	1
		(100)	0	(57)	(14)	(14)	(14)
Zutphen[a]	OK	864	67	155	268	294	94
		(100)	(8)	(18)	(31)	(34)	(11)
	CHD	14	1	5	5	2	0
		(100)	(7)	(36)	(36)	(14)	0
Serbia	OK	1,565	529	235	104	395	302
		(100)	(34)	(15)	(7)	(25)	(19)
	CHD	17	3	3	0	6	5
		(100)	(19)	(19)	0	(38)	(25)
Japan	OK	1,005	157	103	89	250	406
		(100)	(16)	(10)	(9)	(25)	(40)
	CHD	5	0	1	0	1	3
		(100)	0	(20)	0	(20)	(20)

a. At Zutphen many men smoke pipes or cigars. Smoking data are lacking for one man at entry who had CHD.

$p = 0.03$). In all cohorts combined, 32 of the men with coronary heart disease had never smoked; had they been like their fellows in the same cohorts without the disease the expectation would be 73.8 men (chi-square = 14.23).

Also interesting in table 3.3 is the fact that more of the men with CHD had stopped smoking than would be expected to match the rest of the men. Among 102 American men with CHD who had smoked, 46 had stopped at the time of the entry examinations; to correspond with the men without CHD the number would be 28.4 (chi-square = 15.85, $p = 0.00007$). It is fair to infer that many had stopped because they knew or feared they had coronary heart disease and were conscious of the warning of their physicians, the American Heart Association, and the U.S. Public Health Service. The Finns with CHD differed little from the rest of the Finns in this respect. Among the Finnish men with coronary heart disease, 13 had stopped smoking; the expectation to match the other Finns would be 11.7 men (chi-square = 0.69). Presumably advice about the dangers of smoking had not impressed men in rural Finland in 1959. Among men with coronary heart disease in the other cohorts, 18 had stopped smoking when they were first examined; to match the men in their cohorts who were judged free of coronary heart disease the number would be 13.7 (chi-square = 1.517, $p = 0.218$). Combining all the men in all cohorts with coronary heart disease, there were 77 smokers who had stopped; to match the men without CHD in their cohorts the number would be 48.2 (chi-square = 24.56; p is vanishingly small, less than 1 chance in 1 million that the disparity would occur by chance).

Other Characteristics

Table 3.4 summarizes eight characteristics of men who at the entry examination were given diagnoses of previous myocardial infarction, angina pectoris with no indication of infarction, or no such diagnosis. Before comparing the coronary men with the men judged free of the disease, it is interesting to consider differences between the men with the two different positive diagnoses.

Among the American railroad men those with angina pectoris averaged 2.4 years older than the men with infarcts, and the difference is associated with $t = 2.02$, which would indicate $p = 0.046$. But before concluding that this is significant in the usual sense, it should be noted that when comparisons are made with eight sets of variables with no prior hypothesis being tested, the probability that any one of these will be significant cannot be estimated so simply. To reach the level of improbability of chance explanation ordinarily represented by $p = 0.05$ requires a value of p approaching 0.01.

Table 3.4. Characteristics of men with and without coronary heart disease at entry (infarction = codes 00, 01, 03, 04; angina pectoris = definite angina pectoris with no evidence of previous infarction; body mass index (BMI) = kg weight/(m height)^2).

Cohort and item	Infarction			Angina Pectoris			All other men		
	N	Mean	SD	N	Mean	SD	N	Mean	SD
U.S. railroad									
Age	90	52.9	4.9	25	55.3	6.4	2,456	49.7	5.7
Systolic BP	90	143.6	21.4	25	151.9	22.7	2,456	138.9	20.7
Diastolic BP	90	90.1	11.4	25	91.0	12.3	2,456	86.0	11.7
Heart rate	90	73.0	13.5	25	74.7	15.4	2,427	72.0	13.4
Cholesterol	88	254.1	54.2	24	251.0	47.4	2,439	239.6	44.9
BMI	89	25.6	3.2	25	25.5	3.1	2,443	25.0	3.2
Skinfold	90	34.2	10.8	25	41.3	15.3	2,441	33.2	12.3
Height	90	173.0	5.6	25	167.4	7.3	2,447	174.1	6.1
Finland									
Age	35	52.3	4.7	22	53.8	5.5	1,620	49.4	5.5
Systolic BP	35	153.4	27.7	22	171.9	27.5	1,620	143.2	20.1
Diastolic BP	35	90.1	11.9	22	94.1	12.9	1,608	85.2	11.8
Heart rate	35	73.2	13.6	22	70.8	13.9	1,610	67.5	13.0
Cholesterol	35	281.6	57.2	22	286.7	52.0	1,614	260.2	51.9
BMI	35	23.1	2.6	22	23.5	1.8	1,576	23.6	3.2
Skinfold	35	19.0	9.0	22	17.8	9.3	1,616	18.4	9.6
Height	35	167.6	5.4	22	167.6	6.0	1,617	169.7	6.2
Other Europe									
Age	52	52.7	4.9	16	52.3	5.7	7,438	49.7	5.4
Systolic BP	52	149.8	26.9	16	145.1	32.8	7,434	138.8	20.1
Diastolic BP	52	90.4	14.8	16	86.7	18.9	7,431	84.8	11.7
Heart rate	52	73.8	14.4	11	65.9	5.5	6,345	71.6	14.0
Cholesterol	52	218.1	57.7	16	223.4	64.4	7,342	200.8	42.8
BMI	52	23.8	3.7	16	25.2	3.0	7,388	24.3	3.6
Skinfold	52	22.7	12.8	16	23.8	19.3	7,415	21.9	11.7
Height	52	170.2	6.3	16	166.4	5.2	7,435	167.9	13.7

Accordingly, the apparent difference in respect to age in the railroad men cannot be claimed to be significant. However, for two variables there does seem to be a real difference between the two kinds of coronary cases in the American railroad men. On the average, the men with angina had skinfolds that were 21 percent thicker than the average for the infarct men, and that difference is associated with $p = 0.01$. The average height of the men with angina was 5.6 cm less than the infarct men, with p less than 0.0001. On the average, the men with angina were significantly fatter and shorter than the men with infarcts.

For the Finns the only interesting contrast between those with angina and those with infarction is the fact that the average systolic blood pressure was 18.5 mm higher in the men with angina; the difference is associated with $t = 2.46$, $p = 0.01$.

Among the other Europeans, the average age of the men with angina was 0.4 years younger than the men with infarction. Considering all three population groups, there is no significant difference in age between the infarct men and those with angina pectoris.

These possible differences in characteristics between men with angina and those with evidence of prior infarction at the entry examination are relatively small compared to differences between men with prevalent coronary heart disease and their fellows with no such diagnosis. It is reasonable, then, to combine the two diagnostic categories to compare men with and men without coronary heart disease.

In all three groups the men with coronary heart disease at entry differed significantly in respect to age, blood pressure, and serum cholesterol concentration from their fellow countrymen without the disease at that time. The coronary men were older: the average difference was 3.7 years for the Americans, 3.5 years for the Finns, and 2.9 years for the other Europeans. The average systolic blood pressure of the coronary men exceeded that of the CHD-free men by 6.5 mm in the Americans, 17.3 mm in the Finns, and 9.9 mm in the other Europeans. In diastolic blood pressure the average excess for the men with coronary heart disease was 4.3 mm in the Americans, 6.4 mm in the Finns, and 4.7 mm in the other Europeans. The average concentration of cholesterol in the blood serum of the coronary men exceeded that of their CHD-free counterparts by 13.8 mg/dl in the Americans, 23.4 mg/dl in the Finns, and 19.8 mg/dl in the other Europeans. These differences have high statistical significance. In terms of risk as gauged from prospective studies, the outlook for the men with prevalent coronary heart disease was substantially worse than that of the other men in the same populations.

All three groups of men are also consistent in failing to demonstrate any relationship between relative body weight, that is, body mass index, and prevalence of coronary heart disease. Among the Americans and the Finns, but not the other Europeans, the men with CHD tended to be significantly shorter than the other men. The Finnish men with CHD had an average heart rate significantly faster than the other Finns, but heart rate was not important in regard to prevalence in the Americans or the other Europeans.

The indication that men with CHD tend to be significantly fatter than the other men, found among the Americans, was not matched in the data on the Finns and the other Europeans, though in both of those groups there was a statistically insignificant tendency in the same direction. If all populations were combined, the result would be to find the men with CHD have an average skinfold thickness only slightly greater than the other men, but that difference has a very high statistical significance.

Physical activity. An analysis of prevalence data that shows associations between the presence of the disease and some other characteristic raises the following question: Do the observed associations indicate an influence of the characteristic on the development of the disease? When it is observed that the prevalence rate increases with age, it is reasonable to infer that age promotes the disease. But with other variables, such as physical activity, it is proper to ask whether the disease itself may not be the cause of the association.

Many men with overt coronary heart disease avoid exertion on that account. Even before diagnosis of the disease, it is possible that relative coronary insufficiency may produce an unwillingness to undertake heavy work or a tendency to seek less activity. Thus, data on prevalence among men with differing activity levels are unlikely to contribute much to arguments about the hypothesis that lack of exercise promotes the disease. Still, it is interesting to look at the information in the present study on the physical activity required at work. No reliable data could be obtained on recreational activity, and, indeed, the great majority of these middle-aged men in the Seven Countries Study never engaged in any recreational program involving substantial physical effort.

Table 3.5 summarizes the data. Among the American railroad men, the prevalence rate of coronary heart disease of the sedentary men was 1.67 times greater than that of the switchmen, an occupational group chosen because it requires at least moderate activity on the job part of every day (chi-square = 9.13, $p = 0.003$). It should be recalled, however, that there were suggestions of a self-selection bias among switchmen, some of whom feared a job change might result from disclosure of disease.

Another group of 391 railroad men belonged to the Brotherhood of Railway and Steamship Clerks, and their jobs required a fair amount of activity. They were recognized at the outset as nonsedentary (Taylor et al. 1967). The prevalence rate in that group was higher than that of the sedentary railroad men. If those men are added to the switchmen for a comparison of relatively active with sedentary men there is no significant difference in the

CHD rates. So the prevalence data on the railroad men provide no clear distinction related to physical activity.

Among the Finns the men of moderate activity had a higher prevalence rate than the sedentary men, but the difference is not statistically significant. However, the men engaged in heavy physical work were sharply different in prevalence from the other two activity classes, less than one-fourth the average prevalence for the sedentary and only moderately active men (activity classes 1 and 2) ($t = 6.06$). For the other Europeans the CHD prevalence rate for the sedentary men was higher than that for the more active men ($t = 4.21$), but there was no significant difference between the man of moderate and those of heavy activity.

As noted above, there is no way of deciding whether the association in Europe of higher prevalence with lower activity reflects an effect of activity per se or of disease limitation of activity. Actually, the situation is more complicated. In the European cohorts, men of different physical activity also differ in socioeconomic respects. Commonly, the income gradient is in-

Table 3.5. Physical activity of occupation and prevalence of coronary heart disease at entry (moderate = work requiring physical activity but not strenuous; heavy = work involving prolonged effort of large muscle masses).

Group	Sedentary	Moderate	Heavy
U.S. railroad			
All men	1,305	875[a]	0
Men with CHD	60	24	0
CHD per 10,000	460	274	0
SE	58	55	0
Finland			
All men	170	252	1,244
Men with CHD	12	22	23
CHD per 10,000	706	873	185
SE	196	178	38
Other Europe			
All men	1,681	2,081	3,743
Men with CHD	25	18	25
CHD per 10,000	149	86	67
SE	30	20	13

a. Among 391 nonsedentary clerks, 21 had CHD, making a rate of 537 per 10,000 (SE = 114). When these are added to the other men of moderate activity, the CHD rate for that activity class of 1,266 men is 355 (SE = 52).

versely proportional to physical activity. The least active men, the professional men and executives, have the highest incomes. This, of course, is apt to be reflected in the mode of life, including diet and smoking habits, in economies where dietary luxury and costly habits are limited by income.

For the American railroad men an inverse association between activity and income is much less clear. Among the 1,305 sedentary men, there were 317 executives whose incomes were higher than the other men, but there were also 920 sedentary clerks with average incomes lower than those of the switchmen. Furthermore, it should be remarked that for the American railroad men diet and cigarette use were not limited by income.

The Ten-year Follow-up

Table 3.6 summarizes the subsequent experience of the men with coronary heart disease at entry. Among the 90 American railroad men with myocardial infarction, 74 were alive at five years, and 54 at ten years. The ten-

Table 3.6. Deaths in ten years from all causes and from coronary heart disease among 245 men aged 40–59 years with diagnoses of CHD at entry (infarct = myocardial infarction, prevalence codes 00, 01, 03, and 04; angina = definite angina pectoris without evidence of old infarction, code 08; O = observed deaths; E = number expected from the experience of all men in the same cohort matched by single years of age).

CHD by cohort	N	All-causes deaths			CHD deaths		
		O	E	O/E	O	E	O/E
Infarct							
U.S. railroad	90	36	12.45	2.89	26	6.27	4.15
Finland	35	20	7.59	2.64	18	3.22	5.59
All other	57	24	8.48	2.83	17	1.92	8.85
Total	182	80	28.52	2.81	61	11.41	5.35
Angina							
U.S. railroad	25	9	4.21	2.14	6	2.00	3.00
Finland	22	12	4.74	2.53	8	1.92	4.17
All other	16	4	1.67	2.40	1	.31	3.23
Total	63	25	10.62	2.35	15	4.23	3.55
All CHD							
U.S. railroad	115	45	16.66	2.70	32	8.27	3.87
Finland	57	32	12.33	2.60	26	5.14	5.06
All other	73	28	10.15	2.76	18	2.23	8.07
Total	245	105	39.14	2.68	76	15.64	4.86

Prevalence of Cardiovascular Disease at Entry | 49

year all-causes death rate of United States railroad men free of CHD at entry was 10.11 percent. Accordingly, in the absence of CHD, the expectation would be 0.1011 (90) = 9.10 deaths, indicating that the penalty of infarction at entry is (90 − 54)/9.10 = 3.96 times the death rate otherwise. But the average age of these men was 52.9 years, whereas that of their CHD-free counterparts was 49.7, so adjustment for age is necessary. There exists a solution of the multiple logistic equation for estimating, for given age, the probability of death in ten years from any cause among American railroad men free from CHD at entry (chapter 6). From that solution we find that, other things being equal, the death rate expected at 52.9 years is 1.32 times that at 49.7. So the corrected expected deaths is 1.32 (9.10) = 12.01, and the ratio of observed to expected deaths (O/E), 36/12.01 = 3.00, shows the penalty, as a multiple of the CHD-free death rate, associated with infarction at entry.

Among the 25 American railroad men with entry angina, 9 were dead in ten years. With no allowance for age, the expected deaths would be 0.1011 (25) = 2.53, and O/E = 3.46. But again allowance is needed for age, the angina men averaging 55.3 years at entry. From the multiple logistic solution from CHD-free men, it is expected that the ten-year all-causes death rate of men aged 55.3 will be 1.64 times that of men aged 49.7. The correct expected deaths, then, is 1.64 (2.53) = 4.15, and O/E = 9/4.15 = 2.17. The mortality excess associated with entry angina is then about 100 (2.17/3.00) = 72 percent that with myocardial infarction.

The same analysis for the Finns shows that for the 35 infarction men and the 22 men with entry angina the ten-year death expectations to match men CHD-free at entry would be 0.149(35) = 5.23 and 0.149 (22) = 3.28, respectively. Since the observed deaths were 20 and 12, respectively, the corresponding O/E ratios are 3.82 and 3.66. But again allowance must be made for average age—52.3 years for the infarct men, 53.8 for men with angina, 49.4 for men without coronary heart disease. Using the solution of the multiple logistic equation for Finns free of coronary heart disease, the expected death rates at ages 52.3 and 53.8 are, respectively, 1.30 and 1.48 times that of Finns 49.4 years old. So the expected deaths among 35 men = 1.30 (5.23) = 6.80 and the correct ratio, 20/6.80 = 2.94; ten-year deaths among the Finns with entry infarction were 2.94 times those of their countrymen with no CHD at entry. The corresponding calculation for the Finns with entry angina is 1.43 (3.28) = 4.85 expected deaths; 12/4.85 = 2.47, the ten-year deaths of the angina men as a multiple of the expectation in the absence of coronary heart disease.

The corresponding analysis of the mortality of the other European men, 53 with myocardial infarction and 16 with angina pectoris at entry, shows that the ten-year age-corrected deaths to match the experience of their fellow countrymen without CHD at entry would be 7.98 and 2.29 deaths, respectively. Actually, 23 of the infarct men and 4 of the men with angina pectoris died, so the ratios of observed to expected deaths are 2.88 and 1.74, respectively.

It is interesting that the ten-year death rate penalties associated with myocardial infarction and angina pectoris are substantially the same in all three population groups. Men aged 40–59 with old myocardial infarction have a ten-year death rate roughly three times that of men of the same age in the same population but without coronary heart disease at the start. And for men with only angina pectoris the ten-year death rate is roughly double that of men without CHD at the start but is otherwise comparable.

Classes of infarcts: differences in prognosis. The term *infarcts* in table 3.6 includes all four diagnostic classes of infarct prevalence, 00, 01, 03, 04, as defined in chapter 2. It can be asked, however, whether the ten-year follow-up shows differences in the prognosis of the several classes of old myocardial infarction. Class 00, which requires major Q waves in the electrocardiogram, is considered to be a harder and more certain diagnosis than class 04, which requires no persistent confirmation in the electrocardiogram. In the present material of 12,763 men, there were 80 men in entry prevalence class 00, and 53 in class 04. In between are 49 men with entry diagnosis of old infarction based on the criteria of classes 01 and 03, which require less striking and specific ECG abnormality than class 00. For these infarct classes the age- and cohort-specific ten-year expected coronary deaths were calculated to correspond to the numbers at risk if the men in those entry prevalence classes had the same experience as all men of identical ages in the same cohorts. Classes 01 and 03 were combined because there was no evidence of a difference between them in the ten-year outcome, and the numbers are small. Figure 3.2 summarizes the comparison between observed and expected ten-year deaths from coronary heart diseases.

For each of the entry infarct prevalence classes the ratio of observed to expected deaths, O/E, shows a very bad outlook, but there are differences in the indicated prognosis. In this respect, classes 00, 01, and 03 are almost identical with more than six times the eventual death rate from coronary heart disease than experienced by all men of the same age in their cohorts. The prospect of death in ten years from coronary heart disease is only about half as bad for the men with an entry diagnosis of old myocardial infarction based on our criteria for class 04.

The difference between the number of observed deaths and those expected to correspond with the experience of all men matched by cohort and

Prevalence of Cardiovascular Disease at Entry | 51

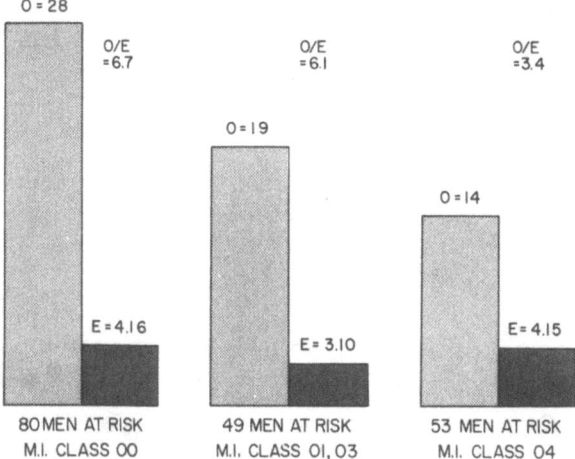

Figure 3.2. Ten-year deaths from coronary heart disease among 182 men given a diagnosis of old myocardial infarction at the entry examination and classified by the criteria used for the diagnosis. O = number of deaths observed; E = number of deaths corresponding to the age- and cohort-specific coronary death rates of all men in those cohorts. M.I. class 00 = prevalence code 00 = Minnesota code 1.1 (major Q waves). M.I. classes 0.1, 0.3 = lesser Q waves plus major T-wave findings (01) or clinical judgment of heart disease of myocardial infarct etiology plus specified ECG abnormalities (03). M.I. class 04 = clinical judgment of definite heart disease and etiology specified as myocardial infarct but without persisting confirmatory ECG changes.

age is highly significant. Consider the greatest difference indicated in figure 3.2, that between the men in myocardial infarction (M.I.) class 00 and those in class 04. In class 00 the total of 28 deaths is made up of 4.16 expected deaths, 23.84 not expected; in class 04 the 14 observed deaths comprise 4.15 expected deaths and 9.85 not expected. These are the numbers for a 2-x-2 contingency table from which we find chi-square = 1.29, $p = 0.26$.

Relationship of prevalence to age. Table 3.4 gives data on mean age of men with angina, with myocardial infarction, and with no such diagnosis at entry, showing that the average age of the men with coronary heart disease is greater than that of the men without disease. More important than this not unexpected finding are details of the relationship of prevalence rate to age. Figure 3.3 shows that the prevalence rate increases more or less linearly with age in both the European and the American men, but that the rate of increase is strikingly different in the two groups.

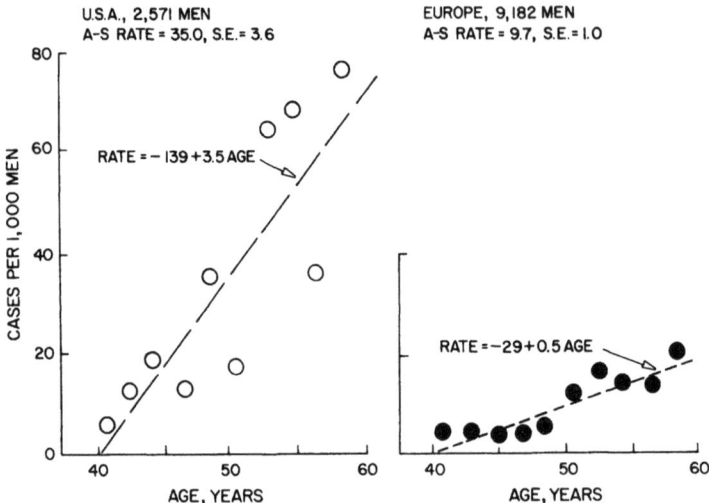

Figure 3.3 Age and the prevalence of old myocardial infarction among American railroad men and among men in the European cohorts. Cases per 1,000 men per two-year age class and the regression of the prevalence rate on age. A-S *rate* = rate per 1,000 men standardized by single years of age.

The age-standardized prevalence rate of myocardial infarction for the Americans is 3.6 times that for the Europeans, the t value of the difference having the extremely high value of 9.24. The prevalence rates for the two groups are not importantly different at the youngest ages, 40–42 years; the great difference for the overall range of 40–59 years is explained by the much greater increase with age for the Americans than for the Europeans. The slopes of the regression lines are 3.5 and 0.47, meaning that the rate of increase with age for the Americans is $3.5/0.47 = 7.4$ times that for the European men.

Figure 3.4 shows the corresponding picture for the prevalence rate of angina pectoris. The difference between the Americans and the Europeans is less striking than in the prevalence of myocardial infarction, but it is still very large. The age-standardized prevalence rate for angina pectoris is 10.6 per 1,000 for the Americans, 4.3 for the Europeans, giving a ratio of 2.5 to 1; this is associated with $t = 3.75$. And again, as in the case of infarction, the prevalence rates of the two groups are not significantly different at the youngest ages; the rise of prevalence rate with age is the important factor. The slopes of the regressions of prevalence on age are 1.54 and 0.81 for Americans and Europeans, respectively, so the increase with age for the Americans is $1.54/0.81 = 1.9$ times that for the Europeans.

These facts show that in reporting the prevalence of coronary heart disease

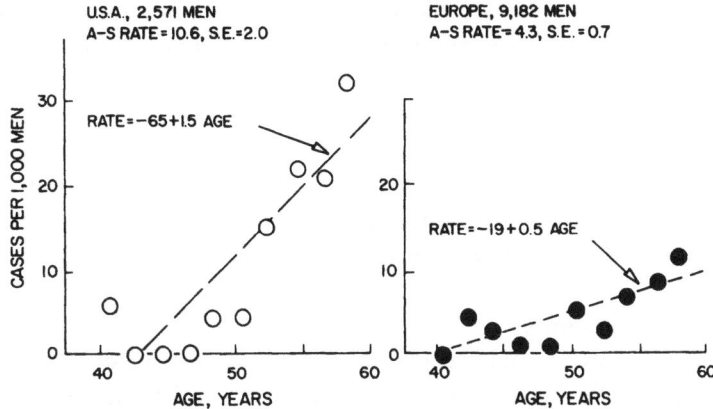

Figure 3.4. Age and the prevalence of angina pectoris as the only evidence of coronary heart disease. Cases per 1,000 men per two-year age class and the regression of the prevalence rate on age. A-S rate = rate per 1,000 men standardized by single years of age.

it is not enough to give the rate for ten-year or broader age classes. To allow comparisons it is essential to have rates standardized by age, preferably by single years of age—at least for two-year classes.

Japanese Men

Five of the 1,010 Japanese men were reported as having coronary heart disease at entry—one at Tanushimaru, four at Ushibuka. The two Japanese cohorts were unique in the Seven Countries Study in not having international teams participating in the entry examinations, a deficiency remedied in follow-up examinations; funds were not available for the costly travel to Japan at the start. However, Dr. Noboru Kimura, head of the Japanese team and director of the Institute for Cardiovascular Diseases, University of Kurume, had received training in cardiology in Minnesota and Los Angeles and had been a member of the international teams conducting our trial surveys in Nicotera, Italy, and Crete in 1957. Several members of Dr. Kimura's team had also had international experience.

The Japanese men labeled coronary at entry were so judged solely on electrocardiographic evidence. Four were given our code 00, corresponding to Minnesota ECG code 1.1 (major Q waves), and one man was given code 01 (Minnesota ECG code 1.2 plus 5.1 or 5.2, that is, lesser Q waves plus major T wave findings). These Japanese men had no angina pectoris or history suggesting infarction, and all were fully employed in nonsedentary work. All were heavy cigarette smokers; one man had hypertension (210/100 mm/Hg in rest); the mean cholesterol was 164 mg/dl of serum. The heart rate in rest was 95 beats per minute in one man; the mean for the other four men was 65 beats per minute.

In the ten-year follow-up examination, one of the Japanese prevalence men died from tuberculosis. The man with entry code 01 was alive and still so coded at the ten-year examination. The other three men, with code 00 at entry, were alive at ten years and showed no evidence, clinical or electrocardiographic, of coronary heart disease.

Other Heart Disease

Table 3.1 gives the numbers of cases and the prevalence rates for definite heart disease other than coronary heart disease. Neglecting the Japanese men for whom the prevalence of all heart disease was relatively trivial, only for the American railroad men and the Finns did coronary dominate the total heart disease picture. Coronary heart disease accounted for 67 percent of all heart disease among the Americans, 60 percent among the Finns, 47 percent among the Dutch, 38 percent among the Italians, 37 percent among the Serbians, 29 percent among the Greeks, and 14 percent among the Croatians.

These figures do not reflect a high noncoronary heart disease (NCHD) prevalence among the Serbs, Italians, and so on; the outstanding feature is the relatively low coronary prevalence in those cohorts. Actually, the prevalence of NCHD was significantly higher among the American railroad men and the Finns than among the other Europeans. The difference in prevalence rate, Finland minus American railroad, 36.8 per 10,000, has $SE = 48.1$, so there is no indication of a real difference. But the difference American railroad minus other Europeans, 64.4, has $SE = 30.2$, $t = 2.13$ and $p = 0.05$. The difference between the Finns and the other Europeans, 101.1 per 10,000, is still more significant, with $SE = 35.9$ and $t = 2.82$, so the probability of chance explanation is only slightly more than 1 in 100.

Table 3.7 gives mean values and standard deviations for eight characteristics measured on 227 men with heart disease other than coronary, omitting the 4 Japanese because the number is too small for significant statistics. As might be expected, the average blood pressure and heart rate of these men is higher than that of the generality of men in their cohorts (compare with table 3.4), but otherwise these men were not remarkable in the characteristics given in table 3.7.

Table 3.8 gives the data on the physical activity of the work these men were doing in the period of the entry examinations. In spite of their heart disease, these men were not much overly represented in the class of sedentary activities. For American railroad men, the prevalence among the seden-

Table 3.7. Characteristics of men with heart disease other than coronary at entry (see table 3.4 to compare with characteristics of other men in the same cohorts).

Item	U.S. RR	Finland	Other Europe
Age			
N	58	44	125
Mean	52.4	49.5	51.0
SD	5.8	5.8	5.7
Systolic BP			
N	58	44	125
Mean	162.2	157.5	153.8
SD	31.2	31.6	29.8
Diastolic BP			
N	58	44	125
Mean	99.9	90.3	91.0
SD	18.4	16.8	17.2
Heart rate			
N	58	44	109
Mean	75.9	78.5	78.1
SD	13.3	19.2	17.4
Cholesterol			
N	58	44	122
Mean	230.4	252.8	194.1
SD	34.3	50.5	46.3
Body mass index			
N	58	44	125
Mean	25.5	23.5	24.5
SD	3.6	3.4	4.1
Skinfolds			
N	57	44	125
Mean	33.9	18.1	22.6
SD	13.1	9.3	12.9
Height			
N	58	44	125
Mean	173.8	169.2	169.0
SD	6.3	7.9	7.6

tary employees was 13 percent higher than among the more active switchmen, but the difference is far from being significant (chi-square = 0.09, $p = 0.76$). In Finland, the prevalence among the sedentary men was only 3 percent higher than among the moderately active men, a difference that could be expected by chance in 94 out of 100 trials ($p = 0.94$). Although the

Table 3.8. Physical activity of occupation and the prevalence of noncoronary heart disease at entry. (moderate = work that requires physical activity but is not strenuous; heavy = work involving prolonged effort of large muscle masses).

Group	Item	Sedentary	Moderate	Heavy
U.S. railroad	N	32	19[a]	0
	Cases/10,000	245	217	—
	SE	42.8	49.3	—
Finland	N	7	10	27
	Cases/10,000	411	396	161
	SE	152	123	47
Other Europe	N	33	32	60
	Cases/10,000	196	154	160
	SE	34	27	21
Japan[b]	N	1	2	1

a. In addition 7 out of 391 nonsedentary clerks had noncoronary heart disease at entry, giving a prevalence of 179/10,000 (SE = 67).
b. Among all men in the Japanese cohorts at entry, 41 were sedentary; 314, moderately active; and 655 heavy workers.

difference between the sedentary and very active Finns shown in table 3.8 looks more impressive, chi-square is only 2.27 and the observed difference would be expected from chance alone in 13 out of 100 trials ($p = 0.132$). The slightly larger difference between the moderately active Finns and their very active countrymen is associated with chi-square = 2.64, $p = 0.104$. For the other Europeans, prevalence among sedentary compared with moderately active men gives chi-square = 0.96, $p = 0.33$, and the comparison of sedentary with the very active men gives chi-square = 0.86, $p = 0.35$. In none of the comparisons, then, is there reason to believe that the habitual level of physical activity is related to the presence or absence of noncoronary heart disease.

Table 3.9 summarizes the smoking habits of the men with noncoronary heart disease at entry. In the cohort of American railroad men, smoking habits seemed to be practically unrelated to the presence or absence of this disease. In Finland, the noncoronary heart disease men were underrepresented among heavy smokers, but the number is small and the difference is not statistically significant. There is a similar trend in Croatia and Serbia, but the numbers are even smaller. Combining the information in tables 3.9 and 3.3, the net picture is that the habit of smoking cigarettes was little influenced by the presence of heart disease in these populations in the period of the entry examinations in 1958–1964. It seems appropriate to

Table 3.9. Smoking status of men with noncoronary heart disease at entry (compare with all men in table 3.3).

					Cigarettes per day		
Cohort	Item	All men	Never smoked	Stopped	<10	10–19	≥20
U.S. railroad	N	58	16	9	2	14	17
	%	100	28	16	3	24	29
Finland	N	44	6	11	16	5	6
	%	100	14	25	36	11	14
Croatia	N	16	4	4	1	5	2
	%	100	25	25	6	31	13
Italy	N	45	8	11	8	9	9
	%	100	17	28	17	19	19
Greece	N	17	3	1	4	5	4
	%	100	18	6	23	29	23
Zutphen	N	16	2	3	8	3	0
	%	100	12	19	50	19	0
Serbia	N	30[a]	7	6	5	10	2
	%	100	23	20	17	33	7
Japan	N	3[a]	0	0	0	0	3
	%	100	0	0	0	0	100

a. Plus one man with no data on smoking.

repeat that the relationship of health to smoking was largely unknown, or ignored, by these men in those years.

Noncoronary Heart Disease: The Follow-up

Table 3.6 shows that among the men with an entry diagnosis of definite old myocardial infarction the follow-up found many of them not only alive after ten years, but on reexamination there was no evidence of the disease except for the entry examination record. Table 3.10 shows that the follow-up picture was similar to the men with definite noncoronary heart disease at entry.

Among 58 American railroad men with entry NCHD, at the five-year reexamination 37 of them were not considered to be suffering from any kind of heart disease, and 4 men had died in the interim, 3 from coronary heart disease, 1 from other heart disease. Although the heart disease status of survivors at ten years is unknown, it is known that only 11 of the original 58 men had died, 6 from coronary heart disease, 3 from other heart disease. Although this rate of 18.96 percent in ten years is 66 percent higher than the

Table 3.10. Ten-year status of men with noncoronary heart disease at entry (heart deaths are from heart disease other than coronary; other deaths are from all other causes; OK = no evidence of any kind of heart disease at ten-year examination; heart = definite heart disease at that time).

Group	N	Age (mean)	Deaths in ten years			Ten-year status[a]		
			CHD	Heart	Other	OK	Heart	Exam
U.S. railroad	58	52.4	6	3	2	37[a]	6[a]	4[a]
Finland	44	49.5	8	7	7	13	8	1[b]
Croatia	16	53.5	3	3	3	4	1	2
Italy	45	51.6	3	7	7	22	2	6[c]
Zutphen	16	52.7	3	0	1	8	3	1[b]
Serbia	31	49.9	1	7	2	19	2	0
Japan	4	56.5	0	2	2	0	0	0

a. For U.S. railroad, five-year status is given.
b. Known to be alive at ten years.
c. One man seen alive at ten years, five Rome railroad men not listed dead by the Italian Ministry of Transportation.

ten-year all-causes rate for all American railroad men, allowance should be made for the fact that the NCHD men averaged 52.4 years old at entry compared with the average of 49.7 years for the other American railroad men. From the regression of all-causes death rate on age for all railroad men, it is calculated that the ten-year death rate for those starting at age 52.4 would be 26.8 percent higher than at age 49.7. The net result is that the observed death rate of the NCHD railroad men is only 31 percent higher than would be expected for all the railroad men at the same age.

In Finland among 44 NCHD men at entry, 22 were dead in ten years, but among the survivors 13 were found to be free from evidence of definite heart disease at the ten-year examination. The 50 percent death rate in ten years is to be compared with the finding of 16.3 percent dead in ten years among all the Finns; NCHD among the Finns was associated with three times the death rate expected in the absence of entry NCHD. Note that no age correction is required because the Finns with NCHD had an average age of 49.5 years and the average for all the Finns was 49.4 years.

As evident from table 3.10, the experience was similar for the men with entry NCHD in the other cohorts. The most extreme finding was with the Greeks. Of the original 17 NCHD men, 13 were alive with no evidence of definite heart disease at ten years. For all cohorts combined, half the men originally labeled definite noncoronary heart disease were not so diagnosed ten years later. On the other hand, the diagnosis at entry was associated with an elevated ten-year death rate, 34.6 percent instead of 11.8 percent for the rest of the Seven Countries Study men. The age correction from age 49.7 for all men to age 52.1 for the NCHD men brings the expected rate at 52.1 years to 15.2 percent. The net result is an all-causes death rate $34.6/15.2 = 2.28$ times that expected in the absence of noncoronary heart disease at entry.

It is not possible here to report details of the representation of various diagnostic categories in the class noncoronary heart disease and the ten-year experience of the men labeled rheumatic heart disease, hypertensive heart disease, and so on at entry. A special case-by-case review of the original examination records is required, and the findings should be separately reported. However, it may be remarked that rheumatic heart disease accounted for 45 percent of NCHD and hypertensive heart disease another 24 percent.

We have considered only the men who received a diagnosis of definite heart disease at entry in which there was agreement between the original examining physician and a consultant. However, a second opinion was not asked for the men given a clean bill of health by the examiner. This suggests that a positive diagnosis was more conservative than a negative one. In other words, some cases of heart disease may have been missed, and the possibility of false negative diagnosis would seem to be greater than the possibility of false positive diagnosis.

The entry prevalence discussed here, both in regard to coronary and noncoronary heart disease, concerns only cases in which the clinicians gave a judgment of definite heart disease. For nearly as many more, the clinicians diagnosed possible heart disease, but it is not proposed here to discuss the details or the subsequent experience of the men labeled as possible heart disease. Those men have not been excluded from the category, free from cardiovascular disease, comprising the basis for the analysis of ten-year incidence of death and of coronary heart disease.

A total of 603 men with no history or clinical evidence of heart disease had electrocardiographic abnormalities not in themselves sufficient to warrant a diagnosis of definite heart disease. These are identified as code 11 and include any of the following Minnesota codes: 1.2, 1.3, 4.1, 4.2, 4.3, 4.4, 5.1, 5.2, 6.1, 6.2, 7.1, 7.2, 7.4, and 8.3. These men were not excluded from the cohort labeled as free from cardiovascular disease at entry, the group of men on whom we have concentrated attention in regard to incidence of death and nonfatal coronary heart disease.

The CVD-free label does not guarantee the absence of cardiovascular disease; it means simply the absence of observed evidence of disease. The inclusion of the men with these ECG abnormalities in the CVD-free cohort allows us to analyze the ECG abnormalities as risk factors in the same way as we treat age, blood pressure, and so on.

A detailed analysis of the separate ECG abnormalities and other ECG characteristics as risk factors is in preparation. Here table 3.11 summarizes the picture in regard to all-causes deaths in ten years. For the combined sixteen cohorts, among the 603 men at risk, 118 were dead in ten years, making a ten-year death rate of 19.57 percent. In contrast, the corresponding death rate for all men in the Seven Countries Study, including these 603 men, was 11.75 percent; for the 12,160 men not coded prevalence 11, the ten-year rate was 11.37. These are crude rates; exact comparison requires allowance for the fact that the men with prevalence code 11 had an average age of 51.35 years, whereas the mean for all men in this study was 49.70 years. This difference should be associated with an increase of 16 percent in ten-year death rate in the absence of code 11 of 13.19 percent. So the mortality associated with code 11 was 19.57/13/19 = 1.48, or 48 percent greater than for the other men.

Table 3.11. Ten-year all-causes death rate of men with nonspecific electrocardiographic abnormalities at entry (code 11) (N is number at risk; base rate is that of all men in the cohort; O/E is rate/base rate).

Cohort	N	Deaths	Rate (%)	Base rate	O/E
U.S. railroad	125	22	18	11.7	1.7
Dalmatia	29	6	21	9.1	2.3
Slavonia	11	12	39	17.8	2.2
Tanushimaru	13	4	31	11.4	2.7
East Finland	21	8	38	18.0	2.1
West Finland	39	8	21	14.8	1.4
Ushibuka	21	5	24	13.9	1.7
Crevalcore	68	16	24	13.7	1.8
Montegiorgio	34	8	24	10.3	2.3
Zutphen	69	11	16	12.4	1.3
Crete	27	3	11	6.1	1.8
Corfu	49	6	12	8.1	1.5
Rome railroad	31	3	10	10.0	1.0
Velika Krsna	22	5	23	12.3	1.9
Zrenjanin	11	0	0	11.6	—
Belgrade	13	1	8	5.0	1.6
Total	603	118	19.6	11.7	1.7

Hypertensive Vascular Disease

As indicated in chapter 2, our code 20, hypertensive vascular disease, requires "finding of hypertensive fundi." As noted in chapter 2, proper funduscopic examination was impossible in some of the cohorts, so caution is necessary in the interpretation of apparent differences among cohorts in the prevalence of code 20.

Men with hypertensive vascular disease but no heart disease or electrocardiographic abnormalities were labeled code 20 in our prevalence code and were excluded from the CVD-free cohort for analysis of subsequent mortality and CHD incidence. There were 121 such men, 67 among the 2,571 American railroad men (2.6 percent, $SE = 0.31$ percent), 25 among 1,677 Finns (1.5 percent, $SE = 0.30$ percent), and 29 among 7,505 other Europeans (0.39 percent, $SE = 0.07$ percent). These differences in prevalence rate are statistically highly significant ($t = 2.44$ for Americans versus Finns, $t = 5.35$ for Finns versus other Europeans, and $t = 10.00$ for Americans versus other Europeans).

In the ten years after entry, from all causes there were 16 deaths among these Americans (23.9 percent, $SE = 5.2$ percent), 8 among the Finns (32.0 percent, $SE = 9.3$ percent), and 9 among the other Europeans (31.0 percent, $SE = 9.3$ percent). Because none of the differences in death rates of the three groups of men with code 20 approaches statistical significance, the code-20 men may be grouped in a comparison with all men without code 20 at entry. The result is that 121 code-20 men had a ten-year all-causes death rate of 27.3 percent ($SE = 4.1$ percent), whereas the 12,642 men not so coded had a rate of 10.9 percent ($SE = 2.8$ percent). The mortality of code-20 men was 2.5 times that of the other men, and the difference is associated with $t = 5.71$.

Intermittent Claudication

In our system men with intermittent claudication without evidence of heart disease with no important electrocardiographic abnormalities and no hypertensive vascular disease were given prevalence code 21. There were only 56 men so coded, and they have been excluded from the CVD-free cohort for analysis of subsequent mortality and CHD incidence. The distribution of these men among the sixteen cohorts seems odd: 0 among 2,582 Greeks and Croatians, 1 among 1,010 Japanese, 3 among the 878 men of Zutphen, 4 among 2,480 Italians, 9 among 2,571 American railroad men, 13 among 1,677 Finns, 12 among 508 men of Zrenjanin, and only 2 among 1,057 other Serbians.

The number of cases is small, and among the differences in prevalence rate only that between the men of Zrenjanin and the other Serbians needs consideration. The rate for Zrenjanin is 12.5 times that for the other Serbians, and the difference, $t = 4.3$. This is interesting because the same team from the University of Belgrade medical school was responsible for the examinations of all three of the Serbian cohorts.

In the ten-year follow-up, 11 of the 56 men with code 21 died (18.0 percent, SE = 4.9 percent), and among 12,702 men not so coded there were 1,489 deaths (11.7 percent, SE = 0.3 percent). The difference is not statistically significant.

"Disappearance" of Coronary Heart Disease

In the report on the five-year experience of the men in the Seven Countries Study it was shown that among 178 men given a diagnosis of old myocardial infarction at entry, 42 were dead in five years but among 136 still alive at that time 47 showed no evidence of coronary heart disease at the five-year examination, a 35 percent rate of spontaneous cure (Keys 1970, p. I-149). Among men with a diagnosis of only uncomplicated angina pectoris at entry, 19 were dead in five years, but among 51 of the men with such angina at entry who were reexamined five years later, 23 (45 percent) had no evidence of coronary heart disease.

The ten-year experience confirmed that the disappearance of signs and symptoms of coronary heart disease is not infrequent. Among 97 European men given a diagnosis of old infarction at the entry examinations, 35 died during the ten-year follow-up, but among 43 survivors who were reexamined at the tenth anniversary, 16 had no evidence of any kind save the entry history of the disease. Among men given a diagnosis of uncomplicated angina pectoris at entry, only one-third of those reexamined after ten years had some manifestations of coronary heart disease (Keys 1978).

Summary

Of 12,763 men aged 40–59 at the entry examinations a diagnosis of cardiovascular disease was made for 658 men (5.2 percent), coronary heart disease being specified for 246 men. Those prevalence cases were excluded from the main analyses of incidence during the ten years of follow-up but were followed in regard to prognosis.

The prevalence rate of coronary heart disease varied from a high of 4.6 percent for the Americans to a low of 0.5 percent for the Japanese and the Greeks. It is shown that these prevalence rates cannot be serious overestimates of the population prevalence, but gross underestimation cannot be excluded when fewer than 90 percent of the men invited appear for examination. Accordingly, the true prevalence in the invited cohort of Americans could be higher than 4.6 percent.

The prevalence of old myocardial infarction in the American men was similar to that reported from other surveys of American white men but was much higher than the prevalence in any other population group in this study. The nearest rate was for the Finns, who had a prevalence 60 percent that of the Americans.

The prevalence of uncomplicated angina pectoris raises questions about the diagnosis such that comparisons among populations are seldom warranted. However, when the same cardiologists make the diagnoses at all ages, the regression of the prevalence rate on age can be calculated. Those calculations show that the slope of the regression of prevalence on age is much steeper for the Americans than for the Europeans.

Compared with their fellows in the same cohort, the men with coronary heart disease at entry tend to be older, to have higher blood pressures, higher serum cholesterol concentrations, and faster resting heart rates, but they were not peculiar in relative body weight, body fatness, or height. The men with coronary heart disease more commonly had stopped smoking but more rarely had never smoked than their healthy counterparts. Understandably, the men with coronary heart disease tended to avoid heavy physical work.

The 129 men with a diagnosis at entry of old myocardial infarction based on electrocardiographic evidence in addition to the medical history had a ten-year death rate from coronary heart disease 6 times that of the other men of the same age in the same cohort. The corresponding coronary death rate of the 53 men with diagnosis of old infarction at entry but without persisting ECG confirmation was half as great, a prognosis substantially the same as that of the 63 men with a diagnosis at entry of only uncomplicated angina pectoris.

Men with hypertensive vascular disease (fundus changes and hypertension but no evidence of heart disease) had an age- and cohort-specific all-causes death rate 2.5 times that of the men with no evidence of cardiovascular disease at entry.

Among 152 men in Europe with a diagnosis of noncoronary heart disease at entry, 62 were dead in ten years, 18 of the deaths being ascribed to coronary heart disease and 24 to other heart disease. Among 58 American railroad men with noncoronary heart disease at entry, only 11 were dead in ten years, 6 of the deaths being certified as caused by coronary heart disease. The better experience of the Americans can be explained by consideration that men with major noncoronary heart disease were not apt to be long-time employees of the railroads.

4 | Ten-Year Deaths

Table 4.1 shows the numbers of ten-year deaths from all causes and from coronary heart disease in each of the sixteen cohorts, the age-standardized ten-year death rates per 10,000 men, the 95 percent confidence limits of those death rates, and the ratio, O/E, of the observed numbers of deaths to those expected from the death rates of American white men matched by single years of age, reported in the U.S. Vital Statistics for 1972 for the first five years of follow-up and for 1967 for the second five years. Details of the calculations are explained in chapter 2.

At entry the American railroad men had been somewhat selected toward health by the fact that they were all full-time workers in an industry with a substantial medical care coverage. Moreover, they lived in the northwest sector of the United States, which, in general, has a lower death rate than the country as a whole. It is not surprising, then, that the all-causes death rate of the American railroad men was substantially lower than the national average for white men of their age. However, the coronary death rate of these railroad men was very little lower than the expectation based on the U.S. vital statistics. This finding is consistent with the common opinion that, at least until now, the availability of a good program of medical care offers little protection against the development of coronary heart disease.

Like their American counterparts, the Italian railroad men were healthy enough at the start to be fully employed, and they too were covered by a system of full medical care as a provision of their employment. Table 4.2 indicates that the Italian railroad men fared somewhat better in all-causes deaths than their American colleagues and very much better in regard to coronary deaths.

The Belgrade cohort, made up of members of the faculty of the Univer-

Table 4.1. Ten-year deaths observed (O) from all causes and from coronary heart disease (age-standardized rates per 10,000, the 95 percent confidence limits of those rates, and the O/E ratio calculated from observed rates and those expected from the rates for white men matched by single years of age in U.S. Vital Statistics life tables for 1962 and 1967).

Cohort	All-causes deaths					CHD deaths				
	O	Rate	95% limits		O/E	O	Rate	95% limits		O/E
U.S. railroad	294	1,153	1,030	1,276	0.77	146	574	484	664	0.92
Dalmatia	61	801	596	1,006	0.60	7	86	16	156	0.16
Slavonia[a]	124	1,652	1,375	1,929	1.17	15	214	106	322	0.34
Tanushimaru	58	1,109	835	1,382	0.63	5	88	7	170	0.15
East Finland	147	1,864	1,597	2,131	1.32	78	992	788	1,198	1.71
West Finland	127	1,479	1,241	1,716	1.00	30	351	228	474	0.57
Ushibuka	70	1,362	1,062	1,662	0.94	4	66	−5	136	0.13
Crevalcore	136	1,381	1,167	1,596	0.94	24	248	151	344	0.40
Montegiorgio	74	1,100	871	1,329	0.73	10	150	61	238	0.24
Zutphen	109	1,218	1,001	1,434	0.84	38	420	297	552	0.71
Crete	42	656	470	841	0.44	1	9	−13	31	0.03
Corfu	43	833	598	1,068	0.56	8	144	43	246	0.25
Rome railroad	77	1,036	820	1,252	0.70	22	290	171	408	0.49
Velika Krsna	63	1,189	908	1,470	0.83	4	80	3	157	0.13
Zrenjanin	60	1,223	940	1,506	0.85	8	152	46	257	0.27
Belgrade	27	594	394	793	0.41	13	288	147	429	0.48
Total	1,507	1,181	1,125	1,237	0.82	410	321	305	337	0.53

a. Includes 24 deaths from tuberculosis.

sity of Belgrade, were also somewhat selected toward health by their full-time employment in a profession that commonly enjoys a relatively low death rate. The ten-year all-causes death rate of the Belgrade professors was only 41 percent of that expected from the U.S. Vital Statistics for white men of the same age. They also fared better than their countrymen in the other four Yugoslav cohorts whose corresponding rates ranged from 60 percent in Dalmatia to 117 percent in Slavonia. Slavonia was remarkable in having 24 deaths from tuberculosis. Without those deaths the all-causes rate for Slavonia would be 95 percent of the expectation for the United States.

Table 4.1 shows that the Greeks had an exceptionally favorable ten-year record for deaths from all causes and were even more notable for their coronary death rate. At the other extreme are the east Finns who had the highest all-causes and coronary death rates in this study. Table 4.1 also shows a substantial difference between the east and west Finns in all-causes deaths and a striking contrast in coronary deaths.

Table 4.1 shows that, except for the east Finns, all of the cohorts in this study had fewer deaths from coronary heart disease than would correspond to the U.S. Vital Statistics on white men of identical age. Moreover, in this respect the coronary death rate of the American railroad men was considerably higher than that for any of the other cohorts except, again, the east Finns. For fourteen of the sixteen cohorts, omitting the Americans and the east Finns, 192 coronary deaths were observed; to match the U.S. Vital Statistics; the number would be 461.3 (O/E = 0.42).

From table 4.1 we may calculate the deaths observed and expected from causes other than coronary heart disease. The result shows that the low coronary rate in Slavonia is much more than compensated for by a very high noncoronary death rate—109 such deaths observed (61.9 expected, O/E = 1.76). The low coronary death rates in Japan, rural Italy, and rural Serbia are associated with death rates from noncoronary causes higher than would be expected from the U.S. Vital Statistics. The net result is to reduce, but not to nullify, the advantage in all-causes deaths. But these data also show that a low coronary death rate is not necessarily associated with an elevated rate of death from other causes. Dalmatia had only 7 coronary deaths with 42.5 expected, and the noncoronary deaths numbered 54 with 59.9 the expected number (O/E = 0.90). For the Italian railroad men the observed and expected noncoronary deaths were 55 and 64.5, respectively (O/E = 0.85). The corresponding figures for Corfu are 35 and 45.3 (O/E = 0.77). And for Corfu with 41 noncoronary deaths observed the expected number is 55.9 (O/E = 0.73).

Table 4.1 concerns all men aged 40–59 at entrance, including the men who were judged to have coronary heart disease at their first examination. That inclusion is necessary, of course, to allow comparison with the U.S. Vital Statistics. But the subsequent deaths of men covered in Table 4.1 are a mixture of fatal outcome of established disease and deaths from new incidence. Any attempt to examine the relationship of risk factors to the follow-up experience is complicated by confusion between characteristics that precede the clinical disease and those that might reflect the established disease. Men who are given a diagnosis of coronary heart disease often avoid strenuous exercise, stop or reduce smoking, and restrict their diet; commonly, there is an urge to change the mode of life, to take medicines, and so on in hope of improving the prospect of survival. This is true also of men who suffer from other heart and cardiovascular diseases. Accordingly, the analysis of the incidence data from this study focuses on the men who were judged to be free of cardiovascular disease at the start, that is, men who were not given a diagnosis of such disease.

Men CVD-free at Entry

Table 4.2 summarizes all-causes and coronary heart disease ten-year death data on the 12,023 men who were judged to be free of cardiovascular disease at entry. The rates per 10,000 are standardized to the age distribution of all men in all cohorts in this study. Again, Slavonia and east Finland are notable for high all-causes death rates; Dalmatia, Crete, and Belgrade are at the opposite end of the scale. And again there are great differences among the cohorts in the coronary death rate, from no death in Crete to 681 deaths per 10,000 in east Finland.

With the data in table 4.2 it is possible, as in table 4.1, to calculate the noncoronary death rates. The result is a range in age-standardized deaths per

Table 4.2. Deaths in ten years from all causes and from coronary heart disease among men without evidence of cardiovascular disease at entry (rates per 10,000 standardized by single years to the age distribution for all cohorts combined).

Cohort	Number at risk	All-causes deaths			CHD deaths		
		N	Rate	SE	N	Rate	SE
U.S. railroad	2,315	219	961	61	97	424	42
Dalmatia	662	58	775	104	6	74	33
Slavonia	680	114	1,553	139	12	174	50
Tanushimaru	504	54	1,052	137	4	71	37
East Finland	728	103	1,511	133	46	681	93
West Finland	806	102	1,270	117	21	251	51
Crevalcore	956	124	1,306	109	28	226	48
Montegiorgio	708	67	1,007	113	8	125	42
Zutphen	845	97	1,134	109	28	317	60
Ushibuka	496	68	1,349	153	3	50	32
Crete	655	38	627	95	0	0	—
Corfu	525	43	847	122	8	149	53
Rome railroad	736	67	964	109	17	247	57
Velika Krsna	487	56	1,136	144	3	71	38
Zrenjanin	476	49	1,129	145	7	155	57
Belgrade	516	21	512	97	9	250	69
Total	12,095	1,280	1,071	28	290	246	28

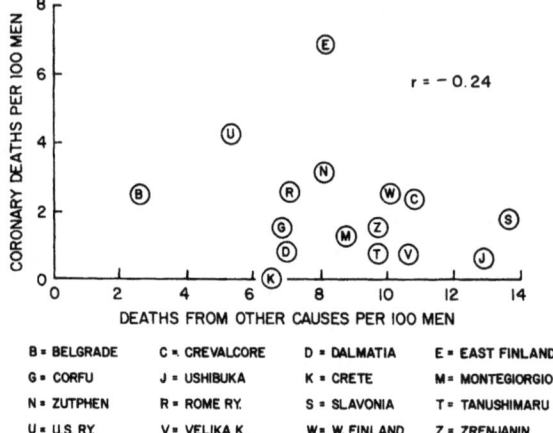

Figure 4.1. Comparison of ten-year age-standardized death rates from coronary heart disease with the rates of death from all other causes. Men free of cardiovascular disease at the entry examination.

10,000 from 262 for Belgrade, 567 for the United States railroad on up to 1,299 for Ushibuka and 1,379 for Slavonia. There is no significant correlation between coronary and noncoronary death rates. The product-moment coefficient of correlation between those two rates is $r = 0.24$, which, for sixteen pairs of rates, has 95 percent confidence limits of -0.66 and $+0.29$. The data are shown in figure 4.1.

The statistical significance of differences in the rates in table 4.2 can of course be calculated from the data in the table. However, the fact that the rates are age-standardized to make them comparable for a fixed age distribution may also slightly distort the picture. A more direct pair comparison could be made by, for example, the Mantel-Haenszel chi-square method to sum up the twenty fourfold tables, one for each of the twenty single-year age classes. Both the Mantel-Haenszel chi-square method and comparisons of age-standardized rates are used in our analysis of differences between pairs or groups of cohorts. But before those analyses are discussed, data are given on two causes of death that seem remote from our interest in coronary heart disease.

Infectious Diseases, Accidents, Poisonings, or Violence

Table 4.3 gives the numbers of deaths in each of the cohorts attributed to infectious disease and to accidents, poisonings, or violence (APV) and the rates of those deaths, standardized by single years of age to the age distribution of all men in all cohorts combined. Of the 72 deaths from infectious

Table 4.3. Ten-year deaths from infectious diseases and from accidents, poisonings, and violence (APV).

Cohort	N		Age-standardized rates per 10,000			
	Inf. dis.	APV	Inf. dis.	SE	APV	SE
U.S. railroad	0	16	0	—	65	16
Dalmatia	9	4	109	40	43	44
Slavonia	25	13	336	68	175	50
Tanushimaru	3	5	55	33	103	45
East Finland	2	11	25	17	137	41
West Finland	8	14	95	33	161	43
Ushibuka	9	6	155	55	114	47
Crevalcore	3	14	33	18	140	37
Montegiorgio	3	2	34	21	20	17
Zutphen	2	4	23	16	43	22
Crete	3	8	36	23	113	40
Corfu	1	3	20	20	69	36
Rome railroad	0	1	0	—	9	11
Velika Krsna	6	6	129	50	111	46
Zrenjanin	0	7	0	—	122	48
Belgrade	0	3	0	—	85	40
Total	72[a]	117	54.3	6.5	90.6	8.4

a. Among 72 deaths from infectious disease 61 were caused by tuberculosis.

diseases, 61 were attributed to tuberculosis, 8 in Dalmatia, 7 in west Finland, 24 in Slavonia, 2 each in Crevalcore, Montegiorgio, Crete, and Tanushimaru, 1 each in Zutphen and Corfu, 7 in Ushibuka, 5 in Velika Krsna, none in the other five cohorts. Of 2,932 Yugoslavs, 37 died from tuberculosis, making a death rate of 126 per 10,000.

A total of 117 men in this study died from accidents, poisonings, or violence in ten years, accounting for 7.7 percent of all deaths in that period. Slavonia had the unhappy distinction of having the highest death rate from this cause as well as from infectious diseases. In general, deaths from APV were more common in rural areas and in men with physically active jobs than in men with sedentary work. These tendencies will be recalled in some analyses in chapter 2 that compare men in different occupations.

American Railroad Men

A major feature in the organization of the study on the American railroad men was the sampling of men by occupation within the industry. This provides a comparison between men with sedentary jobs and men whose work required physical work; the switchmen who work in the railroad yards were selected to represent the latter activity class. Table 4.4 summarizes the ten-year mortality experience of the two activity classes.

Considering all men, including those with diagnoses of cardiovascular disease at entry, there were no significant differences between the sedentary and active men in age-standardized death rates from all causes, from coronary heart disease, or from all forms of heart disease. However, the death rate from APV (almost all accidents) for the physically active men was 4.8 times higher than for their sedentary colleagues, and the difference is highly significant ($t = 3.00$).

The picture for the men free from CVD at entry is somewhat different. The all-causes death rate of the active men was 1.41 times that of the sedentary men, and the difference is highly significant ($t = 2.57$). In regard to coronary deaths, the rate for the physically active men was higher than that of the sedentary men, instead of the reverse difference when all men were considered, but the difference is not significant. The death rates from all heart disease show the same kind of reversal from the picture when all men were considered; the active men free from cardiovascular disease at the start had a higher death rate than the comparable sedentary men, but the dif-

Table 4.4. Ten-year deaths of American railroad men classified by physical activity of occupation (age-standardized rates per 10,000; heart disease deaths include deaths from CHD).

Item	All men			CVD-free		
	Sedentary	Active	Δ	Sedentary	Active	Δ
N	1,305	875	430	1,153	813	340
All-causes deaths	151	95	56	106	83	23
Rate	1,067	1,251	−184	861	1,216	−355
SE	86	112	139	83	115	138
CHD deaths	81	40	41	51	32	19
Rate	581	521	60	419	470	−51
SE	65	75	100	59	75	94
Heart disease deaths	90	45	45	58	36	22
Rate	643	593	50	466	523	−57
SE	68	80	106	62	78	99
APV deaths	4	10	−6	3	10	−7
Rate	29	140	−111	25	159	−134
SE	15	40	37	15	43	41

ference is not statistically convincing. Finally, the disadvantage of the physically active men in regard to deaths from accidents persists when only men CVD-free at entry are considered.

The higher death rate from APV of the physically active men accounts for some but not all of their excess in all-causes deaths compared to the sedentary men. Considering men CVD-free at entry, the age-standardized death rates from all causes except APV were 818 for the sedentary railroad men and 1,057 for the active men. The difference, 1,057 minus 818 = 239 deaths per 10,000, has SE = 132, so $t = 1.81$. This would be significant at about $p = 0.03$ if the hypothesis under test specified the direction of the difference. With the two-tail test we have about $p = 0.06$, close to the convention that $p = 0.05$ is significant.

A third group of 391 American railroad men, the nonsedentary clerks, did not differ significantly from the rest of the railroad men in either all-causes or coronary death. The conclusion, then, is that it is justifiable to combine all of the American railroad men in one group disregarding job activity for comparisons with other cohorts and in the analysis regarding risk factors.

Italian Railroad Men

Table 4.2 showed that for men free from cardiovascular disease at entry the all-causes death rate of the Italian railroad was almost identical with that for the American railroad men, 964 and 961 per 10,000, respectively. However the death rate from coronary heart disease of the Italians was only 58 percent that of the Americans, and the difference is highly significant with $t = 2.5$.

From table 4.2 it can be calculated that the death rate from causes other than coronary heart disease was 33 percent higher for the Italians than for their American counterparts, and that difference too is highly significant. Superficially, at least, it seems as though the Italians had traded an advantage in coronary mortality for an equal disadvantage in other mortality.

The Italian railroad men had a lower all-causes death rate than their rural countrymen in this study, but the difference was significant only in the comparison with Crevalcore where that rate was 35 percent higher. The comparison is 1,306 minus 964 = 343 and SE = 154, so $t = 2.22$. Although the coronary death rate of the Italian railroad men was not significant from that of the men of Crevalcore, it was almost double (198 percent) that of the men of Montegiorgio ($t = 1.82$).

Only a total of 25 coronary deaths are involved in this last comparison of railroad men with the men of Montegiorgio. When the two groups of rural Italians are combined in a comparison with the railroad men, there is no significant difference in death rates from coronary heart disease. For many further analyses it seems reasonable to combine all three of the Italian cohorts.

Unlike American men, many Italian men do heavy physical work. Thus it is possible to classify the Italian railroad men, and also their rural countrymen, into activity classes of sedentary, moderately active, and very active men. The examination of the incidence of death, and also of nonfatal coronary heart disease, in these activity classes will be treated in chapter 11.

Croatia

An area on the Dalmatian coast and another in Slavonia near the Hungarian border were chosen for this study by Professor Buzina and colleagues in Croatia because of reputed differences in the dominant dietary fat: olive oil in Dalmatia, lard in Slavonia. It was thought that such differences might be reflected in the frequency of coronary heart disease. As table 4.2 shows, among men CVD-free at the start, the ten-year coronary death rate of the Slavonians proved to be 2.4 times that of the Dalmatians, but the numbers of such deaths are small, 18 in all, and $t = 1.59$, indicating that the difference could have arisen by chance in about 6 in 100 trials.

The difference in all-causes deaths, based on 172 deaths, is more impressive; the age-standardized rate in Slavonia was twice that in Dalmatia ($t = 4.47$). Much of Slavonia's excessive all-causes death rate is accounted for by 24 deaths from infectious disease and 13 deaths from violence. Omitting these causes of death, the rate for Slavonia is reduced to 1,042 per 10,000; that for Dalmatia, 619. The rate for Slavonia is still 68 percent above that for Dalmatia. It should be remarked that though Dalmatia's all-causes death rate is favorable, and better than that of the United States railroad men, there were 9 deaths in that cohort from infectious disease, 8 of which were from tuberculosis. Croatia's 1,342 CVD-free men, 11 percent of all such men in this study, accounted for more than half of all the deaths from tuberculosis. These were all old infections acquired very likely thirty or more years ago in the days before and during World War II.

East and West Finland

We have already noted that among men CVD-free at the start east Finland was at the top among all cohorts in ten-year coronary death rate and second only to Slavonia in all-causes death rate. It is understandable, then, that east Finland is now the site of perhaps the world's largest intensive anticoronary campaign organized by the Ministry of Health, the Finnish Heart Association, and regional physicians and other health workers. But calculation from the data in table 4.2 shows that in noncoronary deaths east Finland is not nearly as bad among the cohorts of the Seven Countries Study. With a rate of 830 noncoronary deaths per 10,000, east Finland is lower than the corresponding rates for Slavonia, Tanushimaru, Ushibuka, Crevalcore, Montegiorgio, Velika Krsna, and Zrenjanin, and even west Finland, which looked so much better than east Finland when coronary and all-causes deaths were considered.

No single cause accounts for the higher noncoronary death rate in west than in east Finland. Of men CVD-free at entry, 7 died from infectious diseases and 9 from stroke in ten years in west Finland; the corresponding figures for east Finland are 2 and 3. Omitting those two causes of deaths reduces the noncoronary death rate for west Finland to 784 per 10,000; for east Finland, 763. Incidentally, the differences in deaths from infectious diseases and from strokes are not significant.

Rural Italy

Table 4.1 indicates higher all-causes and coronary death rates in Crevalcore than in Montegiorgio among all men, and table 4.2 shows the same kind of difference among men free from evidence of cardiovascular disease at the start. For men CVD-free at entry Crevalcore had 299 more all-causes deaths per 10,000 than Montegiorgio with SE of the difference = 160 and $t = 1.97$. The prior hypothesis was that Crevalcore would fare worse than Montegiorgio because it was supposed that the Crevalcore diet was more atherogenic, or at least more cholesterogenic, than that of Montegiorgio. A one-tail test gives $p = 0.04$. Because the hypothesis concerned coronary heart disease, there might be a question on using a one-tail test for all-causes deaths; a two-tails test gives $p = 0.08$.

The coronary heart disease death rate was 81 percent higher in Crevalcore than in Montegiorgio, but the difference of 101 deaths per 10,000 has $SE = 66$ and $t = 1.53$, which means $p = 0.06$ for the one-tail test appropriate here because of the prior hypothesis.

For one cause of death, lung cancer, there is a better case for concluding that the record is worse for Crevalcore than for Montegiorgio. At Crevalcore ten men died from lung cancer in contrast to only one such death at Montegiorgio. The difference has $t = 2.26$. It is notable that 26 percent of the men at Crevalcore were heavy smokers (twenty or more cigarettes every day) but only 11 percent of the Montegiorgio men were in that smoking category. Among the Crevalcore men who died from lung cancer, seven were heavy smokers, two smoked from ten to nineteen cigarettes a day and one man had never smoked regularly; the one Montegiorgio man who died of lung cancer had been a heavy smoker. Among all Crevalcore men 25 percent had never smoked, whereas 26 percent of the Montegiorgio men were in that category.

Zutphen

The all-causes death rate of men at Zutphen corresponds well with the death rate for all men of like age in the Zutphen area according to the local vital statistics; it is 4.8 percent higher for all the men who entered the study. This slight difference may reflect some preference of men with health problems to accept the invitation; the most common reason given for not joining the cohort was that with perfect health there was no point in having an examination. The death rate from coronary heart disease for the Zutphen cohort was slightly less than that reported for the Zutphen area but slightly higher than for all of the Netherlands, according to the vital statistics.

As table 4.2 shows, the men of Zutphen were in the middle of the distribution for deaths from all causes among men CVD-free at entry, but they were third highest, after east Finland and the United States railroad men, in regard to coronary deaths. But neoplasms were more important as a cause of death than coronary heart disease at Zutphen. Neoplasms accounted for 41 percent of all deaths among all Zutphen men, 44 percent of the deaths among CVD-free men. Lung cancer was held responsible for 39 percent of all the deaths from neoplasms at Zutphen. On the other hand, infectious diseases, accidents, poisonings, and violence accounted for less than 6 percent of all the Zutphen deaths.

Japan

The Japanese cohorts included substantially all men 40–59 in the farming village of Tanushimaru and the fishing village of Ushibuka, on opposite sides of the southern island of Kyushu. The economic conditions are similar in the two areas—modest but no real poverty. In both areas the majority of the men were heavy cigarette smokers and were engaged in work demanding heavy labor. The diets in the two areas were low in fats, with only 8 to 12 percent of total calories provided from that source, and were characterized by very high intakes of rice, vegetables, and fruits. The Ushibuka men commonly ate fish every day, and on the fishing boats an average of a kilogram of fish was eaten raw each day. But the men of Tanushimaru also ate a substantial amount of fresh fish. It turned out, then, that the diets of the two villages were not as dissimilar as had been imagined at first.

Table 4.2 shows that both Japanese cohorts had very low death rates from coronary heart disease. In this respect the Japanese and the Greeks did not differ significantly. In all-causes deaths of men of Tanushimaru were roughly in the middle of the range for the sixteen cohorts, but the fishermen of Ushibuka had the third highest death rate. However, the difference between Ushibuka and Tanushimaru in all-causes deaths proves to be statistically insignificant; for the difference of 297 deaths per 10,000, SE = 208, so $t = 1.43$.

In spite of the common opinion in Japan, and the figures in the older Japanese vital statistics, the experience of the 1,010 men in these two cohorts gives little support to the idea that Japanese are remarkably susceptible to stroke, commonly called "knockdown disease" in Japanese. Among all men the cerebrovascular death rate was 101 per 10,000 (SE = 45) at Tanushimaru, and 169 (SE = 58) at Ushibuka and practically the same for the men CVD-free at entry. The average for the two cohorts combined, 135 per 10,000 (SE = 36), may be compared with the corresponding figures for the other cohorts in this study. Cerebrovascular death rates in the other fourteen cohorts ranged from 32 per 10,000 in Crete to 210 (SE = 66) in Zrenjanin, an average of 118 deaths per 10,000 (SE = 10).

The ten-year experience of stroke mortality in Japan needs comment. In the first place, the southern Island of Kyushu, where the villages of Tanushimaru and Ushibuka are situated, is reported in the Japanese national vital statistics to have a lower death rate from stroke than many areas on the main island of Honshu. A peculiarity in the national vital statistics on stroke mortality is that there are areas of Honshu with extremely high rates of death ascribed to cerebrovascular disease; those areas account for much of the high stroke death rate for Japan as a whole.

The second point of relevance to the stroke mortality rate in Japan is the remarkable decline in recent years in the deaths attributed to cerebral hemorrhage. There is a fall of almost 50 percent from 1950 to 1970 in the age-standardized mortality attributed to that cause. This change was accompanied by a rise in the deaths attributed to cerebral infarction, but even in 1970 the death rate from cerebral hemorrhage was reported to be 50 percent higher than that from cerebral infarction. The popular picture of a very high incidence of stroke in Japan is derived largely from reports on cerebral hemorrhage.

In 1950 the Japanese vital statistics indicated that over 90 percent of all deaths from cerebrovascular disease were due to cerebral hemorrhage. In 1956 we found that death certificates in Japan then almost always attributed sudden unexpected deaths to cerebral hemorrhage. That practice of automatic diagnosis has steadily decreased, and the Japanese national vital statistics indicate the standardized death rate from cerebral hemorrhage in 1970 to be only half that in 1950 with a further decline since 1970. From 1950 to 1970 the Japanese death rate from coronary heart disease doubled in the vital statistics, but even in 1970 the ischemic heart disease death rate was stated to be less than half that of the rate attributed to cerebral hemorrhage.

Finally, it must be emphasized that our calculation of death rate from cerebrovascular disease is based on only 19 such deaths in Japan and 127 among the 11,753 men in the other fourteen cohorts. The confidence limits of the cerebrovascular death rate in our Japanese subjects are, therefore, wide. The upper 95 percent confidence limit for the Japanese men is 248 cerebrovascular deaths in ten years; that figure is 229 percent of the mean rate for the other fourteen cohorts.

Greece

Tables 4.1 and 4.2 show that the ten-year death rates on the Greek islands of Crete and Corfu were notably low for all causes and remarkably low for deaths from coronary heart disease. In our villages on the island of Crete only one man died from coronary heart disease in ten years, and he had the disease at the entry examination. The scarcity of deaths reported from the two Greek cohorts was a cause for concern to the senior investigator. Special interim visits to the villages turned up two deaths on Crete that had been missed in the first years of the follow-up, but thereafter all men reputed to be not dead were verified as being, indeed, alive.

On our first visit to Crete, we were impressed by the large number of very old men who curiously watched the organization and operation of the medical examinations. The ages of these old men, generically called *papou* (grandpa) in Greek, could be verified from the local voting and tax registers and the birth records of the churches, in contrast to the situation with the reputed centenarians of the Caucasus and the "happy Hunza." And we are reminded that around the turn of the century the remarkable genius-eccentric who succeeded Louis Pasteur as director of the Pasteur Institute, Élie Metchnikoff, came to the conclusion that, per unit of total population, there were 20 times more Greek than French centenarians. We can attest to the fact that during the field work of this study it was not uncommon to see men of 80 to 100 and more going off to work in the fields with a hoe.

Serbia

The very low all-causes and relatively low coronary disease death rates of the professors of Belgrade have been mentioned earlier. In all-causes death rate the men of Velika Krsna were practically identical with the men of Zrenjanin, both when all men and when only men CVD-free at the start were compared. In this respect they were in the middle of the range of the sixteen cohorts, better than the men of Slavonia, east and west Finland, Crevalcore, and Ushibuka, practically identical with the men of Zutphen, and poorer than the men in the other eight cohorts. The death rate from coronary heart disease for the men of Zrenjanin was more than double that for Velika Krsna; however, with a total of only ten such deaths in the two cohorts, the difference is not significant. Comparisons between these two cohorts in regard to other causes showed only one difference: there were no deaths from infectious diseases at Zrenjanin, but there were six at Velika Krsna, five from tuberculosis, with age-standardized rates of zero and 129 (SE = 50). By Fisher's exact test of the 2-x-2 table the difference is significant with $p = 0.03$, but the main significance to us is that for most of our purposes it would be best to omit deaths from tuberculosis.

National Groups

The ten-year follow-up showed, as noted earlier, some differences in death rates between cohorts in the same country, notably in Finland. There were less striking differences between the Cretans and the Corfiotes. Among the Yugoslavs, the Slavonians had a high death rate; the Belgrade professors, a low one. But it is interesting to combine the cohorts into national groups and examine the picture by countries (figure 4.2).

In terms of all-causes deaths the Finns are high and the Greeks low, with little difference among the other five groups. The contrasts are much greater for coronary deaths, with Finns and Americans far higher than the others and Greeks and Japanese equally notable for their relative freedom from coronary heart disease deaths.

When the cohorts were organized, it was never suggested that they would be representative of all men in the countries concerned, but it is interesting

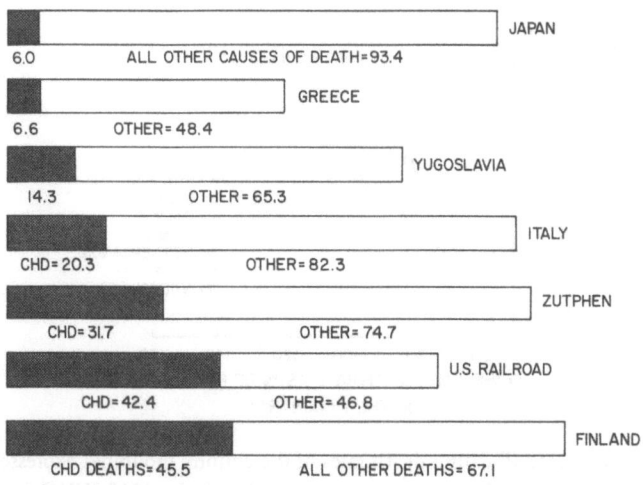

Figure 4.2. Ten-year age-standardized death rates per 10,000 from coronary heart disease and from all other causes, with the cohorts grouped by countries.

to compare, in figure 4.2, the death rates of the national groupings with the death rates in the national vital statistics of the seven countries. A simple comparison of the rates in figure 4.2 with the national rates is not suitable because the available vital statistics concern deaths in particular years of men in five-year age classes. In contrast, the rates in figure 4.2 are for ten years, standardized by single years of age, for men with no cardiovascular disease at entry. The last stipulation was made to avoid possible distortions from differences among cohorts in reasons for refusals to take examinations. As discussed in chapter 3, some men avoided examination to conceal disease, and others saw no point in an examination when they were perfectly healthy, and these reasons for nonparticipation could be differently persuasive in different cohorts.

For the comparison with national vital statistics, the death rates of each national grouping in figure 4.2 were expressed as a percentage of the unweighted mean of the death rates of all seven groups. The death rates in the national vital statistics were similarly expressed as a percentage of the mean of the seven national rates for the year 1965. The comparison in relative all-causes rates is shown in figure 4.3. The correlation coefficient of $r = 0.86$ is highly significant.

The corresponding comparison in regard to death rates for coronary heart disease is shown in figure 4.4. Here the agreement is still better, in part no

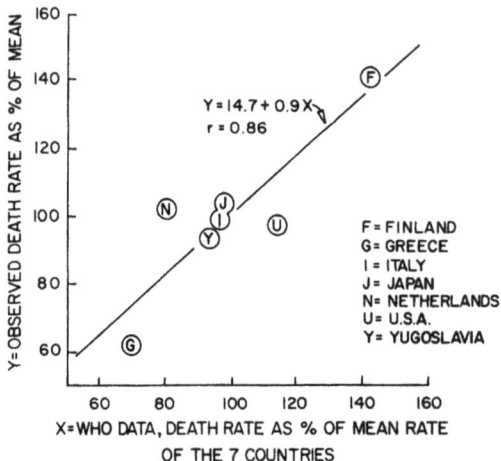

Figure 4.3. Ten-year all-causes death rates of the country groupings expressed as percentage of the mean of the seven rates, compared with the 1965 WHO Vital Statistics rates similarly expressed as percentage of the mean of the seven vital statistics rate.

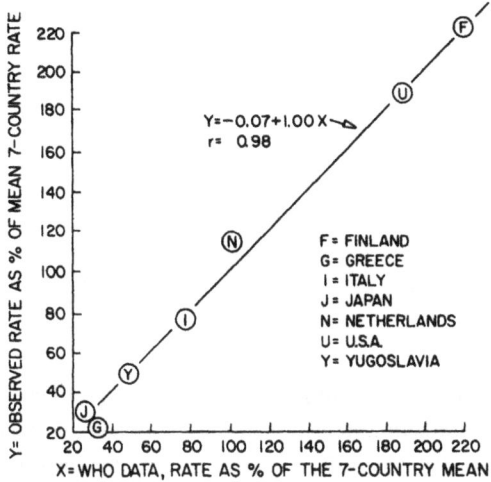

Figure 4.4. Ten-year coronary heart disease death rates of the country groupings compared with the WHO Vital Statistics for deaths from coronary heart disease, rates expressed as percentages as in figure 4.3.

doubt reflecting the much greater range among the groups in coronary than in all-causes death rates, 11-fold (20 to 220 percent) for coronary as compared with 2.3-fold (62 to 140 percent) for all-causes death rate.

Cancer and Other Neoplasms

Among men free from cardiovascular disease at entry, 354 died from cancer and other neoplasms in ten years, 89 of those deaths being attributed to cancer of the trachea, bronchus, or lung. Figure 4.5 shows that the death rates from these diseases differed in major areas of the study. The men of northern Europe had the highest incidence, the United States railroad men the lowest, and the Japanese men had a rate not significantly different from that of the northern Europeans. The difference between the north and the south Europeans would occur by chance in fewer than 1 in 1,000 trials (chi-square = 10.98), and the difference between the southern Europeans and the Americans is only a trifle less impressive (chi-square = 9.37).

The above comparisons concern the total of all deaths from neoplastic diseases. The darker shading in figure 4.5 indicates deaths from cancer of the trachea, bronchus, or lung. These death rates are not significantly different for the Americans and the southern Europeans, but the higher rate for the northern Europeans is extremely significant. Comparison of the northern and the southern Europeans in this regard gives chi-square = 33.16 with one degree of freedom. The difference between the northern and

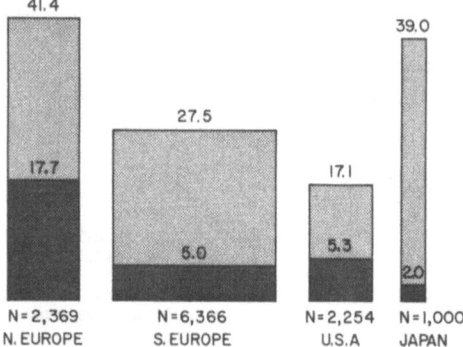

Figure 4.5. Ten-year age-standardized rates of death per 1,000 from cancer and other neoplasms in northern Europe (Finland and Zutphen), southern Europe (Italy, Yugoslavia, Greece), the American railroad men, and the men of Japan. The dark shading indicates deaths from cancer of the trachea, bronchus, or lung.

southern Europeans in cancer of the respiratory system explains almost the entire difference between these two groups of men in the death rate from all neoplastic diseases; the two population groups do not differ significantly in the rate of deaths from neoplasms other than cancers of the respiratory system. The question of a relationship of death from neoplastic diseases and smoking habits will be examined in chapter 9.

Comparison of Cohort Groupings

Besides comparisons by national groupings, the mortality experience in other cohort groups, such as urban versus rural, is instructive. Of the thirteen cohorts in Europe, four may be considered urban—Zutphen, Rome railroad, Belgrade, and Zrenjanin—and the other nine were strictly rural. Also, the men in Europe live in several areas differing in climate, diet, cultural pattern, and living habits. In these respects, the northern Europeans, that is, the east and west Finns and the men of Zutphen, are in obvious contrast to the southern Europeans. Furthermore, the southern Europeans comprise two easily distinguishable groupings, the Mediterraneans and the continental Yugoslavs, that is, the Slavonians and the three cohorts of Serbs who live in a much harsher climate and maintain different customs. The Dalmatians, though Yugoslavs by language and nationality, live along the shore of the Adriatic, a branch of the Mediterranean, and they have many affinities with their Italian and Greek neighbors in regard to climate, mode of life, and diet; they use olive oil instead of the lard and butter used in the rest of Yugoslavia, and they drink wine rather than the beer favored elsewhere in their country. Italians settled on the Dalmatian coast during the many centuries of Roman and later Italian rule which extended through World War I. Finally, the American and the Italian railroad men merit special comparison because of the close similarity of occupation and of socioeconomic status within their respective countries.

Table 4.5 gives, for the various groups, ten-year all-causes and coronary death rates, age-standardized, per 10,000 men free of cardiovascular disease at entry. The last two columns of the table give the numbers of deaths and of survivors calculated from the numbers at risk and the age-standardized death rates. The numbers in the last two columns are used in the chi-square evaluation of the differences between pairs of groups as shown in table 4.6.

For all-causes deaths the rural European rate is 16 percent higher than the urban European rate, and that difference would be expected to occur by chance in only about 1 out of 67 trials.

Table 4.5. Ten-year all-causes and coronary death rates, men without cardiovascular disease at entry, for various cohort groupings (age-standardized death rates per 10,000 and their standard errors; numbers of deaths and survivors calculated from the age-standardized rates and the numbers at risk).

Cohort grouping	Rate	SE	Deaths	Survivors
All-causes deaths				
Rural Europe	1,137	40	707	5,510
Urban Europe	953	58	246	2,321
Rural Japan	1,199	103	120	880
Northern Europe[a]	1,296	69	308	2,071
Mediterranean[b]	953	45	404	3,838
Yugoslavia, inland[c]	1,117	66	240	1,913
U.S. railroad	961	61	223	2,093
Rome railroad	964	108	71	665
CHD deaths				
Rural Europe	206	18	128	5,510
Urban Europe	253	31	65	2,321
Rural Japan	61	25	6	880
Northern Europe	406	41	97	2,071
Mediterranean	135	18	61	3,838
Yugoslavia, inland	164	27	36	1,913
U.S. railroad	424	42	98	2,093
Rome railroad	247	57	18	665

a. East Finland, west Finland, Zutphen.
b. Italy, Greece, Dalmatia.
c. Slavonia, Velika Krsna, Zrenjanin, Belgrade.

Table 4.6. Comparisons of groups for ten-year death rates of men free of cardiovascular disease at entry (chi-square test applied to numbers of deaths and of survivors in table 4.5; group with higher rate given in italics).

Comparison	Chi-square	P
All-causes deaths		
Rural and urban Europeans	5.92	0.015
Rural Europeans and *rural Japanese*	0.33	n. sig.
Northern Europeans and Mediterraneans	8.40	3.8×10^{-3}
Northern Europeans and Yugoslavs	0.36	n. sig.
Yugoslavs and Mediterraneans	4.24	0.04
U.S. railroad and Rome railroad	0.00	—
CHD deaths		
Rural and *urban Europeans*	1.41	0.24
Rural Europeans and rural Japanese	9.56	2×10^{-3}
Northern Europeans and Mediterraneans	45.62	1×10^{-11}
Northern Europeans and Yugoslavs	22.92	1.7×10^{-6}
Yugoslavs and Mediterraneans	0.50	n. sig.
U.S. railroad and Rome railroad	4.42	0.04

Other Studies

Published data on the mortality experience of middle-aged men, followed as in the Seven Countries Study, generally provide little information in a form that allows comparison with the experience of men in the general population or in the present study. However, data from the Framingham study (Dawber, Moore, and Mann 1957) and from Jeremiah Stamler's prospective study (Stamler et al. 1960) on men employed by the Peoples' Gas Company of Chicago can be analyzed for comparison with the mortality of men of the same ages in the general population of the United States.

For Framingham men the all-causes mortality experience was summarized through 1960, covering nine to ten years for most of the men, together with the deaths that would be expected to match the age- and sex-specific death rates for the United States white male population. The men in the Framingham study consisted of men in the community statistical sample, about 80 percent of the total, and volunteers who were enrolled to bring the total number of men to the desired level. The ten-year all-causes death rate of the volunteers was substantially higher than that of the men on the original roster, 96 percent of the deaths expected to match the general population death rates as compared with 76 percent for the men on the original roster. Among the men followed through 1960, 173 deaths were observed; the number expected to match the U.S. Vital Statistics was 220.2, giving a ratio of observed to expected deaths of 0.79. The ten-year experience of the American railroad men in the Seven Countries Study was 293 deaths observed in ten years among 2,571 men at risk. The number of deaths to match the experience of men of the same age as recorded in the U.S. Vital Statistics was 376.7, (O/E = 0.78).

Stamler et al. (1960) reported the mortality of the men in the Chicago Gas Company. So it is possible to make a detailed comparison with the all-causes deaths expected to match the U.S. Vital Statistics death rates for men of the same ages. Among men aged 40–59 at entry who were followed for nine years, there were 142 deaths; the expected number was 166.2 (O/E = 0.85).

Though the Chicago men had a somewhat less favorable mortality experience than the Framingham and American railroad men, the differences among the three studies are small, and all three showed a considerably lower mortality than that of the general American population. This conforms to the general rule that the death rate of groups specifically followed over the years is usually lower than that of persons in the general population calculated from census estimates of persons at risk and death certificates.

Summary

During ten years, 1,507 men died. Coronary heart disease accounted for 410 cases; cancer and other neoplasms, 354 cases; infectious diseases, mostly tuberculosis, 72 cases; and violence, 117 cases. Compared with expectations from U.S. Vital Statistics on white men matched by single years of age, the ratio of observed to expected deaths was O/E = 0.82 for all causes and O/E = 0.53 for coronary deaths, but the ratios varied greatly among cohorts. The men of east Finland had the worst experience, with O/E = 1.32 for all causes and O/E = 1.71 for coronary deaths.

Among American railroad men, the physically active switchmen had a higher all-causes death rate than their sedentary colleagues, but that difference was largely explained by a difference in violent deaths. Among the railroad men free of cardiovascular disease at entry, the sedentary men had a lower coronary death rate than the more active men, but the difference is not statistically significant.

Among 12,095 men free of evidence of cardiovascular disease at entry, the ten-year coronary death rate was less than 75 per 10,000 for the men of Crete, Japan, and Croatia. In contrast, coronary death rates of 250 or more were recorded for east and west Finland, the American railroad men, Zutphen, and Belgrade.

Grouping the cohorts by countries, the all-causes death rates were highly correlated with the rates for men of the same ages reported in the vital statistics of those countries. The corresponding comparison in coronary death rates showed an even higher correlation.

The high all-causes death rate of the men of east Finland is explained by their extremely high death rate from coronary heart disease. Their death rate from noncoronary causes is in the middle of the distribution of the rates of the sixteen cohorts for noncoronary deaths. On the other hand, the very low all-causes death rate of the Greeks is not entirely explained by their relative freedom from coronary heart disease deaths.

The all-causes death rate of the northern Europeans (Finns and Dutch) was significantly higher than that of the Mediterraneans (Italians and Greeks), but did not differ from the Yugoslavs. The American and the Italian railroad men did not differ in all-causes death rate. In all-causes deaths the rate of the rural Europeans was significantly higher than the rates for the urban Europeans and the Japanese.

The coronary death rate of the northern Europeans was significantly higher than the rates of the Mediterraneans, Yugoslavs, and Japanese. The coronary death rate of the American railroad men was significantly higher than that of the Italian railroad men.

For causes of death other than heart disease, the death rate from neoplastic disease is of most interest. That rate was significantly higher for the northern Europeans than for the southern Europeans and the Americans. This is attributed to a death rate from cancer of the respiratory system for northern Europeans 3 times that of southern Europeans and Americans.

5 | Ten-Year Incidence of Coronary Heart Disease

Coronary death is the most dramatic manifestation of coronary heart disease, but other manifestations are also consequential. They are more frequently observed and thus less limited by small numbers in group comparisons and in the examination of associations between the incidence of the disease and characteristics of the individuals concerned.

Table 5.1 summarizes the ten-year coronary incidence data on men who showed no evidence of cardiovascular disease at entry. American railroad men are not represented here because they had no ten-year examinations. We define *hard CHD* as definite myocardial infarction or death from coronary heart disease. There were 351 such cases in the fifteen cohorts, the 193 (290 − 97 American railroad men) coronary deaths covered in table 5.2 plus 158 men who had infarcts but were still alive after ten years. *Any CHD* includes these men and all the men who developed less solid and severe manifestations of the disease—angina pectoris and any of the conditions listed in the incidence code for coronary heart disease in chapter 2. There are 913 men in the any CHD category.

Comparisons of Cohorts within Regions

Table 4.2 suggests a possible difference between Dalmatia and Slavonia in the incidence of the disease as indicated by the coronary death rate. Table 5.1 shows clearly that there was no significant difference between Dalmatia and Slavonia in the ten-year incidence of the disease. The difference between the two cohorts in the age-standardized incidence of hard CHD is 69 cases per 10,000 (SE = 80); of any CHD, −68 (SE = 129). Note that the differences are in opposite directions.

The incidence rate of hard CHD at Ushibuka is 38 percent higher than

Table 5.1 Ten-year incidence of coronary heart disease among men free of cardiovascular disease at entry (age-standardized rate per 10,000).

Cohort	N	Hard CHD			Any CHD		
		N	Rate	SE	N	Rate	SE
Dalmatia	662	13	185	52	40	629	94
Slavonia	680	18	253	60	40	561	88
Tanushimaru	504	8	148	54	20	354	82
East Finland	728	71	1,074	115	201	2,868	168
West Finland	806	45	539	80	129	1,582	129
Crevalcore	956	43	450	67	105	1,080	100
Montegiorgio	708	22	353	69	64	966	111
Zutphen	845	45	513	76	91	1,066	106
Ushibuka	496	11	204	63	23	458	94
Crete	655	2	26	20	13	210	56
Corfu	525	17	337	79	37	686	110
Rome railroad	736	25	357	68	57	786	99
Velika Krsna	487	6	132	52	21	452	94
Zrenjanin	476	12	239	70	37	715	118
Belgrade	516	13	317	77	35	794	119
Total	9,780	351	369.9[a]	19.1	913	943.8[a]	29.6

a. Mean of the cohort rates weighted by the number at risk in each cohort.

the rate at Tanushimaru, but the difference of 56 cases per 10,000 has SE = 83. For any CHD the rate at Ushibuka was 104 cases per 10,000 higher than at Tanushimaru, but SE = 125. In further analyses it is clear that the two Japanese cohorts should be combined as should, also, the two cohorts in Croatia.

In chapter 4 it was shown that the coronary death rate in east Finland was considerably higher than the rate in west Finland. Table 5.2 shows that the difference in favor of west Finland is abundantly clear with any diagnosis of coronary heart disease. The difference in hard CHD rate, more than double in east Finland compared with west Finland, has a value of $t = 3.9$; for any CHD the rate for the east Finns is 1,286 cases per 10,000 higher than that for the west Finns (SE = 2.12, $t = 6.1$).

In chapter 4 it was established that the three cohorts of men in Italy did not differ significantly in age-standardized rate of coronary death among men free from evidence of cardiovascular disease at the outset. From inspection of the data in table 5.1, it is obvious that there is no difference between Crevalcore and Montegiorgio in the rate of coronary heart disease by any

Table 5.2. Numbers of all incidence cases of coronary heart disease and of coronary death or myocardial infarction (hard), the percentage of all cases that are hard, and the 95% confidence limits of those percentages (for comparison, for each region under other regions are given the corresponding figures for the other regions, except Zutphen, combined.)

	Region				Other regions			
	CHD	Hard	%	95% limits	CHD	Hard	%	95% limits
Croatia	86	36	41.9	31.5, 52.3	793	318	40.1	36.7, 43.5
Finland	416	176	42.3	35.7, 48.9	443	178	40.2	35.6, 44.8
Rural Italy	186	78	41.9	34.8, 49.0	673	276	41.0	37.3, 44.7
Greece	59	23	39.0	26.6, 51.4	800	331	41.4	38.0, 44.8
Serbia	112	41	36.6	27.7, 45.5	747	313	41.9	38.4, 45.4
Zutphen	109	59	54.1	44.7, 63.5	859	354	41.2	37.9, 44.5

diagnostic definition. In regard to hard CHD, it is evident from simple inspection that the Italian railroad men do not differ significantly from their rural countrymen, but calculation helps in regard to any CHD. The rate for the rural Italians is 245 cases per 10,000 higher than that for the railroad men (SE = 130, $t = 1.87$). The conclusion is reinforced that for further analyses regarding coronary heart disease in Italy compared with other areas and in examination of the incidence of the disease as related to other characteristics, it is proper to combine the three groups of Italians.

After the successful enrollment and entry examinations of the Crete cohort, it was decided to organize a parallel study on the island of Corfu, considered to be much more "European" and westernized than Crete, so long dominated and ruled from the east. Comparison of Crete with Corfu might show effects of differences in outlook and philosophy, something like the contrast between type A and type B behavior that became popular in 1960. Such a comparison seemed especially intriguing when contrasts in other respects would be minimal in comparing the men of the villages—same race, nationality, and language, similar climate, work, diet, economic status, and medical care. However, on close inspection, the language differs in everyday dialect and accent, Corfu has more rainfall than Crete, and the Cretan diet is higher in olive oil. Undoubtedly there are some other differences between the people of the islands, but similarities still dominate.

In the ten-year outcome, the death rate of the Cretans was lower than that of the Corfiates both from all causes and from coronary heart disease, but the difference is not so impressive statistically as to justify considering it unquestionable. But when the incidence of nonfatal as well as fatal coronary heart disease is examined, as in table 5.1, there can be little doubt that the men of Crete were remarkably favored and did, indeed, differ from their countrymen of Corfu in this respect. In hard CHD the incidence rate on the island of Corfu was 13 times higher than the Cretan rate; the difference in rates, 311 cases per 10,000, has $SE = 74.5$ and $t = 4.2$. The difference in any CHD is 476 cases per 10,000 ($SE = 117.8$, $t = 4.0$). There is no proof, of course, that the difference between Crete and Corfu in susceptibility to coronary heart disease is caused by or even related to a difference in basic philosophy or attitude toward life.

Table 4.2 shows that the Belgrade professors had a much lower death rate from all causes than the other Serbians but had a ten-year age-adjusted coronary death rate of 250 per 10,000 compared with the average of 113 for the other Serbians ($SE = 69$, $t = 1.99$). The death data, then, seem to be fairly convincing that the professors were more prone to the disease or at least to die of it. However, the data in table 5.1 are less positive. For hard CHD the incidence rate of the Belgrade men only has $t = 1.62$ and for any CHD the difference is associated with $t = 1.4$. The suggestion is that although the Belgrade men do not differ very much in incidence the disease is more lethal to them.

Table 5.1 shows that the incidence rate of hard CHD in Zutphen was almost as high as in west Finland, but the incidence of any CHD in Zutphen does not correspond. The rate is only two-thirds as high as in west Finland and, in fact, lower than in Crevalcore, Italy. Zutphen differs from the other European cohorts in the distribution of the coronary cases according to diagnostic category. Hard CHD—death and nonfatal infarcts—accounted for 49.5 percent of all CHD incidence in Zutphen, but for the other Europeans only 36.8 percent of all CHD incidence was represented by hard CHD, ranging from an average of 33.3 percent in Serbia to 39.8 percent in Italy.

A test of the likelihood that chance could account for the difference between Zutphen and the rest of the Europeans can be made with the 2-x-2 contingency table—45 cases of hard CHD and 46 of other CHD in Zutphen versus 287 hard and 632 other CHD in the other Europeans. Chi-square proves to be 12.46 and the probability of chance explanation is less than 5 in 100,000. More detailed analysis shows that a large part of the peculiarity of the Zutphen material on CHD incidence is a relative deficiency of cases of uncomplicated angina pectoris. At Zutphen there were 45 cases of hard CHD and only 20 of uncomplicated angina pectoris; for the other European men there were equal numbers of hard CHD and of angina pectoris, 287 of each. The 2-x-2 contingency table comparing the men of Zutphen with the other European men gives chi-square $= 8.65$ and $p = 0.0033$.

The peculiarity of the distribution of hard CHD versus angina pectoris at

Zutphen could mean that the men of Zutphen are truly different from the other Europeans in their manifestations of coronary heart disease, but it seems more likely that differences in diagnostic custom were responsible. In any case, this contrast is another reason for emphasizing hard coronary heart disease in comparisons between samples. Actually, however, the relative proportion of all diagnoses of coronary heart disease represented by hard CHD was much the same in all of the regions in Europe except at Zutphen. Table 5.2 summarizes the data. Excluding Zutphen there are five regions. Comparing each of those regions with the other four shows no significant differences; the 95 percent confidence limits are overlapping. For Zutphen, however, the lower confidence limit is higher than the upper confidence limit for the other regions.

Incidence Rate of Diagnostic Classes versus CHD Death Rate

Taking coronary death as the ultimate evidence of coronary heart disease, it is pertinent to ask about the relation of its incidence rate to the incidence rates of other diagnostic categories of the disease. For example, our CHD incidence codes 30, 31, 32 were proposed to represent rather solid evidence of nonfatal myocardial infarction. If that supposition is correct and if the natural history of coronary heart disease is similar in the populations covered in this study, we would expect to find a close parallel between the incidence rates of those infarction codes and the death rate from coronary heart disease. Figure 5.1 shows that, in fact, the expectation is fulfilled; in this material the correlation between the two kinds of incidence is $r = 0.88$. It will be noted that in our hierarchical system each man can have only one diagnosis and death takes precedence over nonfatal infarction; if a man has an infarction corresponding to our code 30 (or 31 or 32) and later dies of coronary heart disease within the ten-year follow-up period he is counted as only a coronary death. The regression equation in figure 5.1 shows coronary death to be 1.5 times more common than nonfatal infarction, meaning not merely temporary survival after the acute infarct but survival to the end of the ten years. The least-squares solution of the regression equation emphasizes the lethal nature of the disease.

Our incidence code 34, clinical judgment of myocardial infarction without persistent electrocardiographic evidence of the infarct, proves to be as closely related to the incidence of coronary death as our codes 30, 31, 32, which require electrocardiographic verification. As figure 5.2 shows, the correlation is $r = 0.96$. In that figure the point for the American railroad men, U, was obtained by extrapolation from the five-year data; this may account for the fact that the point for the Americans is the furthermost from the regression line. The inference from comparison of figures 5.1 and 5.2 is

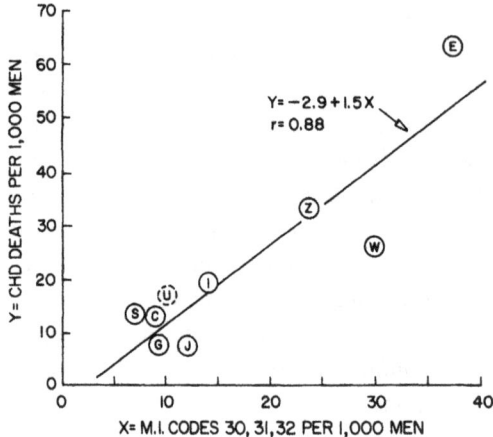

Figure 5.1. Ten-year death rate from coronary heart disease versus the rate of nonfatal myocardial infarction identified by codes 30, 31, and 32. All men free of cardiovascular disease at entry. C = Croatia; E = east Finland; G = Greece; I = Italy; J = Japan; S = Serbia; U = American (extrapolated from five-year data), W = west Finland, Z = Zutphen.

that careful clinical judgment of past infarction may be no less valid than the diagnosis that demands ECG support. But note that the slope of the regression line, 1.14, is less than the slope of 1.5 in figure 5.1. This suggests that the ultimate lethality of our incidence category 34 is less than that of infarct categories 30, 31, and 32.

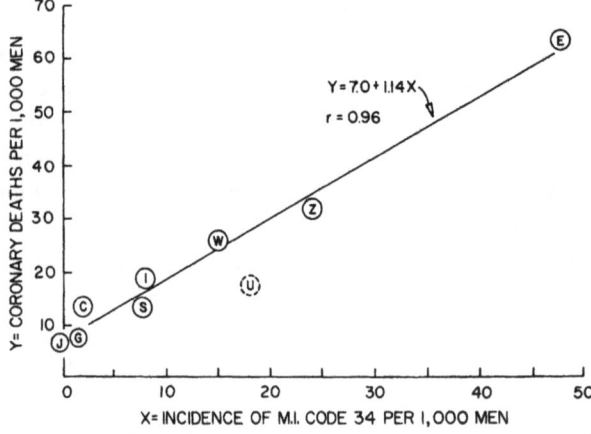

Figure 5.2. Ten-year death rate from coronary heart disease versus the rate of nonfatal infarction code 34. Groups as in figure 5.1.

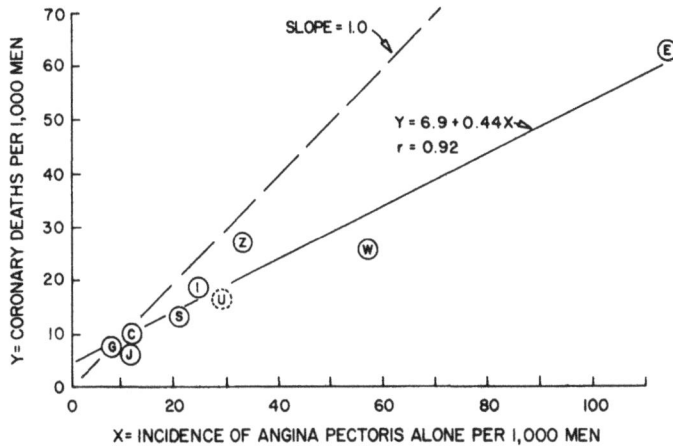

Figure 5.3. Ten-year coronary death rate versus the rate of incidence of angina pectoris as the only evidence of coronary heart disease. All men free of cardiovascular disease at entry. Groups as in figure 5.1.

The relationship of the incidence rate of angina pectoris alone to the coronary death rate, shown in figure 5.3, is particularly interesting. The correlation is high, $r = 0.92$, but the slope is only $b = 0.44$. The inference seems clear: in these populations the frequency of coronary death is closely related to the frequency of angina alone without other evidence of the disease in the ten-year period, but such angina with long survival is about twice as common as coronary death. Here again the value for the Americans is an extrapolation from five-year data.

In our classification of diagnoses of coronary heart disease codes 35, 36, and 37 are based on specified changes in the electrocardiogram from normal at entry; small Q waves, T, and ST abnormalities that were not present before. These codes have been suggested to mean possible infarction, coronary insufficiency, and so on, but the incidence is not significantly related to the incidence of death from coronary heart disease. This is evident from the data summarized in figure 5.4. The correlation, $r = 0.24$, is far from being statistically significant with so few degrees of freedom.

Finally, in our series of diagnostic categories we have code 39, meaning major unexplained arrhythmias. In men of these ages it seemed reasonable to suggest that such arrhythmias could mean coronary heart disease without other manifestation. Figure 5.5 shows that whatever may be the cause or explanation of such arrhythmias their incidence rate as isolated phenomena is unrelated to the incidence rate of coronary death in the populations concerned. This conclusion may be qualified by noting that relatively few men

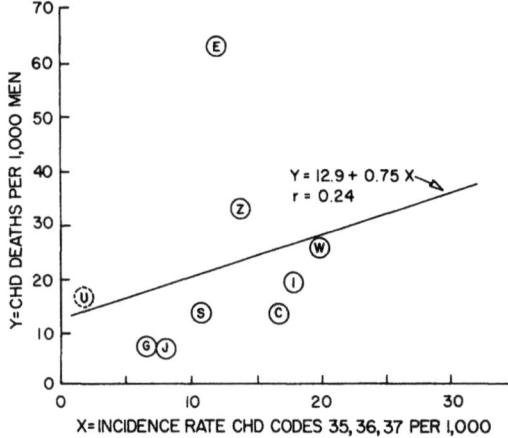

Figure 5.4. Ten-year death rate from coronary heart disease versus incidence rate of coronary heart disease inferred from codes 35, 36, and 37 (identified by nonspecific changes in the electrocardiogram from the entry record). Groups as in figure 5.1.

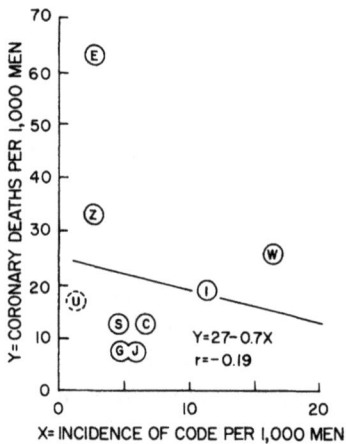

Figure 5.5. Ten-year death rate from coronary heart disease versus incidence rate of unexplained arrhythmias, code 39, all men free of cardiovascular disease at entry. Groups as in figure 5.1.

were given a diagnosis that would place them in code 39. Conceivably, the failure to find a relationship might reflect a lack of numbers; at the five-year examinations only 26 men were coded 39; the ten-year examination added 51 more men.

Summary

The incidence of coronary heart disease was classified as to type of manifestation. Hard CHD is death from coronary heart disease or nonfatal myocardial infarction. Any CHD includes all diagnoses of the disease. During ten years, among 9,780 men in Europe and Japan with no cardiovascular disease at entry, 913 men were given a diagnosis of any CHD, of which 351 were hard. The age-standardized rates ranged from the east Finns with 29 percent of any and 11 percent of hard to the Cretans with 2 percent any and only 0.3 percent hard.

Comparing incidence rates of cohorts in the same regions, there was no significant difference in Croatia between Dalmatia and Slavonia, in Japan between Tanushimaru and Ushibuka, and in Italy among Crevalcore, Montegiorgio, and the Rome railroad men. But in Greece the men of Corfu were more susceptible than the men of Crete, and in Finland the incidence rate in east Finland was almost double that in west Finland. In Serbia the incidence in Belgrade and in Zrenjanin was similar, but the incidence among the men in the farming village of Velika Krsna was only about half as great.

In Zutphen 54 percent of the incidence cases were hard, but in the other areas of Europe hard CHD accounted for only 37 to 42 percent of all incidence. A relative deficiency of cases of uncomplicated angina pectoris diagnosed at Zutphen accounted for the peculiarity, presumably reflecting a difference in diagnostic criteria.

The age-standardized incidence rate of the several diagnostic categories of coronary heart disease in the different regions were compared with the corresponding coronary death rates, which were taken as the ultimate evidence of the disease. The incidence rates of our diagnostic categories of old myocardial infarction, which require electrocardiographic as well as medical history evidence (our codes 30, 31, and 32), corresponded closely with the coronary death rates in the regions ($r = 0.9$). The incidence rates of old infarction diagnosed on the basis of history only (our code 34) was no less highly correlated with the coronary death rate. The rate of the incidence of uncomplicated angina pectoris was equally well correlated with the coronary death rate, but the slope of the regression of death rate on the incidence of angina pectoris was relatively flat. The interpretation of this last fact is that the incidence of angina pectoris with long survival is relatively high.

The incidence rate of coronary heart disease diagnosed only on the basis of nonspecific electrocardiographic changes and questionable medical history (our codes 35, 36, and 37) was not significantly correlated with the coronary death rate. The same was true for the diagnosis of coronary heart disease based only on the appearance of major arrhythmias (our code 39), but this latter lack of correspondence might reflect small numbers. Only 29 men, previously normal, were coded 39 at five years, and 51 more were added at ten years. These findings emphasize the need to insist on hard criteria in epidemiological studies on coronary heart disease.

Age and incidence rate. The influence of age on the rate of incidence of coronary heart disease is so large that reports on the incidence rate for an age range can be seriously misleading. It should be emphasized that all incidence rates here have been standardized by single years of age. In chapter 4 we showed the importance for death rates of considering single years of age and the errors that may arise when rates of death are reported only for ranges of age. The need to consider single years of age for the rate of incidence of coronary heart disease is similar.

Table 5.3 summarizes analyses of data on the ten-year incidence of coronary death or myocardial infarction in Finland and in the Mediterranean area (Italy, Greece, and Dalmatia) and from the Pooling Project (Pooling Project Research Group 1978, table 17E). For each group the solution of the bivariate logistic equation for the experience of that group was used to calculate the incidence, the independent variables being age and the mean blood pressure of the group at entry. Systolic pressure was used for Finland and the Mediterranean groups; diastolic pressure was used for the pool of five studies (Framingham, Albany, Chicago Western Electric, Chicago Gas Company, and Tecumseh, Michigan).

Table 5.3. Effect of a difference of one year of age on the ten-year incidence per 1,000 men of coronary death or myocardial infarction. (Results of calculations with solutions of the bivariate multiple logistic with age and blood pressure as independent variables. In the calculations, for each group the blood pressure was fixed at all ages as the mean of the group aged 40–59 at entry. The coefficients for the five-study pool were published in 1978 by the Pooling Project Research Group in table 17E.)

Group	Age	Incidence	Age	Incidence	One-year change
Finland	45	56.8	46	59.7	5.0%
Finland	55	91.9	56	96.3	4.8%
Mediterranean	45	18.8	46	19.9	5.9%
Mediterranean	55	32.4	56	34.2	5.6%
Five-study pool	45	26.2	46	27.9	6.3%
Five-study pool	55	48.0	56	51.0	6.1%

The effect of a year of age on the incidence rate of major coronary heart disease is similar in all three groups. For all three groups combined, a difference of one year of age at entry is associated with a difference of 5.6 percent in ten-year incidence. An increase of ten years of age at entry is associated with an increase of 72.4 percent in the incidence rate.

6 | Age

Age as a risk factor for coronary heart disease has been variously treated in epidemiological studies. Though age is the most readily ascertainable continuous variable that is obviously related to both prevalence and incidence of the disease, it has often been treated as a discontinuous variable, and its role as a risk factor has not been explicitly emphasized. For example, the incidence rate is commonly reported for an age range, sometimes as great as twenty years, without details of the age distribution. Comparisons of incidence rates in different groups are not infrequently made without proper age standardization.

Ideally, age standardization should be by single years of age. Even an age grouping as fine as five years may lead to serious error because of the implicit assumption that, other things being equal, the risk is the same for all ages within the group. For example, age 49 would be considered to be associated with the same risk as age 45. Actually, from our multiple logistic solution for the five-year incidence of myocardial infarction or coronary death (Keys et al. 1972b), calculation shows that for American railroad men the risk at age 49 years was 27.8 percent greater than at 45 years, when other significant variables were identical. For the European men the corresponding calculation indicates the risk at age 49 was 36.7 percent greater than for men otherwise the same but four years younger. For the 6,854 American men in the pool of five studies, the corresponding analysis of the data on the incidence of myocardial infarction or coronary death in ten years, men aged 40–59 at entry, gives almost exactly the same result as in the American railroad men in the calculation with the data reported by the Pooling Project Research Group (1978). For men 49 years old at entry with the values of diastolic blood pressure, serum cholesterol, smoking habit, and relative body weight at the mean entry values for those variables, men enter-

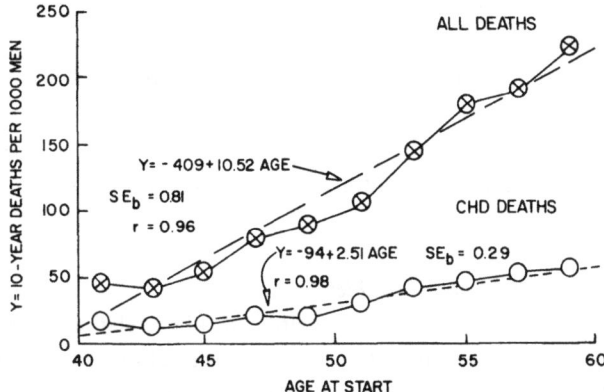

Figure 6.1. Relation of ten-year death rate from all causes and from coronary heart disease to age at the start of the follow-up. All cohorts combined by two-year age classes. SE_b is the standard error of the slope, b, of the regression. N = 12,763.

ing at 49 are indicated to have 28.1 percent higher incidence of infarction or coronary death than men entering at age 45.

Although we used standarization by single years of age, for comparison among cohorts no serious errors would result if age were disregarded. Aside from the men in the Belgrade cohort who averaged 47.8 years at the entry examination, the mean ages of the men in all the cohorts ranged only from 49.0 (east Finland) to 50.7 years (Tanushimaru).

Ten-year Death Rate

Figure 6.1 summarizes our findings on the relationship between the ten-year death rate and age at the start of the follow-up. Of the 12,763 men, 1,512 died in ten years, 413 of the deaths being attributed to coronary heart disease. The least-squares equation for the regression of coronary deaths per 1,000 men, y, on starting age, x, is: $y = -94 + 2.51 x$ (SE of the slope = 0.29). The corresponding equation for all-causes deaths is: $y = -409 + 10.52 x$ (SE of the slope = 0.96). The death rate increases with age much faster for all-causes than for coronary deaths.

Figure 6.1 suggests that although the relationship of all-causes death rate with age is fairly well fitted with a straight line, the relationship is actually curvilinear. A similar relationship is indicated by the U.S. Vital Statistics for the age range 40–70 of American men. A tendency to curvilinearity is less clear in the present data on age and coronary death rate, but curvilinearity is not ruled out. For all-causes deaths, and possibly for coronary heart disease deaths, it appears that a model with death rate as a linear function of age is not ideal for men of these ages; the importance of age as a risk factor may be underestimated, at least over some age ranges.

In any event the analysis of the present data with the linear model indicates that a man aged 59 is 15 to 20 times more likely to die in ten years than a 40-year-old man in the same population. For coronary death the risk of the 59-year-old man is around 8 or 10 times that of the man age 40 at the start.

Correlation with Other Variables

Table 6.1 gives product-moment coefficients of correlation between age at entry and other characteristics of the men recorded at that time. Systolic and disastolic blood pressure in rest were positively correlated with age in all cohorts, but the correlations were not statistically significant in Dalmatia or, for diastolic pressure, in Zutphen. Systolic blood pressure was more closely correlated with age than was diastolic pressure, and the mean difference is

Table 6.1. Coefficients of correlation between age and other variables recorded at the entry examination.

Cohort	S BP	D BP	Smoking	Chol.	BMI	Skinf.	Pulse
U.S. railroad	0.212[a]	0.111[a]	−0.103	0.050	−0.016	0.027	0.063[a]
Dalmatia	0.056	0.022	0.072	−0.008	−0.076	−0.072	−0.001
Slavonia	0.187[a]	0.093[b]	0.033	0.000	−0.065	−0.049	−0.001
Tanushimaru	0.333[a]	0.263[a]	−0.070[b]	−0.075	−0.093[b]	−0.006	−0.014
East Finland	0.257[a]	0.114[a]	−0.094	−0.038	−0.042	−0.018	−0.022
West Finland	0.244[a]	0.178[a]	0.015	0.044	0.003	0.012	−0.109[a]
Ushibuka	0.239[a]	0.188[a]	−0.088[b]	0.029	−0.033	—	0.036
Crevalcore	0.299[a]	0.127[a]	−0.037	0.025	0.005	−0.002	0.002
Montegiorgio	0.262[a]	0.155[a]	−0.036	0.039	0.012	0.051	0.017
Zutphen	0.125[b]	0.037	−0.169[a]	−0.051	−0.084	0.000	−0.097[a]
Crete	0.196[a]	0.083[b]	−0.046	0.126[a]	0.045	−0.055	−0.068
Corfu	0.158[a]	0.078	−0.009	−0.014	0.006	−0.033	−0.092[a]
Rome railroad	0.161[a]	0.090[b]	−0.076[b]	0.052	−0.081	−0.079	−0.019
Velika Krsna	0.287[a]	0.163[a]	0.008	0.088[b]	0.055	−0.014	−0.024
Zrenjanin	0.330[a]	0.199[a]	0.008	0.059	−0.056	−0.016	—
Belgrade	0.281[a]	0.206[a]	−0.139[a]	0.135[a]	−0.061	−0.015	—
Mean	0.227	0.132	−0.046	0.023	−0.036	−0.018	−0.022
S.E.	0.019	0.016	0.016	0.015	0.010	0.009	0.014

a. $p = 0.01$ or less that the correlation is not zero.
b. $p = 0.05$.

statistically highly significant—(0.227–0.132) divided by the standard error of the difference (0.0248) = 3.83.

Aside from blood pressure, the other variables in table 6.1 show only very small correlations with age, though statistical significance is indicated for smoking and age (negative) in five cohorts and for resting pulse rate and age (negative) in four. It should be noted, however, that the correlations in table 6.1 refer only to men limited to the age range of 40 through 59 years. It is well known that at younger ages serum cholesterol and relative body weight are positively correlated with age.

The coefficients of correlation in table 6.1 are useful in examining the question as to whether chronological age, by itself, is an independent risk factor or whether it increases risk through its effect on other risk factors. Among the variables considered in table 6.1 only blood pressure is importantly related to age. In other words, these data offer no basis for suggesting that age may work its evil through blood cholesterol, smoking habits, relative weight or body fatness, or the resting pulse rate. By the same token it is indicated that any risk that may be associated with these variables is essentially independent of age.

As to blood pressure, the correlation with age is statistically very highly significant, but on the average only 5 percent of the variance of systolic pressure is accounted for by age. And age accounted for less than 2 percent of the variance of the diastolic pressure in the average of all sixteen cohorts. We conclude, therefore, that the large influence of age on the incidence of coronary heart disease and of death in this material is almost wholly independent of the other variables considered in table 6.1.

Comparability of the Cohorts

Aside from some men not considered in this book, the age range of the men in the Seven Countries Study was restricted to 40 through 59 years when the rosters of eligible men were compiled. At the entry examinations and the start of the follow-up, a few men had graduated out of the 59-year class, but unless they proved to be more than six months over age they were retained in the study in their roster age class of 59. Similarly, a few men had graduated out of the 40-year roster class, so in some of the cohorts the 40-year class at entry contained very few men. This accounts for the fact that in the combined age distribution of all men in this study the entry class of age 40 in table 2.4 contains fewer than half as many men as in any other single year class.

Table 6.2 shows the means and standard deviations for the entry age for the sixteen cohorts. The range of the means is from 47.80 in Belgrade to

Table 6.2. Age of men at entry.

Cohort	Mean	SD	Cohort	Mean	SD
U.S. railroad	49.83	5.76	Montegiorgio	49.58	4.98
Dalmatia	50.60	5.03	Rome railroad	49.72	5.29
Slavonia	50.43	5.32	Zutphen	50.05	5.51
Tanushimaru	50.72	5.75	Crete	49.24	5.45
East Finland	48.99	5.55	Corfu	49.81	5.69
West Finland	50.05	5.47	Velika Krsna	49.92	6.17
Ushibuka	50.01	5.61	Zrenjanin	49.21	5.35
Crevalcore	49.99	5.15	Belgrade	47.80	5.68

50.72 at Tanushimaru, but aside from Belgrade the lowest mean is 48.99 years in east Finland. It would seem, then, that for many purposes age could be disregarded in comparisons among the cohorts, Belgrade excepted. However, calculation from the regression equation in figure 6.1 shows that on the average the all-causes death rate at entry age 51 is 9 percent greater than that at age 50. For death from coronary heart disease the corresponding difference is 2.5 percent. These considerations reemphasize the importance of insisting on age-standardization by single years and the danger of simplifying analyses by using age classes covering five or, still worse, ten years.

Incidence Rate

In chapters 4 and 5 it was shown that among the cohorts there were important differences in the ten-year age-standardized incidence rates of death and or coronary heart disease. The question arises, then, as to whether the cohorts differed in regard to the force of age as a risk factor. Since both age and blood pressure are powerful risk factors and are significantly correlated in all cohorts, it is essential to allow for blood pressure in examining the relation between incidence rate and age. For a given area we solve the bivariate logistic equation with age and systolic blood pressure as the independent variables, first with all-causes deaths and then with hard CHD as the dependent variable. Then, for given blood pressure, the estimated probability of the events in ten years can be calculated for selected ages for the cohort or area in question. The results, calculated in the same way for different areas, provide the basis for comparing those areas in regard to the independent aging effect.

Figure 6.2 shows the findings for rural Finland and rural Italy. For all-causes deaths the rate at age 40 is over 50 percent higher for the Finns than for the Italians, but at age 60 the rates for the two groups are almost iden-

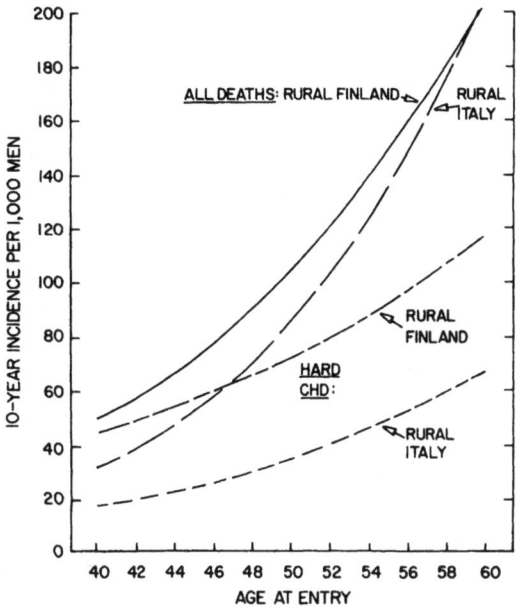

Figure 6.2. Relation of ten-year incidence of hard coronary heart disease (myocardial infarction or coronary death) and of all-causes death to age at entry for rural men aged 40–59 and free of cardiovascular disease at the start in Finland and Italy. The bivariate logistic solutions for incidence versus age and systolic blood pressure were used to calculate the incidence at different ages with blood pressure held constant at the mean pressure of the group recorded at entry.

tical; in twenty years the Italian men catch up, so to speak, with the Finns. The illustration in figure 6.2 is the expression of the fact that the coefficient for age in the bivariate logistic equation proved to be 0.0797 for the Finns, 0.0998 for the Italians. No great emphasis should be given to this difference, however, because when account is taken of the standard errors of the coefficients it appears that the difference between the estimated coefficients could occur by chance in about 1 out of 7 trials.

In regard to the incidence of myocardial infarction or coronary death (hard CHD), the analysis indicates a great difference between the Finns and the Italians at all ages with no suggestion of a differential effect of age.

Summary

For apparently healthy men, age is the most important of the risk factors, both for the incidence of coronary heart disease and for death from all causes. In only very small part is the risk of age related to other risk factors. In this study age had only a trivial correlation, averaging less than $r = 0.05$

in the sixteen cohorts for relative body weight, obesity (skinfold thickness), serum cholesterol, cigarette smoking, and resting pulse rate. The correlation with resting arterial blood pressure in the sixteen cohorts averaged at entry is $r = 0.23$ for systolic and $r = 0.13$ for diastolic pressure.

Because the risk increases substantially with each year of age, all incidence rates have been standardized by single years to the distribution of age of all men in the Study. The age distribution differs only trivially from that of white men in the United States. It is shown that comparisons of incidence rates among populations can be grossly misleading if age groups are used, especially with groups as coarse as ten years.

Considering all 12,763 men aged 40–59 at entry, the least squares regression of all-causes ten-year death rate per 1,000 men, y, on entry age, x, is $y = -409 + 10.52x$. This means that for men in their mid-forties, a difference of one year of age is associated with a 16 percent difference in death rate, whereas for men in their mid-fifties a difference of one year of age is associated with a difference of 6.2 percent in death rate. The corresponding regression of coronary death rate on age is $y = -94 + 2.51x$. For that cause of death a difference of one year in the mid-forties was associated with a difference of 13 percent in death rate; for men in their mid-fifties the difference in death rate associated with a difference of one year of age was 5.7 percent.

The ten-year incidence rate of death varied greatly among the cohorts, especially for death from coronary heart disease. In order to estimate the force of age itself in the incidence, the bivariate logistic equation was solved with age and systolic blood pressure as the independent variables and the ten-year age-standardized incidence rate as the dependent variable. For the incidence rate of all-causes deaths the coefficient found for age with the data on the Finns proved to be very similar to that found with the data on the Italians. The same procedure applied to the incidence of hard CHD (coronary death or myocardial infarction) also indicated that the force of age itself was almost the same in the two areas in spite of the great difference in the incidence rates.

7 | Blood Pressure

Insurance companies have long emphasized hypertension as a major "impairment" and have recognized this in the rates charged for life insurance. However, in setting premium rates, insurance companies commonly treat the arterial blood pressure as a discontinuous variable, classifying the great majority of policy applicants as "standard risks" who pay the same premiums at given starting age regardless of blood pressure so long as it does not exceed some limiting level. Major independent prospective studies on the incidence of heart disease also treat blood pressure as a discontinuous variable when they report the incidence rate for classes of blood pressure, for example for quintiles of the blood pressure distribution. Lately, however, the relationship of follow-up incidence to the blood pressure at entry is commonly presented as a regression with the implicit assumption that such relationship as may exist is linear; the impression is thereby conveyed that the risk of heart attack or death rises continuously with blood pressure. This is in contrast to the old tradition in clinical medicine of a dichotomy—sick or not sick, normal or abnormal. Physicians are concerned about degrees of hypertension, but the main distinction is between normotension and hypertension, with endless argument about where to draw the line. This is essentially the viewpoint of insurance medicine. This chapter is concerned with these questions as seen from the vantage point of ten years of follow-up of contrasting populations without the limitations of a qualitative approach.

Comparisons of blood pressure among the cohorts is tempered by the fact that, in spite of efforts to standardize the conditions and methods, absolute comparability could not be guaranteed; there were some differences between the places of examination in regard to air temperature and noise level, and there may have been small differences among the cohorts in the average

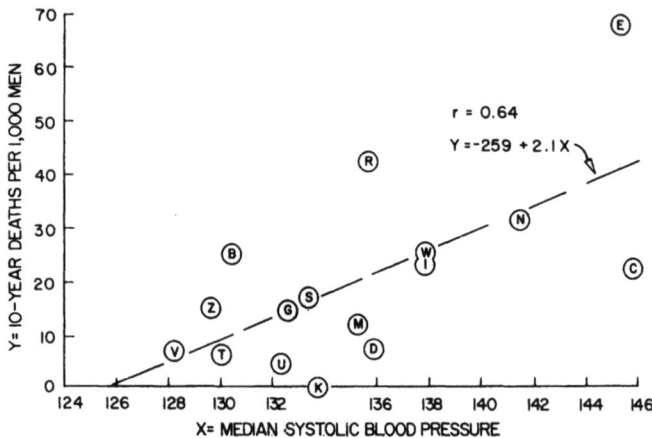

Figure 7.1. The ten-year age-standardized coronary death rates, men without evidence of cardiovascular disease at entry, of the sixteen cohorts versus the median systolic blood pressures of those cohorts at entry. B = Belgrade; C = Crevalcore; D = Dalmatia; E = east Finland; G = Corfu; I = Italian railroad; K = Crete; M = Montegiorgio; N = Zutphen; R = American railroad; S = Slavonia; T = Tanushimaru; U = Ushibuka; V = Velika Krsna; W = west Finland; Z = Zrenjanin.

time between any cigarette smoking or physical activity and the measurement of blood pressure after at least five minutes of rest in the supine position following the medical history interview and the physical examination. Variations among the cohorts in these respects would, of course, tend to obscure such relationships as there might be between true blood pressure characteristics of the cohorts and their subsequent experience of disease and death. Still as figure 7.1 shows, an important relationship emerged from the ten-year experience.

The ten-year age-standardized coronary death rates of the cohorts were correlated with the median systolic blood pressure of the cohorts at entry with $r = 0.64$. This one measurement of blood pressure at the start accounts for 41 percent of the variance in coronary death rate. The similar analysis with the median diastolic pressure as the independent variable shows a relationship to the ten-year mortality that is not significantly different. No difference of significance from the relationship shown in figure 7.1 was found when the independent variable was the percentage of the men in the cohort who, at the entry examination, were labeled hypertensive because the diastolic pressure was 95 mm or higher.

Correlation with Other Variables

In all cohorts there was a high correlation between systolic and diastolic blood pressures, ranging from $r = 0.7$ to $r = 0.8$, closely similar to the findings of other major studies on men of these ages. W. B. Kannel, Joseph T. Doyle, Oglesby Paul and Jeremiah Stamler kindly made available to us data tapes on their studies at Framingham, Albany, and Chicago. For men aged 40 through 59 the coefficient of correlation between systolic and diastolic blood pressures in that material is $r = 0.78$. Such a high correlation does not mean, however, that one pressure can be safely estimated from the other; around 40 percent of the variance in diastolic pressure remains unaccounted for by the systolic pressure. The question of diastolic versus systolic pressures as predictors of risk will be examined later. For the moment we shall concentrate on the systolic pressure.

Table 7.1 summarizes the correlations in the entry examination data between the resting systolic blood pressure and seven other characteristics. Except for cigarette smoking, the correlations are positive in every one of the cohorts. For smoking, the correlation is negative for all cohorts except Tanushimaru where $r = +0.022$ which, for 499 pairs of measurements, is not significantly different from zero or, for that matter, from a value of $r = -0.05$. All of the mean coefficients of correlation shown in table 7.1 are significantly different from zero, the values ranging from $t = 6.2$ for smoking to $t = 11.9$ for age.

The correlations between these variables and the diastolic blood pressure are generally similar to those with systolic blood pressure. However, the mean coefficient of correlation of age and diastolic pressure is highly signifi-

Table 7.1. Correlation between resting systolic blood pressure and other variables recorded at entry in men free of coronary heart disease (mean r = average coefficient of correlation; lat./lin. = sum of bicristal and biacromial diameters divided by height; N columns show consistency of cohorts in coefficient sign).

Item	Mean r	SD	Minimum	Maximum	N+	N−
Age	0.227	0.076	0.056	0.330	16	0
Body mass index	0.214	0.097	0.059	0.384	16	0
Sum of skinfolds	0.209	0.093	0.097	0.409	15	0
Lat./lin.	0.107	0.039	0.023	0.149	12	0
Serum cholesterol	0.133	0.075	0.072	0.261	16	0
Resting pulse rate	0.203	0.078	0.099	0.327	14	0
Cigarette smoking	−0.091	0.057	−0.147	0.022	15	1

cant with $r = 0.132$ ($t = 8.2$), but this coefficient is smaller than for the correlation of age with systolic pressure. The difference between the two means for the correlation coefficient, $0.227 - 0.132 = 0.095$, has SE $= 0.0248$, so $t = 3.83$. The conclusion is that in this material systolic pressure is significantly more closely related to age than is diastolic pressure. On the other hand, the body mass index seemed to be somewhat more closely correlated with diastolic than with systolic pressure with $r = 0.261$, SD $= 0.097$, for the mean of the coefficients for diastolic in comparison with $r = 0.214$ for systolic pressure. However, the difference, 0.047 has SE $= 0.033$ and is not statistically significant.

Ten-year Death Rate

Among variables considered in table 7.1, age is the most highly correlated with blood pressure. Since age itself is a major risk factor for both all-causes and coronary deaths, allowance must be made for it in examining the relationship of mortality to blood pressure. One way of doing this is to express the blood pressure of each man in terms of its place in the distribution of pressures of men of the same age in the same cohort and to examine the number of deaths in the decile classes of those age- and cohort-specific arrays.

Figure 7.2 shows the distribution into decile classes of systolic blood pressure of the American railroad men who had been judged free of coronary heart disease at the entry examination and who died in the ten-year follow-up. Since the number of men at risk in each decile was almost exactly the same, in the absence of a relationship between blood pressure and death rate

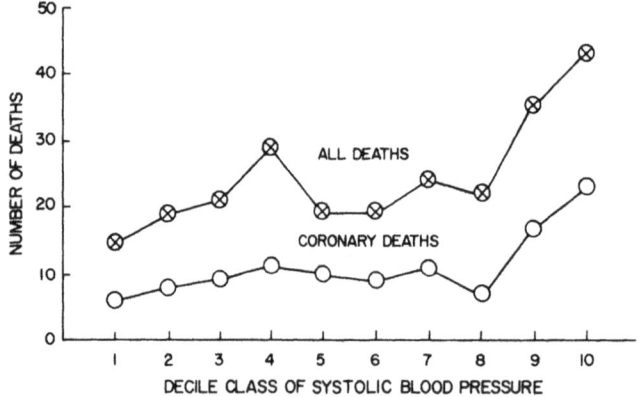

Figure 7.2. American railroad men aged 40–59 and free of coronary heart disease at entry. Deaths in ten years in the decile classes of resting systolic blood pressure.

the points in figure 7.2 would be randomly distributed about horizontal lines passing through the mean for all ten decile classes. Actually, there is a sharp upward trend from the eighth to the tenth decile for both coronary and all-causes deaths. From the first to the seventh decile, there is no statistically significant upward trend in the death rate from all causes and from coronary heart disease. But the men in the ninth decile class suffered 153 percent of the coronary death rate for all deciles combined, and the men in the tenth decile class had double the average coronary death rate of all railroad men who were CHD-free at entry.

Persons unaccustomed to concentrating on the distribution of values in an array will ask about the blood pressures corresponding to the decile classes in Figure 7.2 The cutting points are given in the appendix, but it may help to point out here that the cutting point for the ninth decile was 146 for men initially aged 40–44 and rose steadily with age to 163 for men aged 55–59 at entry. The point to emphasize here is that for the American railroad men no relationship to risk of death in ten years could be found for the men in the lower 80 percent of the distribution. However, being in the top 10 percent of the distribution of men otherwise apparently in full health meant double the average likelihood of dying in ten years.

Figure 7.3 shows the corresponding picture for all men in the Seven Countries Study. The trend is similar to that shown for the American railroad men—no significant relationship between systolic pressure and ten-year deaths for most of the men at risk and then a steep rise in the rate with decile class. The death rate for the men in the eighth decile class had no

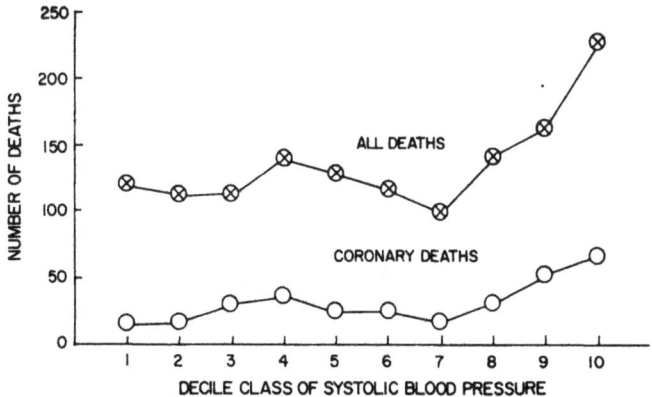

Figure 7.3. All men in the Seven Countries Study aged 40–59 and free of coronary heart disease at entry. Deaths in ten years in the decile classes of resting systolic blood pressure.

more risk than the men in the fourth class. But the 10 percent of men in the top decile class had 207 percent the average coronary death rate of the men in all decile classes; among the men in the top quintile class there were 122 coronary deaths, but 66.2 would be the chance expectation, an excess of 55.8 deaths from that cause. From all causes, 276.2 deaths would be expected in the top quintile of systolic blood pressure in a chance distribution, but 394 were observed, an excess of 117.8 deaths of which only 55.8 would be accounted for by the excess of coronary deaths in that class. Clearly, elevated systolic blood pressure was, if anything, a greater risk factor for noncoronary deaths than for deaths from coronary heart disease.

Figure 7.4 shows the picture for diastolic pressure and ten-year deaths among United States railroad men corresponding to figure 7.2 for systolic pressure. The relationships are similar except that the indication of an absence of an effect of the blood pressure on mortality extends through the first six decile classes with a peak in the death rate in the seventh decile class and then a fall in the eighth class. The coronary death rate in the top quintile of diastolic pressure was 171 percent of the average for all diastolic pressure classes. For all-causes deaths there were 76 men in the top quintile; the chance expectation is only 48.8. Excess of coronary deaths accounts for 15.8 or only 58 percent of the total excess of 27.2 deaths above the expectation from a chance distribution.

The corresponding picture for all men in the Seven Countries Study in regard to ten-year mortality and the entry diastolic pressure is given in figure 7.5. Here the ten decile points for coronary deaths do not depart much from a straight line, but there is a jump from the ninth to the top decile. The coronary death rate in the top quintile is 161 percent of chance expectation. For all-causes deaths the role of elevated blood pressure represented by the

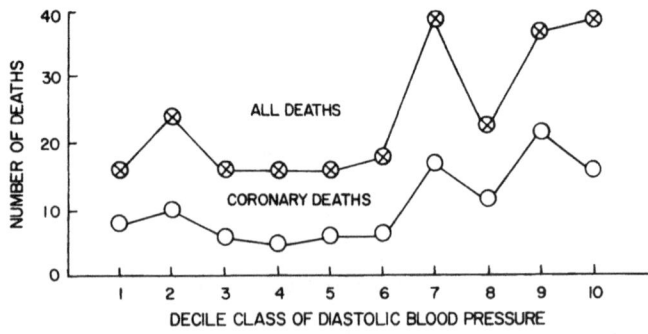

Figure 7.4. American railroad men aged 40–59 and free of coronary heart disease at entry. Deaths in ten years in the decile classes of resting diastolic blood pressure.

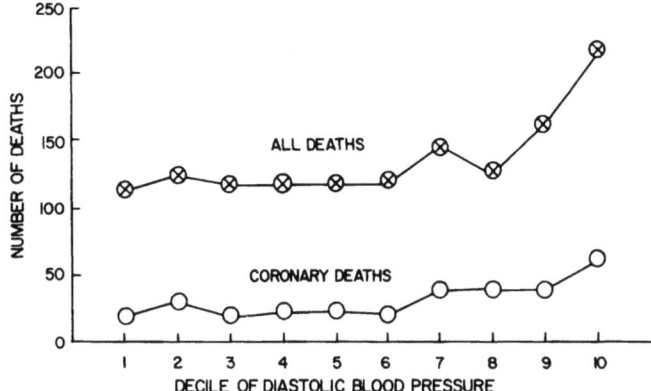

Figure 7.5. All men in the Seven Countries Study aged 40–59 and free of coronary heart disease at entry. Deaths in ten years in the cohort- and age-specific decile classes of resting diastolic blood pressure.

top quintile of diastolic pressure is more impressive. Among men in the top quintile of diastolic pressure at entry 382 were dead in ten years; 275 is the number expected by chance. Of the excess of 107 deaths, 39 are accounted for by the excess deaths attributed to coronary heart disease.

Probability of Death

Figures 7.2–7.5 show that a resting blood pressure in the upper 20 percent or so of the distribution is associated with a much greater risk of death in the next ten years than that faced by the other men in the same cohort and five-year age class. The multiple logistic equation provides another approach to the analysis of the relationship of blood pressure to the risk of death or other incidence with allowance for age as an independent variable. Figure 7.6 gives the solution of the bivariate logistic with the method of Walker and Duncan (1967) applied to the data from 2,246 American railroad men showed no evidence of coronary heart disease at the start of the ten-year follow up. The graph shows the probability of death (all causes) in ten years plotted against the entry systolic blood pressure for various starting ages. At a blood pressure of 200 mm at age 55 the bivariate logistic indicates a 25 percent probability of death in ten years; the probability of death is only 5 percent for a man of 40 with systolic pressure of 160 mm.

Figure 7.7 is the corresponding picture for 1,450 Finns also free of coronary heart disease at the start. The prospect for the Finns is indicated to be somewhat worse than that for the Americans with the same age and blood pressure. With blood pressure of 200 mm at age 55 the probability of ten-

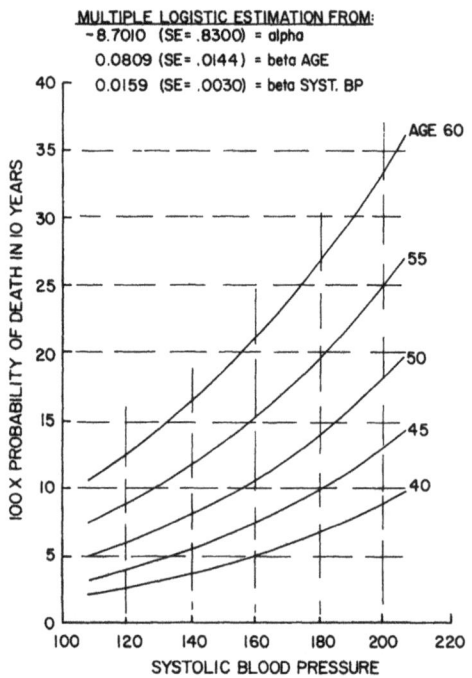

Figure 7.6. American railroad men aged 40–59 and free of coronary heart disease at entry. Coefficients of the bivariate multiple logistic equation for ten-year all-causes deaths versus entry age and resting systolic blood pressure and the application of those coefficients to specific starting ages and blood pressures.

year death (all causes) for Finns is about 32 percent instead of the 25 percent calculated for the American men.

Figure 7.8 is the corresponding picture for 3,321 men in the Mediterranean cohorts of rural Italy, Greece, and Dalmatia. At the high end of the systolic blood pressure distribution and the older ages, the Mediterranean men are indicated to be between the Finns and the Americans in regard to ten-year death rate at equal age and blood pressure. But over most of the range, the Mediterranean men have a relatively low death rate, for example, only 3.5 percent for the man aged 40 with systolic pressure of 160 mm.

A comparison of the indications from the bivariate logistic solutions for the men in the three areas is made in figure 7.9, which concerns men age 50 at the start of the ten-year follow-up. At all blood pressures the outlook is poorest for the Finns. For systolic blood pressures up to about 180 mm, the Mediterraneans had the best record, but the logistic solutions suggest that at around systolic pressure of 190 mm and higher the Americans would do a little better than the Mediterraneans. Of course, the coefficients in the logis-

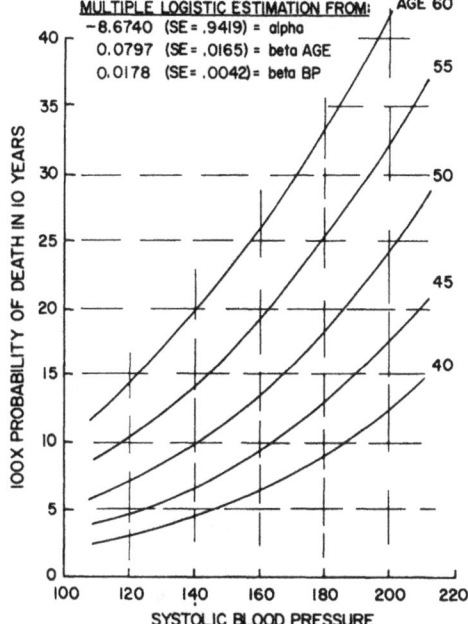

Figure 7.7. Finland, ten-year deaths among men 40–59 and free of coronary heart disease at entry. Multiple logistic coefficients and their application to specific starting ages and blood pressures as in figure 7.6.

tic solutions have fairly large confidence limits. It would appear that over the range 160 to 200 mm systolic pressure the ten-year outlook for the Mediterraneans and the Americans was similar.

Figures 7.6–7.9 summarize ten-year deaths from all causes. Analysis of the relationship of ten-year deaths from coronary heart disease has also been made with the bivariate logistic model, with age and blood pressure the independent variables. Comparison of men starting at age 50 and then free of coronary heart disease is summarized in figure 7.10. At systolic pressures up to about 160 mm the experience of the Finns and the Americans was very closely similar, but at the top of the blood pressure range, the Finns were more prone to die of coronary heart disease. At all blood pressures the Mediterranean men were much less likely to die of coronary heart disease. For starting ages other than 50 the picture is similar—at a given blood pressure, there is little difference between the Finns and the Americans and the Mediterranean men fare better.

In the logistic model both age and blood pressure prove to be major independent risk factors both for deaths from all causes and for coronary heart

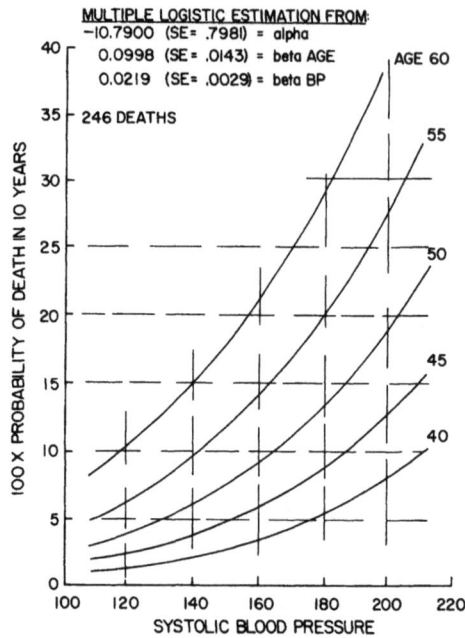

Figure 7.8. Mediterranean men (Italy and Greece), ten-year deaths among men 40–59 and free of coronary heart disease at entry. Multiple logistic coefficients and their application to specific starting ages and blood pressures as in figure 7.6.

deaths; in all analyses the coefficients divided by their standard errors give t values indicating very high statistical significance. When the coefficients are standardized by multiplication with the standard deviations of the variables concerned, it appears that over the range 40 to 60 years at the start, age is more important than the systolic blood pressure for all-causes deaths, but for death from coronary heart disease blood pressure is relatively more consequential. For all-causes deaths in Finland the ratio of the standardized coefficients (age divided by systolic blood pressure) is 1.35; the corresponding ratio for coronary deaths is 0.47. For the American railroad men the respective ratios of the standardized coefficients are 1.51 and 1.03; for the Mediterranean men the corresponding ratios are 1.25 and 0.58.

The solutions to the logistic model are, of course, only mathematical descriptions without necessary implications about cause and effect. Still it is difficult to avoid the speculation that elevated blood pressure does more to promote death from coronary heart disease than death from other causes. But, as shown earlier, a large part of the total of excess deaths associated with elevated blood pressure is not accounted for by an excess of coronary deaths. It could be, of course, that high blood pressure promotes coronary

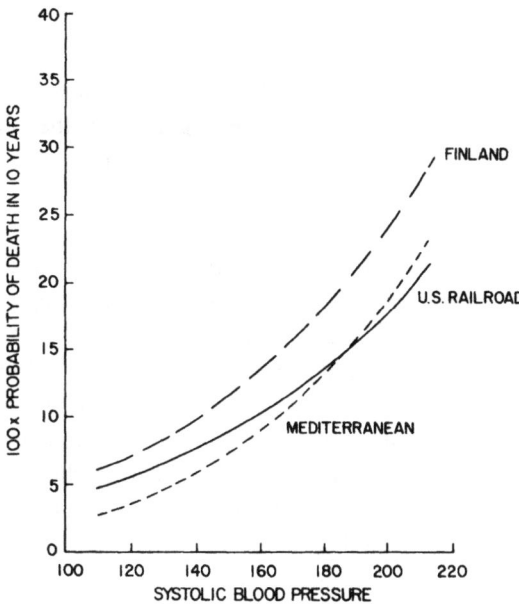

Figure 7.9. Comparison of predictions of the probability of death in ten years, men free of coronary heart disease at the start, from the solutions to the multiple logistic equation for men in the American railroad, in Finland, and in the Mediterranean area to men aged 50 with specified systolic blood pressure at the entry examination.

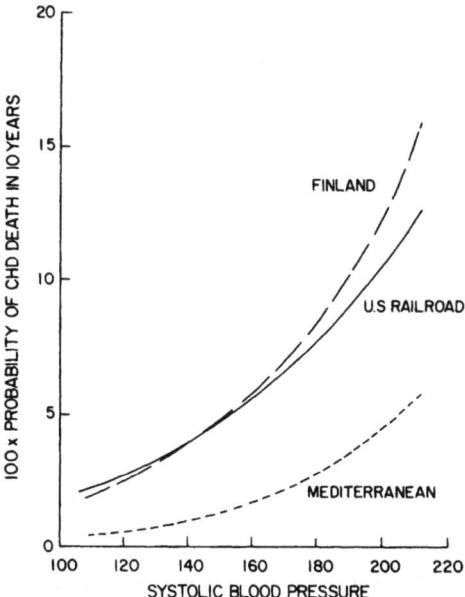

Figure 7.10. Comparison as in figure 7.9 but for probability of death in ten years from coronary heart disease.

heart disease which contributes to death from other causes, the contribution of the coronary heart disease being unrecognized by the physicians who must wrestle with the difficult problem of adjudicating the cause of death.

Incidence Rate

Besides the relationship of blood pressure to the risk of death, it is useful to examine the data in regard to the risk of developing coronary heart disease, fatal and nonfatal. Figure 7.11 summarizes the results with the bivariate logistic model, age and systolic blood pressure as the independent variables, applied to the ten-year incidence of hard CHD—coronary death or nonfatal myocardial infarction—among men free from evidence of the disease at the entry examination. The contrast between the experience of the Finns and that of the Mediterraneans is at least as great as in the case of coronary death and, because the numbers for incidence are larger, the confidence limits of the logistic coefficients are narrower. The analysis summarized in figure 7.11 is based on 112 cases of hard CHD in Finland (1,450 men at risk) and 90 cases in the Mediterranean (3,321 men at risk).

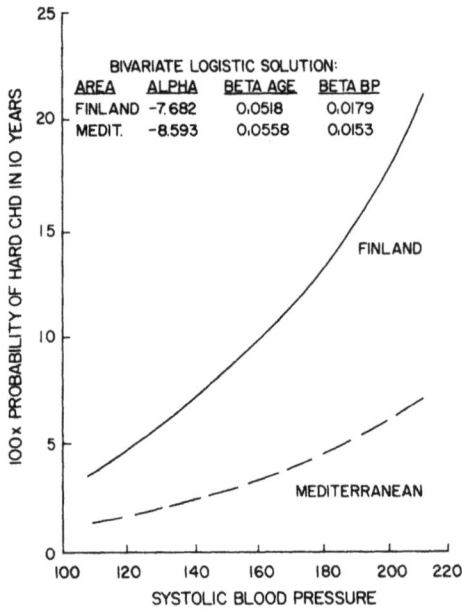

Figure 7.11. Men in Finland and in the Mediterranean areas aged 40–59 and free of coronary heart disease at entry. Coefficients of the bivariate multiple logistic equation for ten-year incidence of myocardial infarction or coronary death and the application of those coefficients to starting age 50 and specified systolic blood pressures.

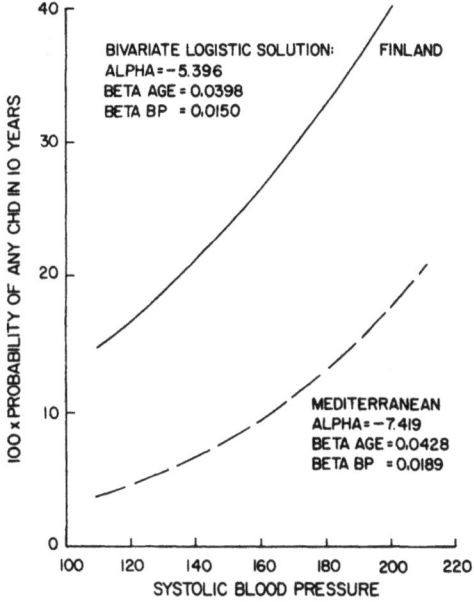

Figure 7.12. Coefficients as in Figure 7.11 but for the probability of developing any diagnostic category of coronary heart disease in ten years.

The incidence of coronary heart disease with any diagnosis of CHD was, of course, much larger—315 cases in Finland, 241 in the Mediterranean—all among men without signs of the disease at the start of the ten-year follow-up. Figure 7.12 shows the bivariate logistic solutions for Finland and the Mediterranean and their application to men aged 50 at entry with systolic blood pressures ranging from 110 mm to around 200 mm. The contrast is, again, extreme. It is not possible to provide corresponding material for the American railroad men because the ten-year follow-up was limited to mortality.

Validity of the Multivariate Model

In the bivariate logistic model, linearity is assumed in the exponent; that is a 10 percent increase in the blood pressure means that the contribution of the blood pressure to the exponent is increased by 10 percent, and so on. The multiple regression equation is another model that can be applied to these analyses, but it also assumes linearity. But figures 7.2–7.5 suggest that the present data do not conform very well to a linear model. Over a large part of the distribution of blood pressures, covering the majority of the men at risk, there is little indication that the blood pressure is a risk factor. The picture is more that of a relationship between blood pressure and risk that

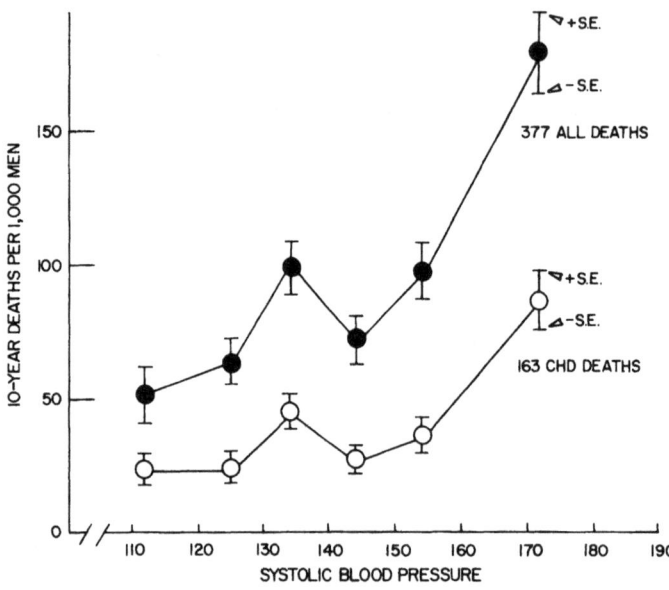

Figure 7.13. American railroad men (2,301) and Finns (1,659) 40–59 years old and free of cardiovascular disease at entry. Age-standardized death rates and their standard errors of men with entry resting systolic blood pressures less than 120, 120–129, 130–139, 140–149, 150–159, 160 or more.

operates only in a range that might be called hypertension. Some readers may object to the use of deciles; they would prefer representation in terms of actual millimeters of blood pressure. As explained earlier, the situation is complicated by the fact that the blood pressure is importantly correlated with age, and age is certainly in itself an important risk factor. A plot of death rate against blood pressure disregarding age is bound to overemphasize the influence of blood pressure. To counter these objections, figure 7.13 summarizes the ten-year death data for 2,301 American railroad men and 1,659 Finns of the same age and similarly free of cardiovascular disease signs at entry. The plot against systolic blood pressure suggests nonlinear relationships. For coronary heart disease there is no significant upward trend for blood pressures under 160 mm. And the men with entry blood pressures above 160 mm were mostly the older men. For example, among the American men aged 55–59 at entry, 21 percent had entry blood pressures of 160 mm or more, but only 6 percent of the railroad men aged 40–44 had blood pressures in that high range; the Finns were similar in this respect.

The present data fully confirm the belief that blood pressure is an important risk factor. The analysis of the data, however, suggest that the assumption of a simple linear relationship between blood pressure and risk is not justifiable. In our experience there is nothing to support the idea that a blood pressure of 120 mm is better than one of 130 mm, or even of 140 mm, in men in the age range 40 to 60.

Differences in Population Comparisons

We have noted marked differences in mortality and the incidence of coronary heart disease among the population samples in the Seven Countries Study, as well as differences in the size of the blood pressure coefficient in the bivariate logistic solutions. The question remains as to what extent the differences in the coronary death rate may be explained by differences in the frequency of hypertension in the cohorts. Figure 7.14 shows the picture for ten-year coronary deaths in the national groups as related to the frequency of hypertension, here arbitrarily defined as a systolic pressure of 160 mm or more. In these population comparisons, age plays little or no role because the populations are so closely matched in age.

Figure 7.14 shows that the frequency of hypertension in the population is by no means the only determinant of the future coronary death rate, although some relationship is evident. The population samples with the lowest frequency of hypertension by this definition were also those with the

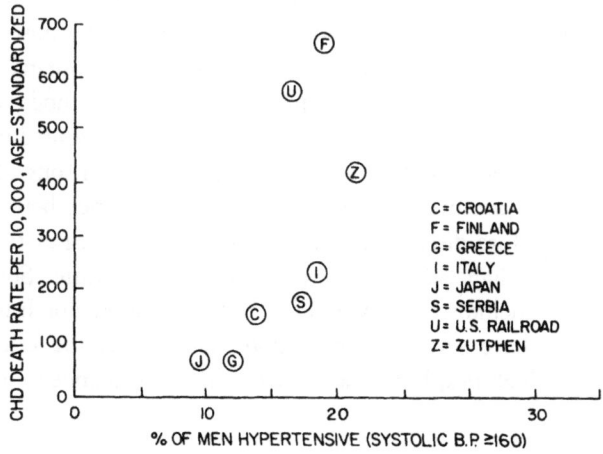

Figure 7.14. Ten-year age-standardized coronary heart disease death rates of men aged 40–59 and free of coronary heart disease at entry plotted against the percentage of men in those cohorts judged then to be hypertensive because of resting systolic blood pressure of 160 mm or greater. C = Croatia; F = Finland; G = Greece; I = Italy; J = Japan; S = Serbia; U = United States; Z = Zutphen.

lowest coronary death rate—Japan (Tanushimaru and Ushibuka), Greece (Crete and Corfu), and Croatia (Dalmatia and Slavonia). Finland is at the top for coronary heart disease death rate and second from the top in the frequency of hypertension. Hypertension is more frequent in east Finland than in any of the other fifteen cohorts, and it also had the highest ten-year coronary death rate.

Systolic versus Diastolic Blood Pressure

Internists commonly consider diastolic to be more informative than systolic blood pressure, partly at least because the diastolic pressure is less affected by temporary emotion. Moreover, as noted earlier, the diastolic pressure is not as highly correlated with age as is systolic pressure. It is agreed that both pressures should be routinely made in physical examinations; such conditions as coarctation of the aorta might well be missed otherwise. But how do the two blood pressures compare in regard to evaluating the future risk of people in population samples?

In the Framingham study the follow-up experience showed that both diastolic and systolic pressure were important factors but that, if anything, the systolic pressure was the better predictor of the later incidence of coronary heart disease (Kannel, Gordon, and Schwartz, 1971). The five-year experience of the Seven Countries Study was in full agreement (Keys et al. 1972; Keys 1975). With the data from the ten-year follow-up, comparison was again made of systolic versus diastolic pressure as risk factors to discriminate men who stayed well from those who died from all causes or from coronary heart disease and from those who developed nonfatal coronary heart disease. The multiple logistic equation and other methods were used in those comparisons. The details of the analysis will be presented in chapter 15. Here it is enough to note that in none of the comparisons of the two measures of blood pressure was there a significant difference between them as predictors of future disease or death, though in some cases the systolic seemed to have a slight advantage over the diastolic pressure. Some intervention studies, including the MRFIT (Multiple Risk Factor Intervention Trial) program, have selected the diastolic pressure as the criterion for selecting men at high risk, but we are unaware of any evidence to justify that choice.

Cause and Effect

Cross-sectional surveys frequently raise the question of cause and effect: Does a characteristic promote a disease or is it simply a reflection of the disease? That question is the reason for emphasizing prospective studies that relate the incidence of a disease to characteristics recorded before the appearance of the disease. But even in such incidence studies, the question of cause and effect may be asked in regard to diseases that make their clinical appearance long after the start of the disease process. Clinical coronary heart disease is commonly an end result of many years of silent atherogenesis, and the question of cause and effect may be asked in connection with the identification of arterial blood pressure as a risk factor.

In experimental animals, raising the blood pressure promotes atherosclerosis. The filtration hypothesis for atherogenesis in man holds that raised blood pressure increases the filtration of lipoprotein-bearing plasma into the intima, and through this kind of mechanism the arterial pressure is an important cause of atherosclerosis. But it is also clear that atherosclerosis in the aorta and the large arteries in general tends to cause a rise in the systolic pressure. Stiff arteries do not yield to the wave of systolic pressure as do young healthy arteries, and this fact must be reflected in the sphygmomanometer reading. So it might appear that atherosclerosis promotes hypertension.

The fact that the systolic blood pressure tends to rise much more with age than the diastolic pressure is commonly interpreted as a result of the progression with age of atherosclerosis in the great arteries. Granting that this may be so, there is good reason for rejecting the suggestion that the relationship between blood pressure and coronary heart disease in the Seven Countries Study is an expression of an effect of atherosclerosis on blood pressure. First, autopsy studies have repeatedly shown a poor correlation between atherosclerosis in the coronary arteries and that in the great vessels. Second, if atherosclerosis were the cause rather than the effect of elevated blood pressure, we would expect that the relationship of the incidence of coronary heart disease to diastolic blood pressure would differ from that to systolic pressure. But this is not the case; systolic and diastolic blood pressures are substantially the same as predictors of the incidence of coronary heart disease or death. The objection that systolic and diastolic pressures are so highly correlated that their effects are very hard to distinguish may be answered in the following way: In spite of the high correlation between the two measures, measuring one pressure leaves unexplained about a third of the variance of the other.

Summary

At entry the resting systolic blood pressure tended to increase with age in all cohorts, and the average correlation between age and systolic pressure is $r = 0.23$. Smaller but statistically significant correlations were found between systolic pressure and body mass index, skinfold thickness, laterality of the skeletal shape, serum cholesterol, and the resting pulse rate. In fifteen out of sixteen cohorts the systolic pressure showed a slight negative correlation with cigarette smoking. The correlation between systolic and diastolic blood pressure ranged from $r = 0.7$ to $r = 0.8$, so measurement of either blood pressure failed to explain around a third of the variance of the other.

In all cohorts the entry blood pressure was a very important risk factor for all-causes death and for the incidence of coronary heart disease in the next ten years. Systolic and diastolic pressures were equally important in this respect. Over a range of 70 to 80 percent of the age-specific blood pressure distribution, there was little or no relation to disease or death in the next ten years, but the incidence rose steeply in the top 20 percent of the blood pressure distribution. An increase in deaths from coronary heart disease accounted for only about half of the excessive death rate of the men in the upper 20 percent of the age-specific blood pressure distribution.

The median blood pressures of the cohorts at entry accounted for 40 percent of the variance among cohorts in the ten-year age-standardized rate of death from coronary heart disease of men with no evidence of cardiovascular disease at the entry examination. The incidence rates of all coronary heart disease, including nonfatal manifestations, were similarly related to the blood pressure characteristics of the cohorts.

The entry blood pressure was more closely related to the subsequent incidence of myocardial infarction and coronary death than to the incidence of softer diagnoses, such as angina pectoris.

In spite of a great difference in the incidence rate of coronary heart disease between southern Europeans, on the one hand, and American railroad men and northern Europeans, on the other, the relative importance of blood pressure for incidence was similar. In all areas the men in the top 20 percent of the age-specific distribution of blood pressure at entry tended to have something like twice the incidence rate of all men in the same area. The several areas were also similar in regard to the relative importance of entry blood pressure as a predictor of ten-year all-causes deaths.

Reasons are given for believing that the blood pressure is causal in regard to the relation between blood pressure at entry and the ten-year incidence of disease and death.

8 | Serum Cholesterol

The concentration of cholesterol in the blood serum is widely recognized as an important risk factor for the incidence of coronary heart disease, at least in populations where that disease is very common, but its significance in other populations and its relevance to mortality has received much less attention. The ten-year experience of the men in the Seven Countries Study provides information on these points, as well as on the more familiar question of the cholesterol in the serum as a predictor of the likelihood of developing coronary heart disease.

The sixteen cohorts in this study differed greatly in the general level of serum cholesterol as well as in mortality and in the incidence of the disease. The distribution of serum cholesterol values in five-year age groups of each cohort are given in the appendix. The general levels are indicated in figures 8.1 and 8.2 in which the median value for each cohort is plotted on the abscissa. The median is perhaps the best single indicator of the general level because the distribution of cholesterol values is skewed to the right. This study concerns cohorts with cholesterol medians of the order of 160 mg/dl (two Serbian cohorts, one cohort in Japan) to medians above 250 mg/dl (Finland). The first question, then, concerns the extent to which the mortality differences among the cohorts may be attributed to, or at least associated with, the differences among the cohorts in serum cholesterol.

Figure 8.1 shows the relation between the median serum cholesterol levels of the sixteen cohorts and the ten-year age-standardized all-causes death rates of the cohorts, considering only the men who showed no evidence of cardiovascular disease at the entry examinations. Though figure 8.1 covers 1,403 deaths among the 12,509 men at risk, the rates for some of the individual cohorts have substantial standard errors, being based on as few as 25 deaths in Belgrade, 42 in Crete, and 43 in Corfu. In any event,

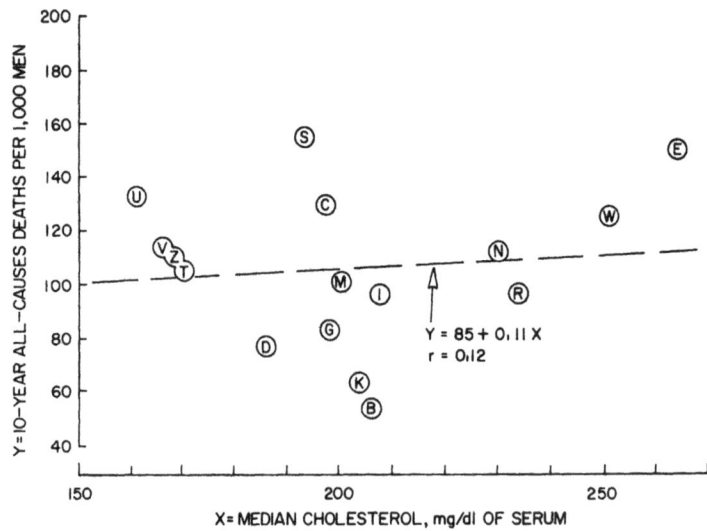

Figure 8.1. All-causes age-standardized ten-year death rates of the cohorts versus the median serum cholesterol levels (mg per dl) of the cohorts. The coefficient of correlation is $r = 0.29$. B = Belgrade; C = Crevalcore; D = Dalmatia; E = east Finland; G = Corfu; I = Italian railroad; K = Crete; M = Montegiorgio; N = Zutphen; R = American railroad; S = Slavonia; T = Tanushimaru; U = Ushibuka; V = Velika Krsna; W = west Finland; Z = Zrenjanin. All men judged free of coronary heart disease at entry.

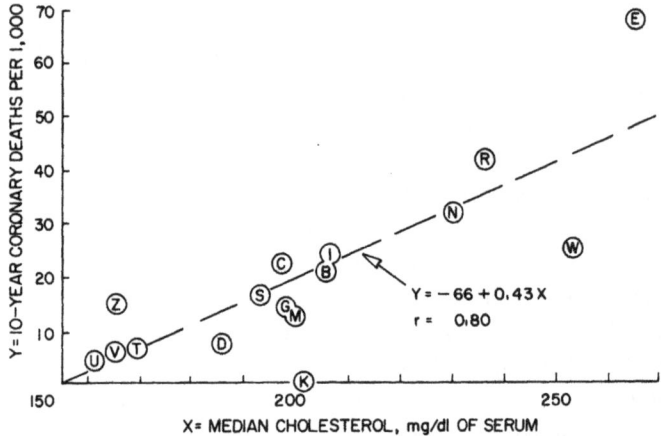

Figure 8.2. Coronary heart disease age-standardized ten-year death rates of the cohorts versus the median serum cholesterol levels (mg per dl) of the cohorts. All men judged free of coronary heart disease at entry. The coefficient of correlation is $r = 0.82$. Cohorts as in figure 8.1.

the coefficient of correlation from these data is $r = 0.12$, a value too small to be considered statistically significant with only sixteen pairs of values. This does not mean that serum cholesterol is therefore unimportant as a risk factor for all-causes death; the conclusion is only that the differences in the all-causes death rates among these cohorts cannot be explained in any consequential part by considering the median cholesterol values of the cohorts. This might well have been expected in view of the fact that in only five of the sixteen cohorts is coronary heart disease a leading cause of death; the five are the two cohorts in Finland and the cohorts in the United States, Zutphen, and Belgrade. In six cohorts, two each in Greece, Japan, and rural Yugoslavia, coronary heart disease accounted for less than 10 percent of all deaths.

When deaths from coronary heart disease are considered, a very different picture emerges, as shown in figure 8.2. The correlation coefficient of $r = 0.80$ between the cohort median cholesterol value and the death rate from coronary heart disease means that 64 percent of the variance in coronary death rate is accounted for by the median cholesterol values of the cohorts. In chapter 4 it was shown that in this material, as in vital statistics for the more developed countries, the population death rate from coronary heart disease is unrelated to the death rate from other causes. So it is of interest to examine the relationship, if any, between the noncoronary death rates of the cohorts and the cholesterol characteristics of the cohorts. When the serum cholesterol median values of the cohorts are related to the rate of death from causes other than coronary heart disease, the result is an indication of a negative relationship with $r = -0.344$. The transformation of r to Z, which has substantially a normal distribution, gives $Z = -0.359$ and the standard error of Z is 0.277. Accordingly, the ratio $Z/SE = 1.30$, indicating that the observed negative correlation could occur by chance in about 1 out of 8 trials.

Ten-year Death Rate

Figure 8.3 shows the distribution of deaths of the American railroad men into the age- and cohort-specific deciles of serum cholesterol at entry. For coronary deaths among these men who were free of evidence of coronary heart disease at entry there is obviously a direct relation to entry serum cholesterol. The men in the top cholesterol quintile had almost 4 times the death rate of the men in the bottom quintile. In a comparison of men in the upper versus those in the lower half of the cholesterol, chi-square = 21.2 with an astronomically large probability against chance explanation. But the coronary death rate does not appear to be related to cholesterol level in the lower five decile classes.

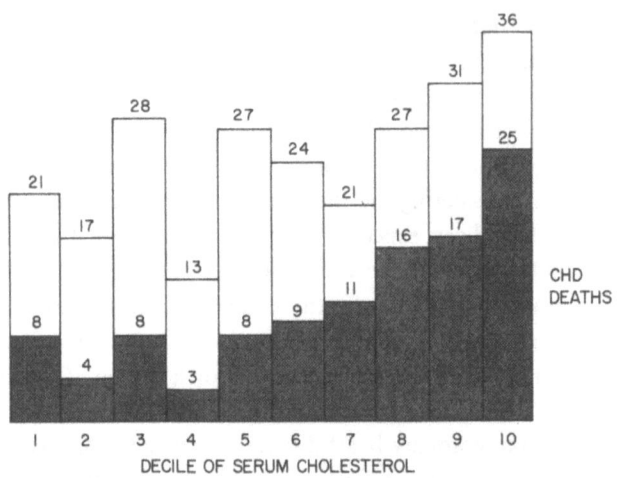

Figure 8.3. Numbers of ten-year deaths of American railroad men, free of coronary heart disease at entry, in the age- and cohort-specific decile classes of entry serum cholesterol level. Figures at the top of the shaded columns show numbers of deaths from coronary heart disease.

The death rate from all causes combined was also directly related to the serum cholesterol concentration at entry; for upper versus lower halves of the cholesterol distribution of all deaths and nondeaths chi-square = 4.66 and $p = 0.03$. This reflects the dominance of coronary heart disease as cause of death in this population sample; among the men with no evidence of the disease at the entry examination, 44 percent of all the deaths in the ten-year period were caused by coronary heart disease. Deaths from causes other than coronary heart disease were not significantly related to the serum cholesterol level; comparing the lower and the upper halves of the cholesterol distribution in this regard gives chi-square = 2.30, $p = 0.13$.

Figure 8.4 gives the corresponding picture for Finland. Coronary deaths are related to entry cholesterol with chi-square = 6.22, $p = 0.013$ when the two halves of the distribution are compared. However, cholesterol at entry was not significantly related to all-causes ten-year deaths; for the two halves of the cholesterol distribution, chi-square = 1.58, $p = 0.21$. In the corresponding comparison of the distribution of deaths from causes other than coronary heart disease there is a highly significant negative relationship (chi-square = 11.22, $p < 0.001$).

The relationship in Italy and Greece between ten-year death rate and the entry serum cholesterol concentration is summarized in figure 8.5. There is a tendency for the all-causes death rate to decrease with increasing cholesterol level. A comparison of the distribution of deaths and nondeaths into

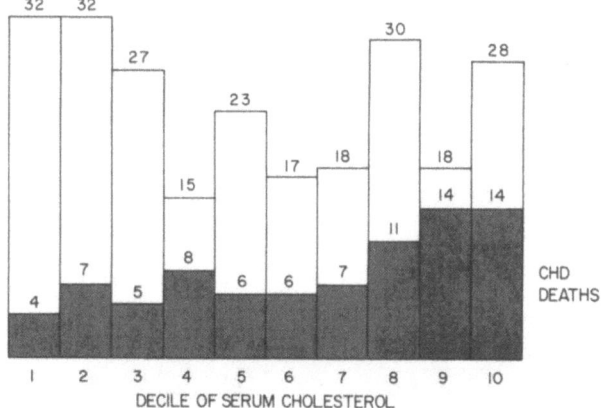

Figure 8.4. Numbers of ten-year deaths of men of east and west Finland, free of coronary heart disease at entry, in the age- and cohort-specific decile classes of entry serum cholesterol level.

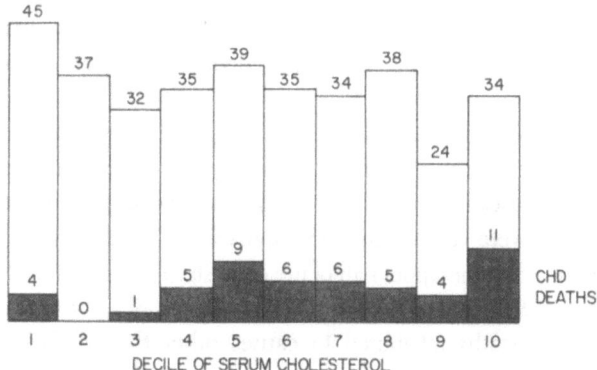

Figure 8.5. Numbers of ten-year deaths of men in Italy and Greece, free of coronary heart disease at entry, in the age- and cohort-specific decile classes of entry serum cholesterol level.

the lower and the upper halves of the cholesterol distribution gives chi-square = 4.25, indicating a probability for chance explanation of $p = 0.039$. On the other hand there is an opposite tendency of the coronary death rate to increase with increasing cholesterol, the comparison of the two halves of the cholesterol distribution giving chi-square = 3.37, $p = 0.066$, meaning that the observed distribution could be expected to occur by chance in about 1 out of 15 trials. It follows, of course, that in the Italian-Greek group there

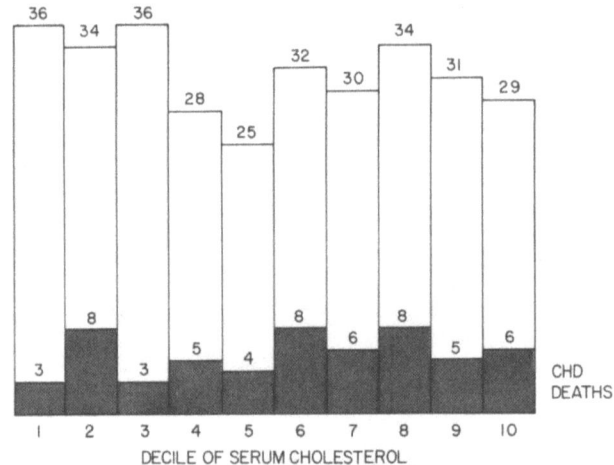

Figure 8.6. Numbers of ten-year deaths of men in Yugoslavia (Dalmatia, Slavonia, Velika Krsna, Zrenjanin, Belgrade) free of coronary heart disease at entry, in the age- and cohort-specific decile classes of entry serum cholesterol level.

was a significant tendency for the deaths from noncoronary causes to fall with increasing cholesterol in the blood serum; chi-square = 4.66, $p = 0.031$.

Figure 8.6 gives the corresponding picture for the men of Yugoslavia who were judged to be free of evidence of coronary heart disease at entry. The numbers of all-causes ten-year deaths in the two halves of the entry cholesterol distribution were very similar, 159 and 156. CHD deaths numbered 23 in the lower and 33 in the upper half of the cholesterol distribution, but the difference is not statistically significant (chi-square = 1.82, $p = 0.18$). The distribution of the deaths attributed to causes other than CHD is also not peculiar in regard to serum cholesterol (chi-square = 0.72, $p = 0.40$).

The corresponding data from Zutphen are given in figure 8.7. Among the Dutch there were 44 deaths in the lower and 52 in the upper half of the cholesterol distribution, but the difference in these all-causes deaths is not statistically significant (chi-square = 0.75, $p = 0.39$). Nor was the death rate from causes other than coronary heart disease related to the entry cholesterol level (chi-square = 1.64, $p = 0.20$). However, lower serum cholesterol at entry was strongly related to a low death rate from CHD with the two halves of the cholesterol distribution giving chi-square = 11.19, $p < 0.001$.

At the entry examinations of the men in Japan there were difficulties in the measurements of cholesterol in the blood serum, and detailed conclusions cannot be drawn about the relationship of entry cholesterol to subsequent death rate. However, the general level of cholesterol in the serum

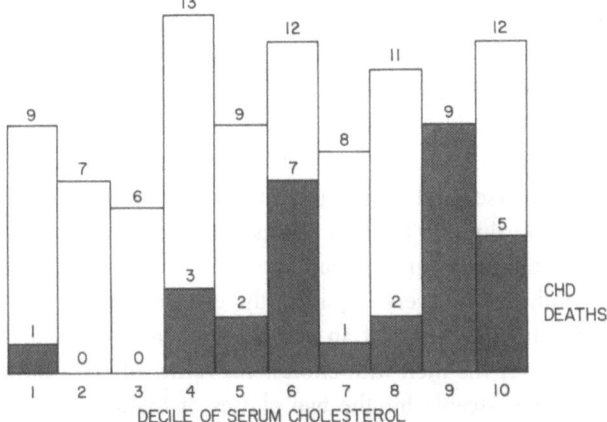

Figure 8.7. Numbers of ten-year deaths of men in Zutphen, free of coronary heart disease at entry, in the age- and cohort-specific decile classes of entry serum cholesterol level.

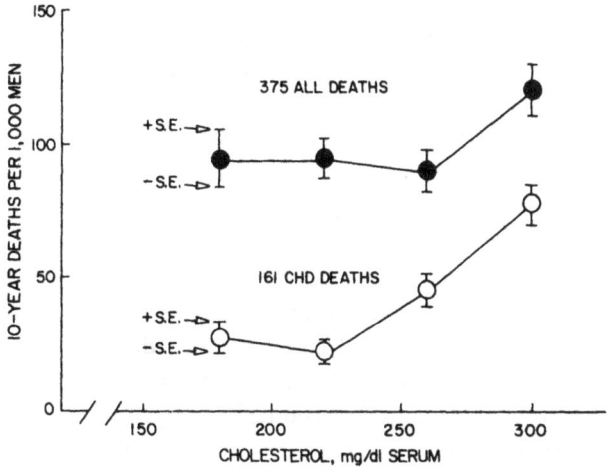

Figure 8.8. Death rates of 2,287 United States railroad men and 1,498 Finns, free of cardiovascular disease at entry, in four serum cholesterol classes.

was very low, the average being less than 170 mg/dl both at Tanushimaru and at Ushibuka, and the ten-year incidence of coronary heart disease included only eight men.

The foregoing analyses of the relationship of death to cholesterol distribution is for men in the same cohort and five-year age class. Figure 8.8 concerns absolute concentrations of cholesterol in the serum and the age-standardized death rate of the American railroad men and the Finns. The men were classified into four groups according to their serum cholesterol values at entry: under 200 mg/dl, 200–239 mg/dl, 240–279 mg/dl, and 280 mg/dl and above. Figure 8.8 shows the death rates from all causes and from coronary heart disease, and their standard errors, plotted against the mean serum cholesterol values for the four classes of concentration. For all deaths, cholesterol appears to be unimportant except for the top cholesterol class where the death rate is very significantly elevated. For coronary heart deaths, there is no indication of an advantage of the men with values less than 200 mg/dl over the men with cholesterol values of 200–229 mg/dl, but the death rate rises steeply for the two classes of higher serum cholesterol level at entry. Note that the men covered in figure 8.8 were free from any evidence of any kind of cardiovascular disease at the entry examinations; the picture is substantially identical for the men who were selected less rigidly, simply excluding those with entry coronary heart disease.

Incidence Rate

Among the men in this study who developed coronary heart disease in the ten-year follow-up, only one out of four had died from that disease at the end of the ten years, so it is important to consider the relationship of entry cholesterol level to the several diagnostic categories of the disease, hard (CHD death or myocardial infarction), angina pectoris only and other diagnoses of CHD as described in chapter 2. In respect to security of diagnosis and importance, distinction may be made between hard and soft diagnoses, the latter including angina pectoris only and all other diagnoses.

Figure 8.9 shows the distribution into the decile classes of cholesterol of the several classes of incidence of coronary heart disease in Finland. Incidence obviously tends to rise with increasing serum cholesterol concentration, and this is almost entirely accounted for by the incidence of hard CHD. Comparing the upper and lower halves of the cholesterol distribution in regard to hard CHD, chi-square = 10.35, $p = 0.001$. For all CHD combined chi-square = 6.94, $p = 0.008$; and for soft CHD chi-square = 0.54, $p = 0.47$.

In Serbia entry serum cholesterol level appears to have been somewhat more important in regard to the risk of developing coronary heart disease in the succeeding ten years (figure 8.10). A comparison of the number of cases and of noncases in the two halves of the serum cholesterol distribution gives chi-square = 7.97 ($p = 0.005$) for hard CHD, 3.88 ($p = 0.049$) for angina pectoris, 3.28 ($p = 0.07$) for other CHD, and 4.64 ($p = 0.03$) for any CHD.

The corresponding data for Zutphen are summarized in figure 8.11. The

Serum Cholesterol | 129

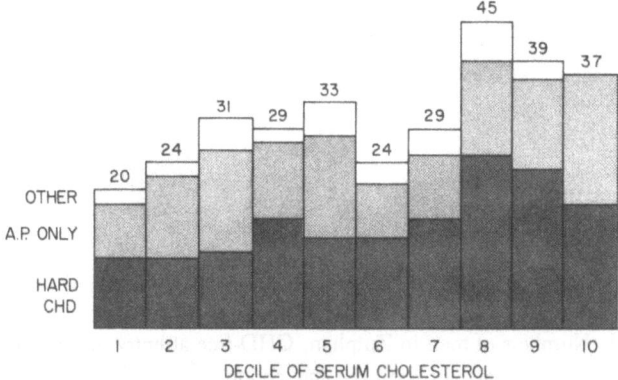

Figure 8.9. Numbers of Finns, CHD-free at entry, with ten-year incidence of coronary heart disease in the age- and cohort-specific decile classes of entry serum cholesterol. *Hard CHD* = myocardial infarction or death from coronary heart disease; *AP only* = angina pectoris only; *other* = all other diagnoses of CHD. Numbers at the tops of the columns are the numbers of men with any diagnosis of coronary heart disease.

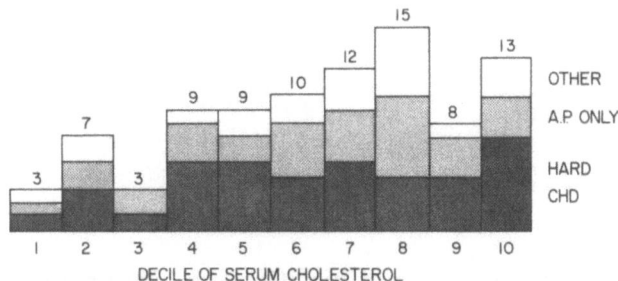

Figure 8.10. Numbers of men in Velika Krsna, Zrenjanin, and Belgrade, CHD-free at entry, with ten-year incidence of coronary heart disease in the age- and cohort-specific decile classes of entry serum cholesterol level.

picture is similar to that found with the men in Finland and in Serbia, showing a clear tendency for the incidence of the disease to rise with increasing entry serum cholesterol level largely but not entirely accounted for by hard CHD. The incidence of hard CHD in the top quintile of cholesterol was 4 times that in the bottom quintile. Comparison of cases and noncases in the two halves of the cholesterol distribution gives chi-square = 11.43 ($p = .001$) for hard, 1.36 ($p = 0.24$) for angina pectoris only, and 6.70 ($p = 0.01$) for any coronary heart disease.

The ten-year incidence findings in Italy and Croatia (Dalmatia and Sla-

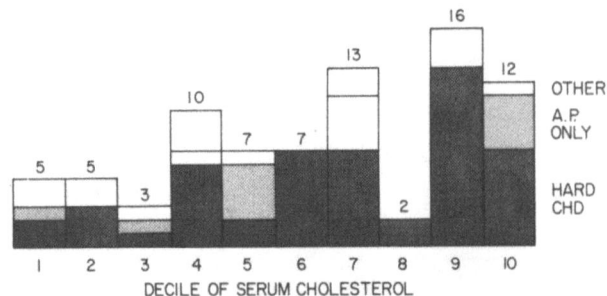

Figure 8.11. Numbers of men in Zutphen, CHD-free at entry, developing coronary heart disease in ten years, in the age- and cohort-specific decile classes of serum cholesterol level at entry.

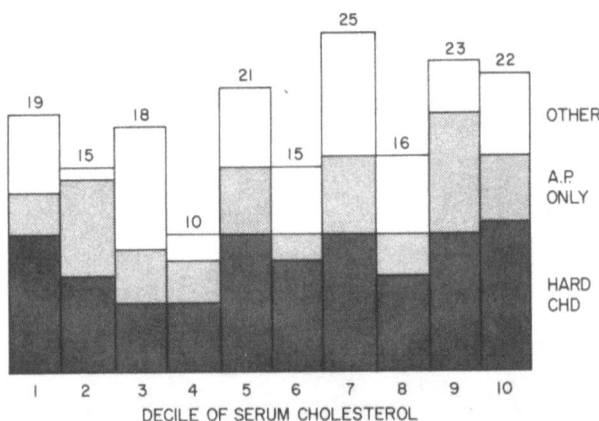

Figure 8.12. Numbers of men in Italy (Crevalcore, Montegiorgio, and Rome railroad), CHD-free at entry, developing coronary heart disease in ten years, in the age- and cohort-specific classes of entry serum cholesterol level.

vonia) are summarized in figures 8.12 and 8.13. In Italy the tendency for the incidence of coronary heart disease to rise with increasing serum cholesterol concentration is smaller than observed in Finland, the Netherlands, and Serbia, and it does not reach statistical significance for any of the categories of coronary heat disease or for all diagnoses combined. In Croatia there is no discernible tendency for the incidence of any category of coronary heart disease to be related to the entry serum cholesterol level.

In Greece (Crete and Corfu) the incidence of any kind of coronary heart disease in ten years amounted to a total of only 37 men among 1,081 men with no evidence of coronary heart disease at entry. The distribution of the

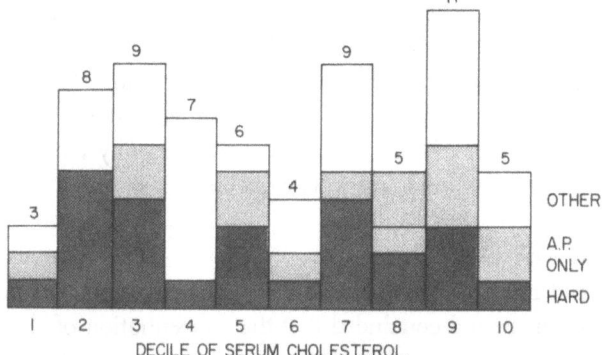

Figure 8.13. Numbers of men in Croatia (Dalmatia and Slavonia), CHD-free at entry, developing coronary heart disease in ten years, in the age- and cohort-specific decile classes of entry serum cholesterol level.

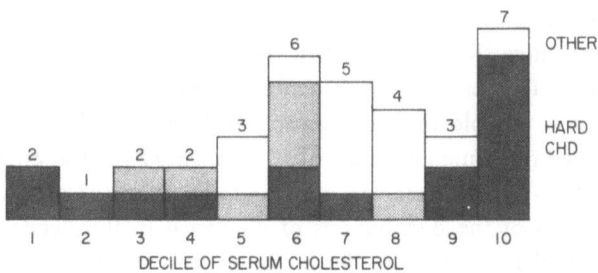

Figure 8.14. Numbers of men in Greece (Crete and Corfu), CHD-free at entry, developing coronary heart disease in ten years, in the age- and cohort-specific decile classes of entry serum cholesterol level. Light shading indicates angina pectoris only.

incidence cases of the several categories of coronary heart disease into the decile classes of cholesterol is shown in figure 8.14. For all diagnoses of coronary heart disease 25 of the Greeks were above the cholesterol median, 12 below (chi-square = 5.64, $p = 0.018$). It will be noted also that out of 16 men with hard CHD, 8 were in the top quintile of the cholesterol distribution, yielding a value of chi-square = 8.71, $p = 0.003$.

The ten-year experience of the Seven Countries Study indicates that the importance of serum cholesterol as a risk factor varies among populations. In populations with a high frequency of coronary heart disease, the incidence of the disease, especially of death and infarction, tends to be directly related to the serum cholesterol level. In populations in which the disease is relatively uncommon, the cholesterol level in the blood seems to have much less, or even no, prognostic significance for middle-aged men. Another rather different generalization can be suggested from the data, namely that at blood serum levels below 220 mg/dl or so, cholesterol is not a significant factor. But neither of these propositions clarifies why serum cholesterol seemed to be relatively important in Greece but not in Italy.

Correlation with Other Variables

Acheson and Baird (1973) analyzed data from the U.S. National Health Examination Survey and concluded that the concentration of cholesterol in the blood serum in that material was importantly correlated with both age and relative body weight, using weight:height, weight:height squared, and ponderal index as measures of relative weight. They define ponderal index as the cube root of the ratio of weight to height, but that has never been proposed by anyone else to be the definition of the ponderal index. In any event the population sample involved covered the age range 18–79 years. Because there is a curvilinear relationship between serum cholesterol and age over that range (Keys et al. 1950), it is grossly inappropriate to use a rectilinear model as was done by Acheson and Baird.

Age is not a variable in our comparisons between cohorts because all cohorts covered the same age range of 40 through 59 years at entry and the mean ages of the cohorts were very closely similar. Nor was age a variable in the examination of the distributions of incidence in the decile classes of entry cholesterol because those decile classes were age-specific. However, the correlation of serum cholesterol with variables of interest is summarized in table 8.1.

Clearly there is no significant correlation between serum cholesterol and age in any of the cohorts. This conforms to the finding many years ago that there is a curvilinear relationship between cholesterol and age of men, and that over the middle-aged range the relationship is flat (Keys et al. 1950). The correlation between serum cholesterol and the body mass index is generally statistically significant because the numbers of pairs of values are large, but the biological significance is trivial. The mean coefficient of correlation, $r = 0.199$, indicates that less than 4 percent of the variance in cholesterol can be accounted for by the body mass index relationship. The findings in regard to cholesterol versus body fatness as indicated by skinfold thickness are almost identical, and the mean value of the correlation coefficient is $r = 0.193$. The correlation between serum cholesterol concentration and arterial blood pressure is slightly smaller, averaging $r = 0.133$, meaning that systolic blood pressure accounts for less than 2 percent of the variance of serum cholesterol. It should be noted that blood pressure is also correlated

Table 8.1. Product moment correlation of serum cholesterol concentration with other characteristics at entry in men free of coronary heart disease.

Cohort	N	Age	BMI	Skinfold	S BP
U.S. railroad	2,313	0.05	0.09	0.09	0.07
Dalmatia	627	−0.01	0.24	0.22	0.26
Slavonia	605	−0.00	0.26	0.22	0.22
Tanushimaru	351	−0.08	0.03	0.04	0.07
East Finland	698	−0.04	0.10	0.03	0.05
West Finland	774	−0.04	0.13	0.10	0.09
Ushibuka	389	0.03	0.09	—	0.11
Crevalcore	887	0.03	0.21	0.23	0.08
Montegiorgio	688	0.04	0.33	0.34	0.19
Zutphen	770	−0.05	0.21	0.18	0.10
Crete	611	0.13	0.28	0.22	0.25
Corfu	513	−0.01	0.25	0.27	0.17
Rome railroad	708	0.05	0.28	0.27	0.24
Velika Krsna	461	0.09	0.26	0.31	0.08
Zrenjanin	482	0.06	0.26	0.29	0.05
Belgrade	516	0.13	0.13	0.09	0.11
Mean		0.023	0.199	0.193	0.133
SE		0.015	0.020	0.025	0.018

with relative body weight and with the sum of the skinfolds, so it is interesting to calculate first-order partial correlation coefficients. In this material the mean correlation between systolic pressure and the sum of the skinfolds is $r = 0.209$. Accordingly, from the values in table 8.1 the calculation gives $r = 0.096$ for the correlation between cholesterol and blood pressure holding skinfold thickness constant, and $r = 0.189$ for the correlation between cholesterol and skinfold thickness holding blood pressure constant. Because the numbers of pairs of values is large, these correlations are statistically significant in the sense that it is very improbable they differ from zero only by chance. Biologically, however, these correlations seem to be of little importance.

Summary

The concentration of cholesterol in the blood serum at entry showed greater differences among the sixteen cohorts than in any of the other risk factors examined. Median serum cholesterol values ranged from the order of 160 mg/dl or less in Serbia and Japan to over 250 mg/dl in Finland. In the sixteen cohorts the mean correlation of serum cholesterol at entry with age was $r = 0.02$; with systolic pressure, $r = 0.13$; with body mass index, $r = 0.20$.

The age-standardized all-causes death rates of the sixteen cohorts were only slightly correlated with the serum cholesterol medians of the cohorts, but there was a highly significant correlation, $r = 0.65$, between median cholesterol and death rate from coronary heart disease. The correlation between the ten-year death rate from causes other than coronary heart disease and the cholesterol medians of the cohorts was $r = -0.34$. The indicated negative relationship could be expected to occur by chance in about 1 out of 8 trials.

In the cohort of American railroad men free from coronary heart disease at entry, the ten-year death rate from all causes was significantly related to the entry serum cholesterol concentration, but the relationship was demonstrated only in the upper half of the distribution of serum cholesterol values. The death rate from coronary heart disease was much more strongly related to the cholesterol level at entry, but again the relationship was clear only with cholesterol values in the upper half of the distribution.

In Finland the ten-year death rate from coronary heart disease was similarly related, with high statistical significance, with the entry cholesterol level, but the cholesterol concentration was not shown to be a significant risk factor for all-causes deaths. For deaths from causes other than coronary heart disease, the data from Finland suggested that serum cholesterol was a negative risk factor. The lowest serum cholesterol concentrations at entry were associated with an excessive ten-year death rate from causes other than coronary heart disease. The bottom 20 percent of the entry cholesterol distribution accounted for 53 out of a total of 151 noncoronary deaths.

At Zutphen the relationship of ten-year mortality to entry serum cholesterol concentration was similar to that found in Finland. The coronary death rate was related with high significance to the entry cholesterol level, but no significant relationship was found with the all-causes death rate. The bottom half of the entry serum cholesterol distribution contributed 38 out of 66 noncoronary deaths, or 58 percent.

In Italy and Greece the tendency of men, free of coronary heart disease at entry, to die from coronary heart disease was somewhat related to the entry cholesterol concentration. Among 51 coronary deaths, 32, or 63 percent, were in the upper half of the entry cholesterol distribution. However, for all-causes deaths there was a tendency for the death rate to rise with decreasing cholesterol concentration at entry. Among 302 noncoronary ten-year deaths, 169, or 56 percent, were in the lower half of the entry cholesterol distribution.

In Yugoslavia, among 2,821 men with no evidence of coronary heart disease at entry, 56 died from coronary heart disease in ten years, and 33 of them, or 59 percent, were in the upper half of the entry serum cholesterol distribution. However, for all-causes deaths, entry cholesterol level was not indicated to be a significant risk factor. The data suggest that entry cholesterol could be a negative risk factor for noncoronary death in Yugoslavia.

In Japan, neither all-causes nor coronary deaths were related to entry cholesterol level, but there were only 7 coronary deaths.

For the ten-year incidence of nonfatal plus fatal coronary heart disease, the entry serum cholesterol level was a significant risk factor in Finland, Zutphen, Greece, and Serbia but not in Croatia or rural Italy. The incidence of nonfatal coronary heart disease among the American railroad men in the second five years is unknown, but the incidence in the first five years was definitely related to the entry cholesterol concentration.

From the evidence it appears that the serum cholesterol concentration is an important risk factor for the incidence of coronary heart disease at levels of perhaps 220 mg/dl or more. At levels below 200 mg/dl, decreasing cholesterol concentrations tend to be associated with increasing rates of noncoronary death.

9 | Smoking Habits

The cohorts in the Seven Countries Study differed in smoking habits as well as in subsequent death rate and incidence of coronary heart disease. Table 9.1 summarizes the men's reports of their smoking habits at the time of the entry examinations. In all of the

Table 9.1. Smoking habits of the men, recorded at entry, as percentages of all men in each cohort.

Cohort	Never Smoked	Stopped	Cigarettes per day		
			<10	10–19	≥20
U.S. railroad	21	21	6	28	24
Dalmatia	30	12	7	28	23
Slavonia	27	13	9	32	19
Tanushimaru	16	13	2	26	43
East Finland	16	15	8	30	31
West Finland	21	20	15	29	15
Ushibuka	15	7	8	32	38
Crevalcore	25	12	18	27	18
Montegiorgio	26	15	28	21	10
Zutphen	7	17	31	34	11
Crete	24	19	10	17	30
Corfu	25	12	13	28	22
Rome railroad	19	15	11	25	30
Velika Krsna	41	11	9	25	14
Zrenjanin	19	18	7	36	20
Belgrade	41	16	4	15	24
Mean	22.4	15.9	11.7	27.3	22.7

cohorts only a minority of the men had never smoked regularly, and in all but two—Velika Krsna and Belgrade—more than half of the men were cigarette smokers when they entered the study. Moreover, only a small proportion of the smokers averaged fewer than ten cigarettes a day at that time. Except at Zutphen, almost all of the smokers used only cigarettes. At Zutphen many men smoked pipes or cigars, but the majority of those men also smoked cigarettes. Only cigarette smoking will be considered in the examination of the relationship of smoking to the follow-up experience because the numbers of pipe and cigar smokers are too few to warrant analysis.

At Velika Krsna and Belgrade 41 percent of the men had never smoked regularly, but in all of the other cohorts such never-smokers were less common. The percentage of men who were heavy smokers, regularly using twenty or more cigarettes a day, varied from only 10 percent of the men of Montegiorgio, Italy, to 43 percent of the men of Tanushimaru, Japan. The first question, then, is to what extent, if any, the differences among cohorts in smoking habits were reflected in the rates of death and incidence of coronary heart disease in the ten-year follow-up.

Figure 9.1 shows the age-standardized all-causes ten-year death rates of

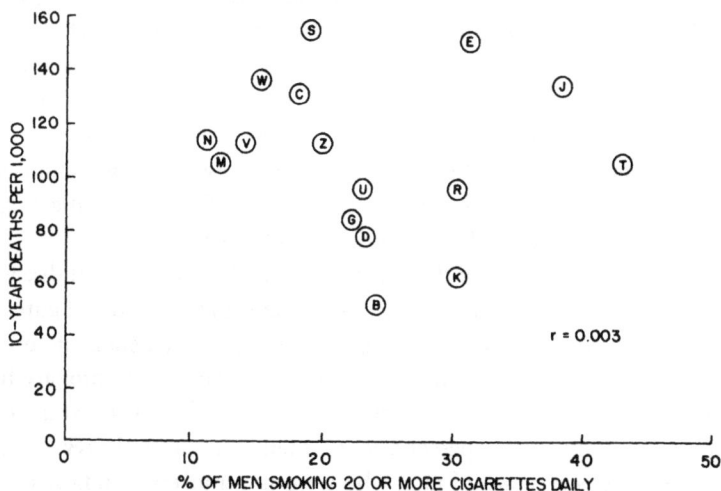

Figure 9.1. Deaths from all causes versus smoking habit among men free of cardiovascular disease at entry. Age-standardized ten-year rates of the men in sixteen cohorts versus percentage of the men in those cohorts smoking twenty or more cigarettes daily. B = Belgrade; C = Crevalcore; D = Dalmatia; E = east Finland; G = Corfu; J = Ushibuka; K = Crete; M = Montegiorgio; N = Zutphen; R = Rome railroad; S = Slavonia; T = Tanushimaru; U = U.S. railroad; V = Velika Krsna; W = west Finland; Z = Zrenjanin.

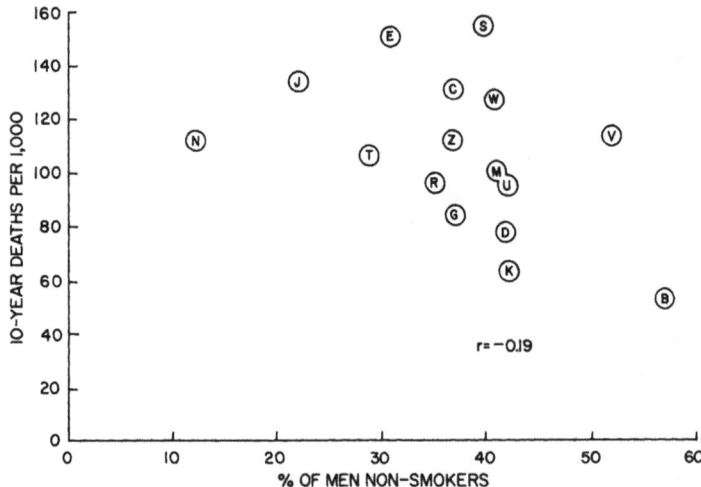

Figure 9.2. Ten-year all-causes death rates versus percentage of the men in the cohorts who were nonsmokers at entry. Cohorts as in figure 9.1.

the cohorts for men free of cardiovascular disease at entry plotted against the percentages of men in those cohorts smoking twenty or more cigarettes daily. There is no suggestion of any relation between death rate and the frequency of heavy smoking. Figure 9.2 shows the all-causes death rates plotted against the percentage of men in the cohorts who were nonsmokers. The slight negative correlation of $r = -0.19$ depends almost entirely on the contribution of the men of Belgrade, but in any case that correlation is far from being statistically significant; a value of $r = 0.497$ is required for significance at the 5 percent level with 14 degrees of freedom.

Data on the relationship of the incidence rate of coronary heart disease to the smoking habits of the men in the cohorts are summarized in figures 9.3 and 9.4. These concern the ten-year age-standardized incidence rate of hard coronary heart disease—myocardial infarction or death from coronary heart disease—for men without evidence of any cardiovascular disease at the entry examination. Neither the percentage of men who were heavy cigarette smokers nor the percentage of men who were nonsmokers is indicated to be related to the cohort incidence rate of hard coronary heart disease.

The lack of any relationship between the cohort incidence rates of disease and death and the characteristics of those cohorts in respect to cigarette smoking must not be overinterpreted. The findings simply show that the differences among the cohorts in the incidence rates of coronary heart disease and of death from all causes are not explained by, or related to, the differences among the cohorts in their smoking habits. However, that negative

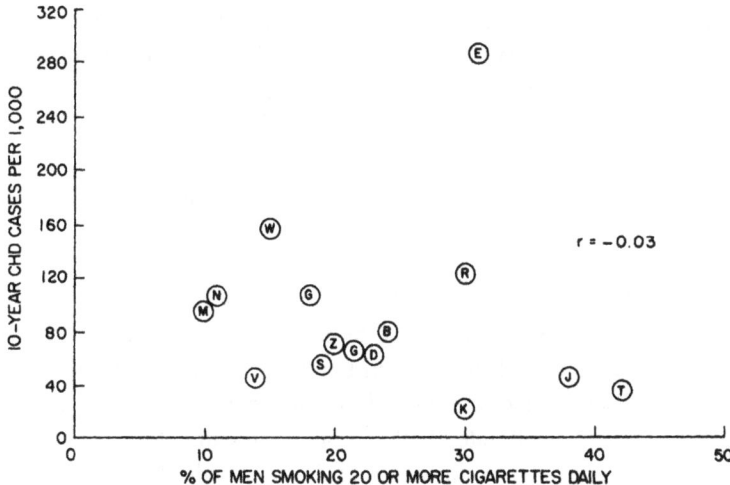

Figure 9.3. Ten-year incidence rate of coronary heart disease in fifteen cohorts versus percentage of the men in those cohorts who were smoking twenty or more cigarettes at entry. Cohorts as in figure 9.1.

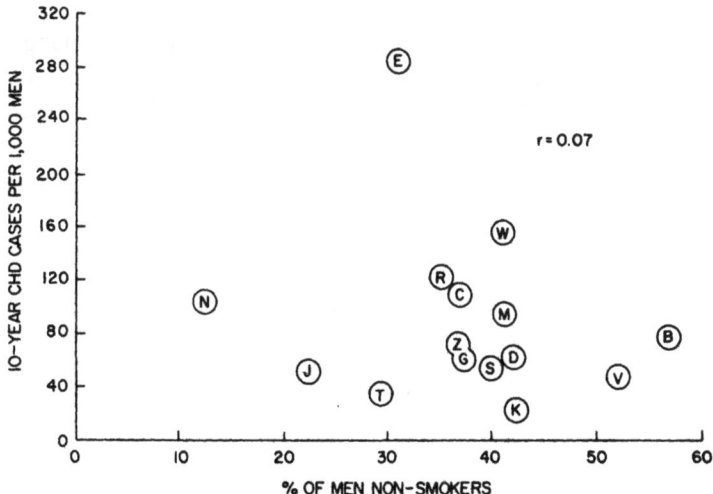

Figure 9.4. Ten-year incidence rate of coronary heart disease in fifteen cohorts versus percentage of the men in those cohorts who were nonsmokers at entry. Cohorts as in figure 9.1.

result does not necessarily rule out smoking as a risk factor promoting heart disease and premature death. Evaluation of smoking as a risk factor within a given population sample requires analysis of the follow-up experience of the men in that sample classified by their individual smoking habits. That analysis, summarized in the following sections, shows that smoking is indeed an important risk factor both for coronary incidence and for all-causes death.

Ten-year Death Rate

In the northern European cohorts (east and west Finland and Zutphen), among 2,369 men with no evidence of cardiovascular disease at the entry examination, there were 198 deaths in ten years. Figure 9.5 shows the age-standardized death rates of the men classified according to smoking habit at entry. The lowest death rate, both for all-causes and for coronary heart disease deaths, pertained to the group of 357 men who had never smoked; their all-causes and CHD death rates were less than half the rates for the men who had stopped smoking or who smoked fewer than ten cigarettes daily. Among smokers the death rate rose progressively with the average number of cigarettes smoked. Note that in figure 9.5 the width of the bars is proportional to the number of men at risk in the smoking category concerned.

In Yugoslavia in ten years 295 men died from all causes among 2,797 men, initially CVD-free; this is the experience of the combined cohorts of Dalmatia, Slavonia, Velika Krsna, Zrenjanin, and Belgrade. Figure 9.6

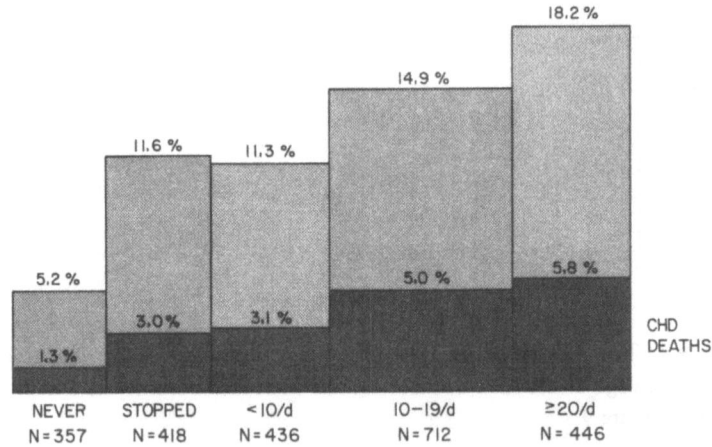

Figure 9.5. Age-standardized ten-year death rates from all causes and from coronary heart disease of men in northern Europe (east and west Finland and Zutphen) classified by smoking habit at entry. All men free of cardiovascular disease at entry.

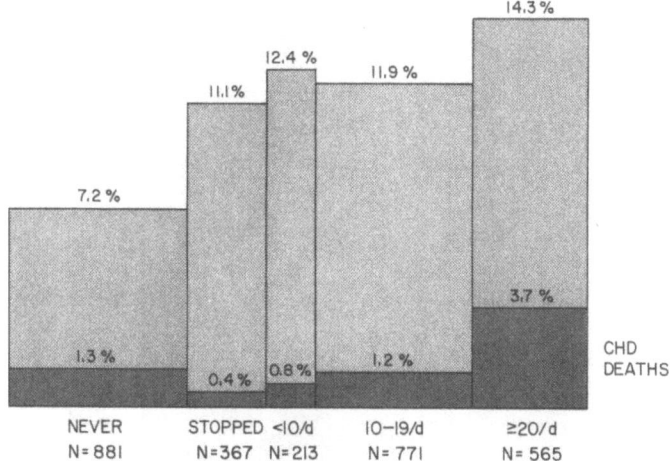

Figure 9.6. Age-standardized ten-year death rates from all causes and from coronary heart disease of men in Yugoslavia (Dalmatia, Slavonia, Velika Krsna, Zrenjanin, and Belgrade) classified by smoking habit at entry. All men free of cardiovascular disease at entry.

shows the death rates of these men classified by their smoking habits at entry. The 881 men who had never smoked regularly had the lowest all-causes death rate, only a trifle more than half the death rate of the 565 men who customarily smoked twenty or more cigarettes daily. Although this is a highly statistically significant difference, it is less impressive than that found in the follow-up of the men in the northern European cohorts. The death rate for coronary heart disease was highest for the Yugoslavs who were heavy smokers, but there were no significant differences in the other smoking categories.

Figure 9.7 shows the corresponding data for the 3,551 Italians and Greeks with no evidence of cardiovascular disease at entry. While there is some indication of a relation between smoking habits and the ten-year death rates, that relationship is smaller than observed in the Yugoslavian data and far less striking than observed in the men in the northern areas of Europe. When smokers are compared with nonsmokers, the all-causes death rates are 10.29 and 8.96 percent, respectively. The probability of finding such differences by chance are $p = 0.19$ for all-causes deaths and $p = 0.27$ for coronary deaths; the differences between smokers and nonsmokers in death rates do not approach statistical significance.

Figure 9.8 is the corresponding picture for 219 deaths in ten years among 2,315 American railroad men free from cardiovascular disease at entry. The mortality rate was not significantly different for men who had stopped smok-

142 | Seven Countries

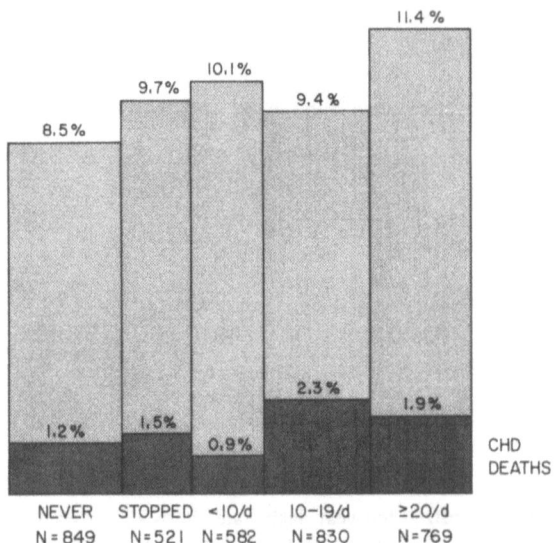

Figure 9.7. Age-standardized ten-year death rates from all causes and from coronary heart disease of men in Italy and Greece (Crevalcore, Montegiorgio, Rome railroad, Crete, and Corfu) classified by smoking habit at entry. All men free of cardiovascular disease at entry.

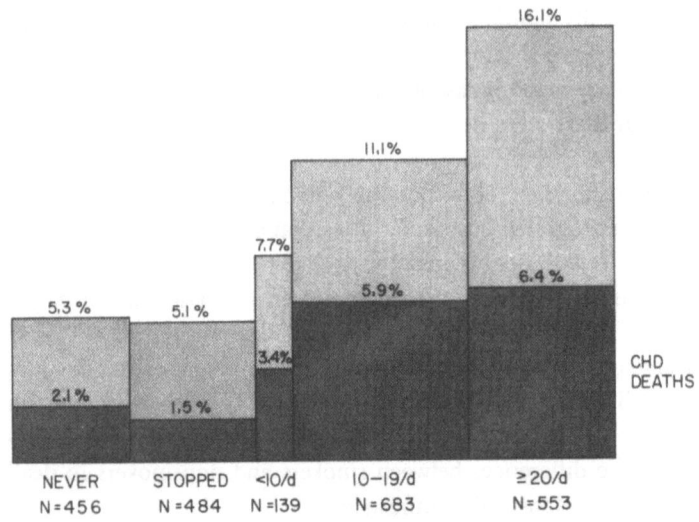

Figure 9.8. Age-standardized ten-year all causes and coronary death rates of American railroad men classified by smoking habit at entry when free of cardiovascular disease.

ing as compared with men who had never smoked regularly, but both all-causes and coronary death rates rose progressively with amount of smoking. For men smoking twenty or more cigarettes daily both the all-causes and the CHD death rates were more than 3 times those for nonsmokers of the same age. Statistically, the relationship of mortality to cigarette smoking of the railroad men is highly significant. For example, the comparison of smokers versus nonsmokers in regard to death rate from coronary heart disease gives chi-square = 22.7!

Figures 9.5 through 9.8 suggest a linear relationship between smoking and mortality in each of the areas, but with substantial differences among the areas in the gradient of mortality with smoking. It seems appropriate, then, to examine the data with the model $y = a + bx$, where y is the age-standardized death rate and x is the smoking habit represented on the following scale: 0, never smoked; 1, stopped smoking; and 2, 3, and 4, regular smokers using, respectively, under ten, ten through nineteen, and twenty or more cigarettes daily.

Figure 9.9 shows the results for all-causes deaths in northern Europe,

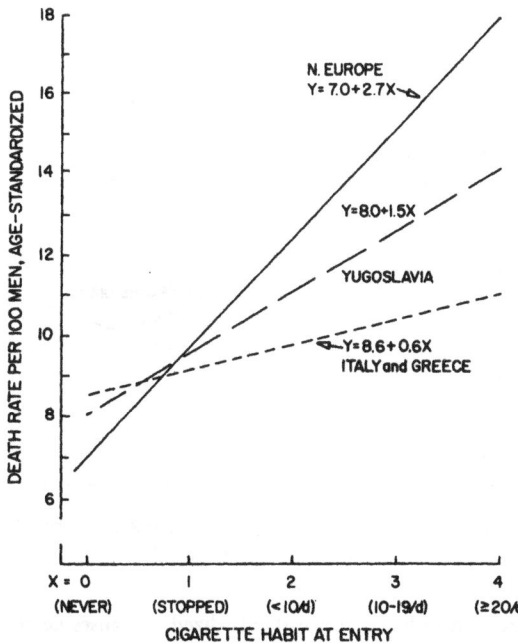

Figure 9.9. Regression of ten-year age-standardized all-causes death rate, Y, on smoking class, X, for men in northern Europe, Yugoslavia, and Italy and Greece. All men free of cardiovascular disease at entry.

Yugoslavia, and Italy plus Greece. The least-squares solutions of the regression equation indicate no significant mortality rate differences among the areas for the nonsmokers and for those who had stopped smoking. The slope, b, is almost 4 times greater for northern Europe than for Italy and Greece, with Yugoslavia intermediate.

Figure 9.10 shows the least-squares regressions of mortality on cigarette smoking for the American railroad men and the Japanese men of Tanushimaru and Ushibuka. For the Japanese men the slope of the regression of all-causes death rate on smoking habit is not significantly greater than zero while for the American men the slope, $b = 2.95$, is greater than that for the men in northern Europe. For the Japanese men, the lowest age-standardized ten-year death rate, 973 per 10,000, was that for the 396 heaviest smokers (twenty or more cigarettes a day) but the difference from the highest rate, 1,379 per 10,000, observed in the 284 men smoking ten to nineteen cigarettes a day, is not statistically significant ($p = 0.10$). Furthermore, comparison of Japanese smokers with nonsmokers in regard to ten-year all-causes deaths gives chi-square $= 0.008$ ($p = 0.93$).

Figure 9.10 also shows, for the Americans, the regression on smoking of

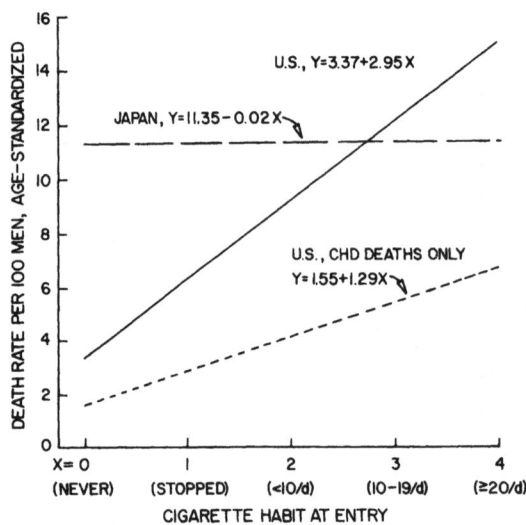

Figure 9.10. Regression of ten-year age-standardized all-causes death rate on smoking class of United States railroad men and of men in Japan (Tanushimaru and Ushibuka). For U.S. men only, regression of coronary heart disease death rate on smoking class. All men free of cardiovascular disease at entry.

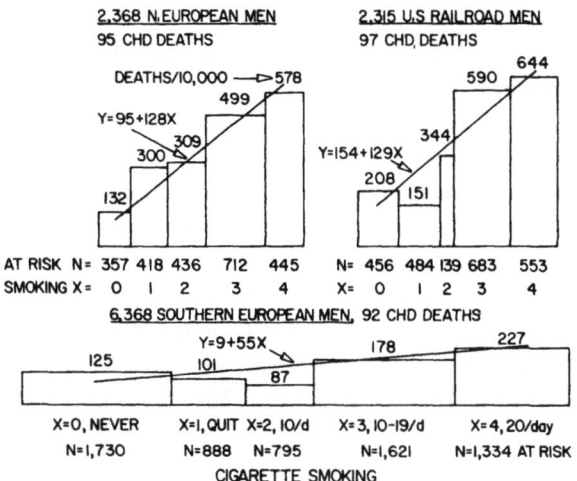

Figure 9.11. Ten-year age-standardized death rates from coronary heart disease among men free of cardiovascular disease at entry and classified by cigarette smoking habit at that time. The width of the bars is proportional to the number of men in each smoking class. Scales are the same for all three populations. The regression lines of death rate, Y, on smoking, are shown.

the death rate from coronary heart disease; that slope, although highly significant, is less than half as great as the slope of all-causes deaths on smoking in the same American cohort. Deaths from coronary heart disease among the Japanese men were too few to warrant regression analysis.

The contrasts between regions in the importance of smoking as a risk factor for coronary heart disease are shown in figure 9.11, which covers 284 coronary deaths among 11,051 men in Europe and the United States who showed no evidence of cardiovascular disease at the start of the ten-year follow-up. The men of northern Europe and the Americans do not differ in the rise in the coronary death rate with cigarette smoking; in both areas the least-squares solutions of the regression equation indicate that men smoking twenty or more cigarettes a day are 3.5 to 4 times more prone to coronary death in ten years than their fellows of the same age who are nonsmokers.

The men in southern Europe—Italy, Greece, and Yugoslavia—differ strikingly in this respect. The slope of the least-squares regression line is not convincingly different from zero. And when the smokers are compared with nonsmokers in southern Europe in regard to coronary deaths, chi-square = 2.0, meaning that the observed difference could be expected to occur by chance in about 1 out of 7 trials. Similar chi-square tests of the men in northern Europe and the American men indicate differences that are highly significant; for the Americans the result is chi-square = 11.6 (1 degree of freedom)!

Death from Neoplasms

In all of the populations the smokers had excessive all-causes deaths compared with the nonsmokers, but except in the United States, most of the excess deaths were attributed to causes other than coronary heart disease. Cancers and other neoplasms were frequently the cause of death in this study. Among 12,011 men with entry data on the major risk factors and free of cardiovascular disease at the outset, 361 were dead from neoplasms in ten years, and the crude ten-year death rate is 301 per 10,000 with 24.4 percent of those deaths attributed to cancer of the trachea, bronchus, or lung.

The relation of death from neoplastic disease to smoking habit in northern and southern Europe is summarized in figure 9.12. The results of an analysis with the linear regression model are summarized in figure 9.13. The slopes of the regression lines for all-causes deaths are not importantly different for the two areas of Europe, but the intercepts differ greatly. The analysis indicates that, independent of smoking habits, the age-standardized rate of death from neoplastic disease is much greater in the samples of men

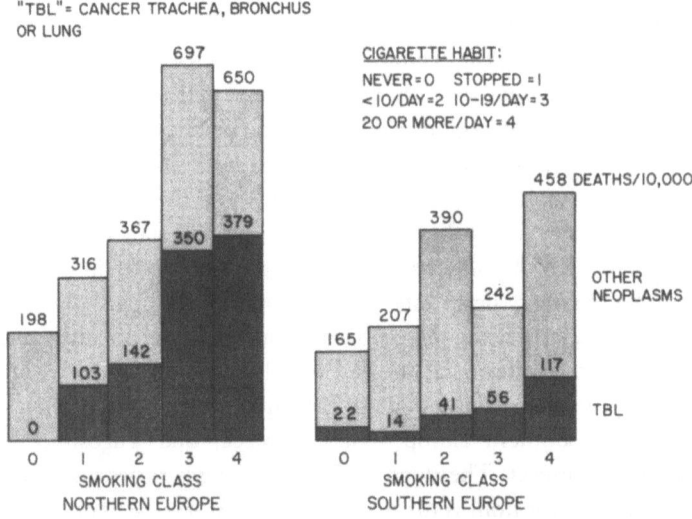

Figure 9.12. Neoplastic disease, ten-year age-standardized death rate of men in northern Europe (east and west Finland, Zutphen), and of men in southern Europe (Italy, Greece, Yugoslavia). All men free of cardiovascular disease at entry. Dark shading identifies death rate from cancer of the respiratory system.

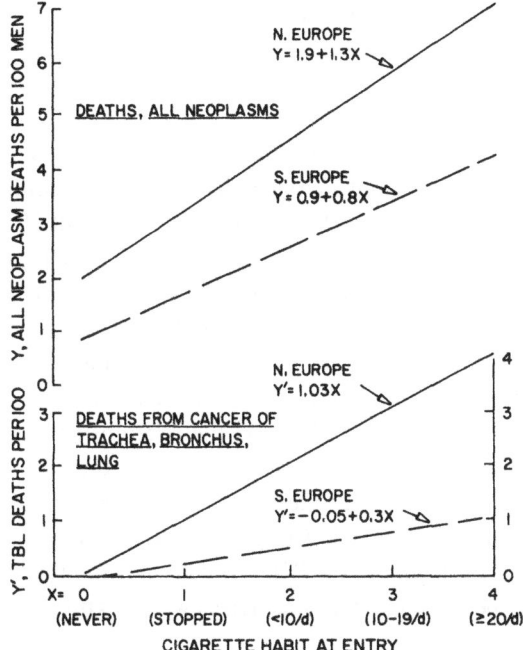

Figure 9.13. Regression of ten-year age-standardized death rate from neoplastic disease on smoking class of men in northern and in southern Europe. Upper regressions concern deaths from all neoplasms; lower regressions are for deaths from cancer of the respiratory system.

in northern than in southern Europe. On the other hand, for deaths from cancer of the trachea, bronchus, or lung, the intercepts of the regression lines do not differ, but the slope is much greater for northern than for southern Europe. It would appear that for the men in Italy and Greece cigarette smoking less often caused cancer of the respiratory system than for the men in Finland and the Netherlands. In this connection it should be remarked that in the study areas of northern and southern Europe, air pollution is minimal.

Compared with nonsmokers, deaths from causes other than coronary heart disease or neoplasm were unduly frequent among smokers in northern Europe, Yugoslavia, and the United States but not in southern Europe. This latter exception corresponds to the finding noted above that, in general, cigarette smoking seems to be a much less important risk factor in southern Europe than in the United States and in the other areas of Europe. The ten-year follow-up in Japan failed to show any significant differences between smokers and nonsmokers in regard to any cause of death. The two areas studied in Japan, Tanushimaru and Ushibuka, are notably free of air pollution.

Incidence Rate

The examination of the relationship in each area of the incidence of coronary heart disease to smoking habits has so far been confined to deaths from that disease. But CHD deaths represented only about 20 percent of the total incidence of coronary heart disease in these men. Here we shall examine the incidence of all coronary heart disease in the men, free of cardiovascular disease at entry, classified by smoking habit, distinguishing between hard CHD, CHD death or myocardial infarction, and soft CHD, all other CHD diagnoses, including angina pectoris alone.

For northern Europe figure 9.5 shows the relationship to smoking of 95 CHD deaths. Figure 9.14 is the corresponding picture for 342 incidence cases of CHD. For hard CHD the incidence rate rises progressively with smoking class, but the slope is less impressive than that for the CHD death rate. For other (soft) diagnoses of CHD the data show no relation to smoking habit. In this respect the rate for nonsmokers was insignificantly higher than that for smokers.

For Yugoslavia figure 9.6 shows the relationship of 38 CHD deaths to

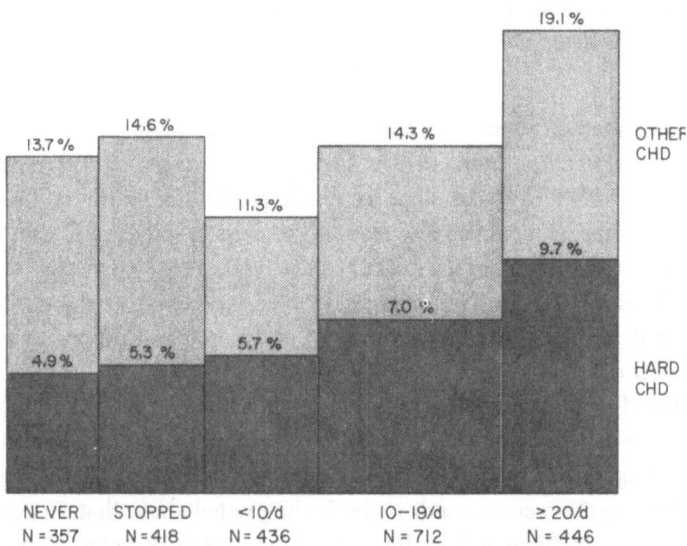

Figure 9.14. Age-standardized ten-year incidence rate of coronary heart disease of 2,369 men in northern Europe (east and west Finland and Zutphen) classified by smoking habit at entry and then free of cardiovascular disease.

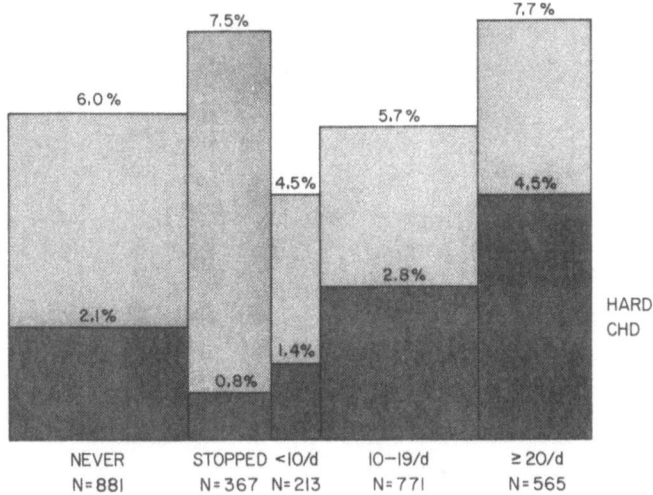

Figure 9.15. Age-standardized ten-year incidence rate of coronary heart disease of 2,797 men in Yugoslavia (Dalmatia, Slavonia, Velika Krsna, Zrenjanin, and Belgrade) classified by smoking habit at entry and then free of cardiovascular disease. Diagnostic categories as in Fig. 9.14.

smoking habit. Figure 9.15 gives the corresponding picture for 177 incidence cases, 62 of which were hard CHD. Among the smokers the rate of incidence of hard CHD rose steeply with the number of cigarettes smoked habitually, but the rate for the men who had never smoked was actually higher than that for the men who had stopped smoking or who smoked fewer than ten cigarettes daily. However, this latter peculiarity is not statistically significant. The 2-x-2 contingency table is made up of 14 hard cases among 881 men who had never smoked, 6 cases among 580 men who had stopped or used fewer than ten cigarettes daily. Chi-square = 2.62, and the observed distribution could arise by chance with $p = 0.18$. The ten-year incidence of soft CHD in Yugoslavia was unrelated to smoking habit as recorded at the entry examination.

Figure 9.16 gives the corresponding picture for Italy and Greece. Although there is some indication of a tendency for the incidence of hard CHD to rise with smoking class, this is not statistically convincing with any analysis. For example, in the comparison of smokers with nonsmokers, the ten-year incidence of hard CHD was 3.39 percent for smokers, 2.26 percent for nonsmokers (chi-square = 2.99, $p = 0.084$). For soft CHD the incidence rate was lower for smokers than for nonsmokers, 3.30 versus 3.50 percent, respectively.

For none of the European areas was there any significant relation between

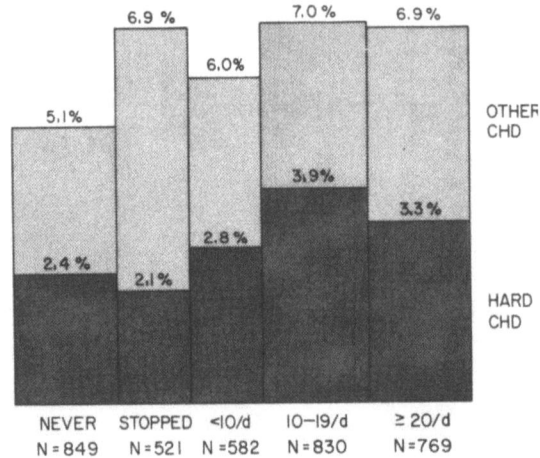

Figure 9.16. Age-standardized 10-year incidence rate of coronary heart disease of 3,551 men in Italy and Greece (Crevalcore, Montegiorgio, Rome railroad, Crete, and Corfu) classified by smoking habit at entry and then free of cardiovascular disease.

smoking and the ten-year incidence rate of soft CHD, but it is of interest to compare the areas in respect to the relationship in each area of hard CHD incidence to smoking habits. Figure 9.17 shows the regressions, $y = a + bx$, where y = incidence of hard CHD and x = smoking class. The slope of the regression in Yugoslavia is double that in Italy and Greece but only half that in northern Europe. Roughly, at least, these values for the slope, b, indicate the relative importance of smoking habit as a risk factor for the incidence of myocardial infarction or death from coronary heart disease in ten years of men initially without evidence of any cardiovascular disease and aged 40 through 59 at the start of the follow-up.

In the absence of ten-year reexaminations of the American railroad men it is not possible to report on their ten-year incidence of nonfatal coronary heart disease. The data on ten-year coronary deaths were reported earlier in this chapter. Here we examine the relationship of CHD incidence to smoking habits as found in the first five years of follow-up of these Americans, following the same format used in this chapter for showing the ten-year experience in the other areas. Figure 9.18 is a summary for 162 incidence cases of CHD in 2,254 American railroad men free of evidence of the disease at the start of the five-year follow-up. Among the 162 cases, 20.5 percent represented hard CHD, a proportion similar to that observed in the other areas of the Seven Countries Study.

As in the experience of the European groups, the relationship of smoking

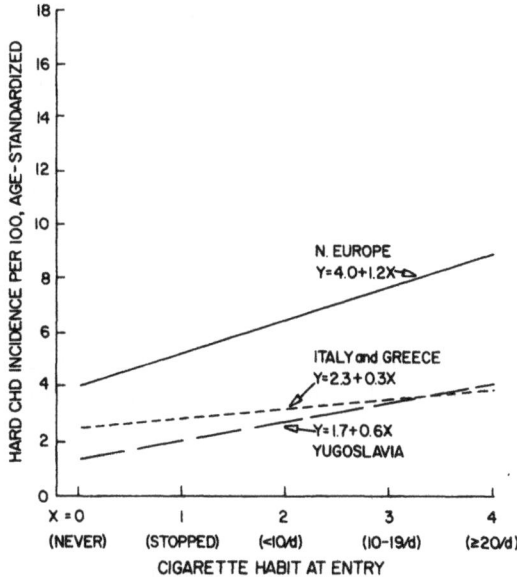

Figure 9.17. Regression of age-standardized ten-year incidence rate of hard CHD on smoking class of 8,717 men free of cardiovascular disease in northern Europe at entry (east and west Finland, Zutphen) in Yugoslavia (Dalmatia, Slavonia, Velika Krsna, Zrenjanin, and Belgrade), and in Italy and Greece (Crevalcore, Montegiorgio, Rome railroad, Crete, and Corfu).

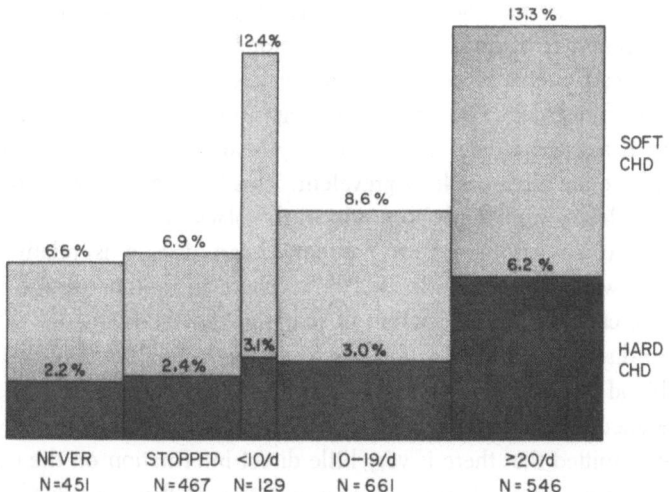

Figure 9.18. Five-year incidence per 100 men according to smoking class in 2,254 American railroad men free of cardiovascular disease at entry.

habit to hard CHD in the American men is much more important than that to soft CHD incidence. Soft CHD is not related to the amount of smoking, the highest incidence rate being that for the men smoking fewer than ten cigarettes a day, 9.3 percent in five years, compared with 5.6 percent and 7.1 percent, respectively, for the men smoking ten to nineteen and twenty or more cigarettes a day. However, the incidence of soft CHD was 6.6 percent for all smokers combined and only 4.5 for nonsmokers (chi-square = 4.53, $p = 0.033$). For hard CHD the linear model seems appropriate to the data and the least-squares solution is: $y = -1.69 + 1.88x$, and the standard error of the slope is 0.043. This is in agreement with all other analyses in indicating that smoking habit is more important as a risk factor for the incidence of hard CHD in the American men than in other groups in the study.

Regional Differences

The ten-year seven countries findings are that cigarette smoking was much less of a risk factor, less predictive of heart attacks and premature death, in southern Europe and Japan than in the United States and northern Europe. It would be too much to extrapolate the experience of these cohorts to the general populations of the areas concerned, but we are unaware of any good epidemiological evidence that the general populations do not differ in something like the same way as found in these cohorts. Still, regardless of the extent to which the seven countries results may apply to whole populations, the area differences observed raise important questions. Although there are no ready answers, several factors are suggested.

The importance of smoking as a risk factor for myocardial infarction and coronary death seems to be related to the frequency of the disease in the population concerned. The slope of the regression of incidence rate on cigarette use is steepest where severe coronary heart disease is most common, flattest where the disease is least prevalent. This is in keeping with the observation that heavy smoking is common in the black and colored populations of South Africa among whom coronary heart disease is relatively rare (Bronte-Stewart, Keys, and Brock 1955). There is another parallel in that these differences in the association of smoking and the frequency of coronary heart disease are linked to differences in the general level of cholesterol in the blood serum in the populations studied. This suggests, in turn, parallel differences in the frequency of severe coronary atherosclerosis, though it must be admitted that there is very little direct information on the epidemiology of atherosclerosis. Perhaps it is enough to note that the risk of having a heart attack and dying from coronary heart disease is increased much more by smoking when the serum cholesterol concentration is high than when it is low. An obvious mechanism to propose is that smoking may trigger the heart attack by increasing the irritability of the myocardium when its blood supply is already compromised by severe coronary atherosclerosis. This concept, emphasizing a more immediate than a long-term effect of smoking on the heart, is supported by indications in this and other studies that former smokers may be little or no more at risk of heart attacks than persons who had never smoked regularly.

This concentration on cholesterol, atherosclerosis, and coronary heart disease does not explain the fact that in the Seven Countries Study smoking was as great a hazard for premature noncoronary deaths as for coronary deaths. Even when allowance is made for deaths from cancer of the respiratory system, there is a large excess of deaths associated with cigarette smoking in the United States and in northern Europe but not in southern Europe or Japan.

Several other suggestions may be proposed to account for the difference between areas in the danger of cigarette smoking. There is no reason to think that differences in the manner of smoking may be involved. In all areas almost all cigarette smokers inhale at every puff, and from ordinary observation the depth of inhalation in the several areas seems to be much the same. From unsystematic but repeated observations over many years only two common differences between the areas in the manner of smoking stand out. American men discard half-smoked cigarettes far more often then we have observed in the other areas of this study. In Italy especially, the custom is to smoke the cigarette to a very short butt. In Italy and some other areas another peculiarity is keeping a partly smoked, unlit cigarette in the mouth to be relit from time to time as opportunity or inclination arises. This may reflect the lack of addition to the cigarette by the manufacturer of chemicals that keep the cigarette alight even when it is not being puffed.

A lifetime exposure to cigarette smoke, not the number of cigarettes smoked daily, could be important, but there is little indication that differences in this respect could help explain the differences between areas in smoking as a risk for the succeeding ten years after entry into the study. Cigarette smoking was established as a common habit of men in all of the areas many years before the start of this study. In personal visits to Japan as early as 1923 widespread heavy cigarette smoking, even by young boys, was obvious. During World War II differences among some of the areas were imposed by shortage of tobacco in the countries with no local tobacco production. In Finland and the Netherlands cigarettes were in very short supply during the war years and immediately afterward. In contrast, the Greeks, Italians, and Yugoslavs were self-supplied with their native-grown tobaccos, subject to wartime limitations of labor and transport. The Japanese too had their customary tobacco grown in their southern islands and, until the closing period of the war, in Taiwan. In the United States the trend of increasing per capita consumption of cigarettes was accelerated, not interrupted, during the war. Such information as is available about the long-time exposure to cigarette smoking would not seem to clarify the differences among the areas of the Seven Countries Study in smoking as a risk factor. The northern Europeans who had a major interruption in smoking over some years in the 1940s, matched the American railroad men in regard to the importance of smoking as a risk factor in the experience of the 1960s. For the southern Europeans who were not cut off from tobacco during the war, and therefore had a longer history of relatively uninterrupted smoking, cigarette smoking in the 1960s seemed to be much less of a risk factor. So a major question remains unanswered.

The incidence rates of men with different smoking habits must not be overinterpreted. For example, it is true that the ten-year data on the Japanese men fail to give any evidence that the all-causes death rate is related to smoking habits. At entry, 255 of the Japanese were nonsmokers, and 31 of them died in ten years; 496 smoked at least twenty cigarettes every day, and 61 were dead in ten years. The respective deaths per 1,000 were 121.6 and 123.0, and the difference is nowhere near being significant, with standard errors of 20.5 and 14.8, respectively.

The data fail to show a difference, but they also fail to show there is no difference. The 95 percent confidence limits of the two death rates are 81.5 and 161.7 for the nonsmokers, 94.1 and 151.9 for the heavy smokers. So it would be quite possible that the population rate for the heavy smokers could be, say, 50 percent higher than that of the nonsmokers. All that can be fairly concluded from these data is that the risk of death associated with smoking in Japan is probably smaller than in the United States or in northern Europe.

Probability of Death

The data summarized in figures 9.5 through 9.18 offer strong evidence that smoking habit recorded at entry is a much more important risk factor for the Americans and northern Europeans than for the southern Europeans and the Japanese. However, the implications are so important that the differences among the areas in the ten-year experience should be carefully examined in terms of probabilities. For example, although striking differences are shown in the graphs in figure 9.11, the question arises as to the extent those differences could be ascribed to chance. One approach is to examine these data with the chi-square test.

Among, 1,375 smokers in the American railroad group without evidence of coronary heart disease at entry, 79 men died from coronary heart disease during ten years of follow-up and 18 of 940 nonsmokers died from that disease. There can be no doubt that the American smokers were more prone to die than their nonsmoking fellows. But what is the probability that the risk associated with smoking is different in other population samples? One approach to the question is to use the chi-square test in a comparison of the numbers of deaths observed among the smokers and the number that would be expected from the experience of smokers versus non-smokers in other populations. For example, in southern Europe among 2,618 nonsmokers 31 men died from coronary heart disease in ten years, and among 3,730 smokers 61 men died from coronary heart disease, making a ratio of rates of 1.37 to 1. If the experience were proportional in the American railroad group, the expectation for the smokers would be $1.37(18)(1375)/940 = 36.07$. Hence chi-square is calculated as $(79-36.07)^2/36.07 = 51$. So the coronary death rate of the American smokers far exceeds the expectation based on the experience of the southern Europeans and the projection from the death rate of the American nonsmokers; the odds against chance explanation are astronomical. These calculations are based on the crude data; however, when age-standardized data are used the results are substantially identical (chi-square = 51.3).

From the graphs in figure 9.11 it would seem that a similar comparison between the northern and the southern European men in regard to the penalty of smoking would yield much the same result as in the case of the Americans, but this is not the case. Among 775 nonsmokers in northern Europe, there were 22 coronary deaths in ten years; among 1,593 smokers there were 73 coronary deaths. The calculation then is: $1.37(22)(1953)/775 = 61.95$ for the number of deaths expected among the smokers to correspond with the experience of smokers versus nonsmokers in southern Europe. The chi-square value is then $(73-61.95)^2/61.97 = 1.97$, indicating no significant difference. The explanation of the apparent discrepancy is visible in figure 9.11; a major difference is shown between the Americans and the Finns in the coronary death rates of the ex-smokers. Men stop smoking for many different reasons and may well represent different kinds of persons in different populations. It can be argued then that when ex-smokers seem to depart widely from a common trend, as they do in figure 9.11, it is unwise to group never-smokers and ex-smokers in a single category of nonsmokers. The analysis of smokers versus never-smokers starts with the fact that of 315 northern Europeans who had never smoked regularly 6 died of coronary heart disease in ten years. The projection from the experience of the southern Europeans is 42.78 expected coronary deaths for the northern European smokers and 73 observed deaths (chi-square = 21.35).

The analysis of smokers versus never-smokers in the American men compared with that for the southern Europeans yields 42.52 deaths expected and 79 observed (chi-square = 31.3). So both for the American and the northern European men, the risk of coronary death is increased by smoking far more than for the southern Europeans, and the odds against a chance explanation are extremely great.

Comparisons limited to smokers and nonsmokers may be less relevant than comparisons of the slopes of the regression lines in figures 9.9–9.11, but for the latter it is essential to estimate the standard errors of the slopes. For each case there are five sets of rates, each based on substantial numbers of deaths and of men at risk, and account must be taken of those numbers in calculating errors. Consider the 533 United States railroad men smoking twenty or more cigarettes daily, among whom 36 died from coronary heart disease. Since all of the men at risk are equivalent in regard to the smoking variable, it can be suggested that each of the men who died represented $553/36 = 15.36$ men at risk and that, in effect, the overall death rate of men in that smoking category represents 36 sets of rates of $1/15.36 = 0.0651$, or 651 per 10,000 men. (Age standardization accounts for the discrepancy from 644 shown in figure 9.11). Following this reasoning the rates for the railroad men of 208, 151, 344, 590, 644 are based on values of $N = 9, 7, 5, 40$, and 36, respectively. These are rounded age-standardized numbers, the corresponding numbers of deaths not age-adjusted are 10, 8, 6, 38, and 35, respectively. Taking the values of X for the smoking classes as 0, 1, 2, 3, and 4, respectively, the least-squares regression gives 129 for the slope using the age-standardized figures, 128 for the nonadjusted values, with a standard error of 4.5 in both cases.

Applying the same approach to the ten-year coronary heart disease deaths in northern Europeans, the result is slope $b = 128$ with a standard error of 2.7 for the age-standardized values. Without such standardization the slope is 107, $SEb = 2.6$. Whereas the age-standardized results show the slopes of the regression of coronary death rate on smoking to be substantially identical for the Americans and the northern Europeans, comparison using the nonstandardized data indicate a steeper slope for the Americans, $128 - 107 = 21$ with a standard error of the difference of 5.3 and $t = 21/5.3 = 4.0$.

The corresponding solution of the regression equation for the southern Europeans gives slope $SEb = 1.8$. In any case the probability estimate is that the observed difference between the slopes for the Americans and the northern Europeans compared with that for the southern Europeans would occur by chance with extreme rarity, and the t value is of the order of 10 or more.

All of the foregoing analysis regarding probabilities concerns the incidence of coronary heart disease death among men free of evidence of cardiovascular disease at the start of the ten-year follow-up. The all-causes deaths as related to smoking can be analysed in the same way. For Italy and Greece combined, as illustrated in figure 9.9, the slope of the regression of all-causes death rate on smoking is $b = 56$, $SEb = 2.2$. In contrast, for the northern Europeans the slope of all-causes deaths versus smoking habits is 271 with $SE = 5.0$, and the odds against chance explanation of the difference between the slopes are astronomically great, t on the order of 30. For the Yugoslavs the slope is 151 and its standard error $= 3.7$. The indication, therefore, is that the slope of the regression of all-causes deaths on smoking habit is higher for the northern Europeans than for the Yugoslavs, which, in turn, is higher than for the Italians and Greeks, with all of the differences highly significant. Note that all these slopes and their standard errors refer to rates per 10,000 men.

For Japan the slope of the regression of all-causes deaths on smoking is $b = -2$ with age-standardization, -9 without, and $SEb = 10$. In contrast (figure 9.10) are the findings on the relation between the ten-year all-causes deaths and smoking habits of the 2,315 American railroad men judged to be free of cardiovascular disease at entry. In terms of incidence per 10,000 men the slope is $b = 295$; $SE = 5.9$.

For comparisons of the population groups in the relationship between the incidence of coronary heart disease and smoking habits, the corresponding calculations can be made with the data given in figures 9.14–9.16 and 9.18. Data for the estimation of the significance of differences in the death rates from neoplastic diseases are given in figure 9.12 for northern and for southern Europe. For the United States railroad men the regression of the death rate from all neoplasms on smoking habit has slope $b = 52$, $SEb = 5.5$. The corresponding analysis for the men of southern Europe gives slope $b = 64.8$, $SEb = 3.7$. The difference in slope between the Americans and the southern Europeans, 12.8, has $SEb = 6.6$; the value $t = 1.93$ suggest the likelihood of a significant difference. For the men of northern Europe the regression of ten-year death rate from neoplastic disease on smoking habit at entry shows, for the rate per 10,000, $y = 192 + 129x$ where x is the smoking class; the standard error of the slope $= 4.8$. The indication is that the risk of dying from neoplastic disease rises much more steeply with smoking in northern Europe than in either the United States or in southern Europe.

Deaths attributed to neoplasms of the respiratory system are too few for detailed comparisons, 42 such deaths in northern Europe, 32 in southern Europe, 13 among the Americans, 2 among the Japanese. For ten-year deaths per 10,000 men from neoplasms of the respiratory system, the regression on smoking habit is $y = -4.5 + 27x$, with $SEb = 2.4$ for southern Europe, $y = 0.3 + 103x$ with $SEb = 6.4$ for northern Europe. This indicates a much greater influence of smoking on respiratory cancer development in northern than in southern Europe, with the t value for the difference more than 10.

The outcome of these estimations of probabilities is to confirm the conclusion that cigarette smoking is a much more important risk factor for the American and northern European men than for the men of the same age in southern Europe and Japan, and that difference in risk applies to deaths from all causes, from coronary heart disease, and from neoplasms, and to the incidence of coronary heart disease.

Summary

Except in two Serbian cohorts, at entry more than half of the men in this study were cigarette smokers, almost all smoking at least ten cigarettes daily. Pipe and cigar smoking was very rare except at Zutphen. The Dutch commonly also smoked cigarettes. This analysis concerns only cigarette smoking.

Smoking habits in the cohorts were examined in four ways: the percentage of men who had never smoked, those who were nonsmokers at entry, those who currently smoked twenty or more cigarettes daily, and the average number of cigarettes smoked a day for each cohort. No relationship was found between any of these smoking characteristics and the ten-year incidence rates of all-causes deaths, coronary death, or any diagnosis of coronary heart disease in the cohorts.

The relationship between individual smoking habits and their ten-year experience varied greatly among the cohorts. Among the American railroad men, cigarette smoking was a major risk factor for both all-causes and coronary death, but there was no difference between the men who had never smoked and those who had stopped. The death rate of nonsmokers was about a third of that of the men smoking twenty or more cigarettes daily, and the disproportion was roughly the same for coronary and for other deaths.

The experience of the Finns and Dutch was similar except that the death rate of the men who had never smoked was only about half that of the men who had stopped smoking at least a year before entry. In Yugoslavia, the heavy smokers had more than twice the coronary death rate of the other men, but there were no significant differences in the death rates of men who had never smoked, those who had stopped, and those who smoked ten to nineteen cigarettes a day.

In Italy and Greece, cigarette smoking was a relatively minor risk factor. The ten-year all-causes death rate of heavy smokers was only 27 percent higher than that of the nonsmokers. For deaths from coronary heart disease the corresponding difference was 45 percent.

Japan had the highest proportion of heavy smokers in this study, 41.5 percent smoking at least twenty cigarettes every day. However, the ten-year mortality could not be shown to be related to smoking habits of these Japanese. It is notable that in ten years only 7 of the 1,000 Japanese men died from coronary heart disease.

The incidence of nonfatal plus fatal coronary heart disease was related to smoking habits in northern Europe, but there was no significant difference in the incidence among men who had never smoked or who had stopped, or those who were light smokers. The incidence of hard CHD (coronary death of nonfatal infarction) among 446 heavy smokers was almost double that among 775 nonsmokers. The incidence of other diagnoses of coronary heart disease in northern Europe was unrelated to smoking habits.

In Italy and Greece the ten-year incidence of hard CHD among 769 heavy smokers was 43 percent higher than among 1,370 nonsmokers, but the incidence of all other diagnoses of coronary heart disease was unrelated to smoking habits.

Among 565 heavy smokers in Yugoslavia, the incidence rate of hard CHD was 2.6 times that among 1,248 non-smokers, and there were no significant differences among men who had never smoked, who had stopped, or who were light smokers. For 106 men with other (soft) diagnosis of coronary heart disease in ten years, no relationship with smoking habits was found.

For the American railroad men the incidence of nonfatal coronary heart disease in the second five years of follow-up is unknown, but the five-year finding was that the incidence of hard CHD among 546 heavy smokers was almost three times that of 918 nonsmokers, and the incidence of other coronary diagnoses was double. The experience of the railroad men who stopped smoking was not significantly different from that of the men who had never smoked regularly.

Both in northern and in southern Europe the ten-year age-standardized rate of death from neoplastic disease rose roughly linearly with cigarette smoking. Deaths from cancer of the trachea, bronchus, or lung accounted for most of the relationship. In northern Europe the death rate of smokers from cancer of the respiratory system was 8 times that of the nonsmokers. In southern Europe the death rate of smokers from that cause was 4.6 times that of nonsmokers. Apart from smoking habits, the northern Europeans were more prone than the southern Europeans to die from cancer of the respiratory system.

These comparisons of incidence rates of men of different smoking habits should be tempered by consideration of the standard errors of the rates. The data on the Japanese fail to show a relation of death rate to smoking habit. It is also true that these data do not rule out the possibility that the population rate of Japanese heavy smokers could be substantially higher than that of the nonsmokers.

10 | Overweight and Obesity

Before coronary heart disease was credited as being a major cause of death, American insurance companies, led by the Metropolitan Life Insurance Company, were pointing to overweight as a serious impairment associated with undue probability of premature death. Insurance company actuaries published tables showing the average body weight of persons of given height, age, and sex who had applied for life insurance from some companies, and overweight was calculated in terms of percentage departure from those averages. From the mortality experience of policy holders it was concluded to be justifiable to charge extra premiums to insurance applicants who were grossly overweight according to the standard tables. With recognition that coronary heart disease was the leading killer in the United States, it was assumed that overweight promotes the disease, though the insurance actuaries did not provide any convincing data in confirmation. Still, relative weight was the first variable proposed for control in efforts to prevent heart attacks.

Serious defects and limitations in the life insurance material on overweight and mortality have been pointed out repeatedly (Keys 1954, 1955a, b; Keys and Blackburn 1963; Keys et al. 1967; Seltzer and Mayer 1965; Seltzer 1966) and at least some of the insurance companies have abandoned the view that each pound of weight adds to the risk of coronary heart disease and premature death. One of the leading insurance companies reported that in the actuarial follow-up no appreciable increase in mortality was found at any level of overweight less than 25 percent of the average weight for given height and age (Hutchinson 1961). In general, insurance companies demand an increased premium because of overweight only in extreme cases—when the body weight is more than 25 or 30 percent above that of the average applicant of the same sex, age, and height. This means that relative weight is of interest to the insurance companies in only a very small proportion of the applicants. For the men in the present study only about one out of thirty of the American railroad men might be asked to pay extra insurance premiums because of overweight.

The picture has been confused by the common assumption that relative body weight is a good measure of obesity or body fatness. Actually, body fatness and relative weight are not closely correlated except at the extremes, and to some extent overweight and body fatness reflect metabolic opposites. Most football players are lean but overweight because their exercise builds a large muscle mass; sedentary men are often obese without being overweight, excess fat being counterbalanced by a deficit of muscle. For the men in the Seven Countries Study the mean product-moment coefficient of correlation between relative body weight and fatness as indicated by the sum of skinfold thickness was $r = 0.77$. If the men who represent the 5 percent who are most overweight are excluded, the correlation falls to $r = 0.5$.

In this material there is a significant correlation between relative weight and the skeletal form as represented by the index of laterality/linearity. We have measured this as the height divided by the sum of the biacromial and bicristal diameters; in the seven countries material the mean coefficient of correlation between these two measures at entry is $r = 0.422$. There is also a small correlation between the index of laterality and the sum of the skinfolds, with mean $r = 0.222$. Allowing for this latter correlation the partial correlation between relative weight and the index of laterality/linearity is $r = 0.40$. In other words, at constant fatness estimated by skinfold thickness, there is still a very significant correlation between relative weight and skeletal shape. The corresponding partial correlation between relative weight and skinfold thickness holding laterality/linearity constant is $r = 0.76$.

What this means is that relative weight alone accounts for about 58 percent of the variance of skinfold thickness, and the skeletal form alone accounts for about 16 percent (the square of $0.4 = 0.16$). So relative weight is not a very good measure of fatness as represented by skinfold thickness in this total material. If the extremes of the relative weight distribution are omitted, say the 5 percent of men at each end of the overweight-underweight distribution, there is only a very low correlation between relative weight and fatness. For 90 percent of the men, then, it is grossly inaccurate to infer relative obesity from relative weight.

Measures of Relative Weight

The foregoing calculations have been made with the body mass index as the measure of relative weight; the conclusions about relative weight as a measure of fatness are the same with other measures of relative weight. Relative weight is often expressed as a percentage of the weight corresponding to height and age in tables giving the averages for insurance applicants, though the latter refer to weight "as commonly dressed" and height with shoes. Moreover, the tables refer to persons applying for insurance in past years, so there are questions about possible changes over the years in clothing weight and shoe height. The insurance company tables of "desirable weight," once called "ideal weight," are essentially the averages for young applicants, but there is no mention of age. The three "frame" or "build" types specified in the tables are based on no measurements or estimates; they are essentially the tertiles of the distribution of weights at given height.

The concept of ideal weight standards disregarding age was developed by the late Dr. Louis Dublin, then chief actuary of the Metropolitan Life Insurance Company. He argued that after growth in height is finished in the early twenties, he could see no good physiological reason why growth in weight should continue. But the fact is that in substantially all civilized populations weight does continue to increase until middle age, commonly reaching a peak at around 50 years. Accordingly, when overweight is estimated as a percentage of ideal or desirable weight, age may be a confounding variable, and effects attributed to overweight may actually relate to age as a concealed variable. In one major follow-up study, a table of diastolic blood pressure versus weight as a percentage of desirable weight was interpreted as showing the ill effect of increasing weight, ignoring the fact that increasing age was more likely the controlling variable (Paul 1971).

Relative weight refers to weight independent of height. In the insurance company tables relative weight is the observed weight as a percentage of the average weight of persons of given sex and age of the same height who applied for insurance policies from certain American companies some ten to thirty years earlier. That arbitrary standard relates only to a very special population at a particular period in the past. For many purposes an index of relative weight with fixed physical meaning is preferable. The simple ratio of weight divided by height is sometimes used, but unfortunately it proves to be correlated with height. The ponderal index, the cube root of weight over height, or the similar Rohrer index, the weight divided by the third power of height, have been more widely used, but are also not fully independent of height (Keys et al. 1972c). The body mass index, the body weight divided by the square of the height, is not significantly correlated with height and seems to be the best simple index of relative weight; the BMI is the index used in the present analysis, as it was in the analysis of the experience in the first five years of the Seven Countries Study. The BMI has been selected as the best index of relative weight for standard tables in Great Britain (Kemsley, Billewicz, and Thomson 1962).

Although the estimation of relative obesity or body fatness is troublesome, skinfold thickness is generally agreed as giving a reasonable approximation, especially when skinfolds are measured at more than one site. For this purpose we have used the sum of the thicknesses over the triceps muscle at the midpoint of the upper arm and that over the tip of the scapula. As noted above, this measure of obesity is correlated with relative body weight, but relative weight accounts for less than 60 percent of the variance of skinfold thickness.

Differences among the Cohorts

Keys et al. (1967) published details of the distributions of relative body weight and of the sum of the skinfold thicknesses at entry. In both measures there were wide variations among the sixteen cohorts. The mean body mass index was over 25.5 in three cohorts—Rome railroad men, Belgrade and Crevalcore—and under 22.5 in three—Velika Krsna and the two Japanese cohorts. The American railroad men were fourth highest in relative body weight. The range of mean values for the sum of the skinfolds was much greater, with the men of Belgrade and the Americans averaging over 32 mm, but mean values under 18 mm were observed in six cohorts—both Japanese, both Greek, and both Croatian cohorts.

The question of a relationship between ten-year death rate from all causes and from coronary heart disease and the characteristics of the cohorts in respect to relative weight and body fatness is examined in figures 10.1 through 10.4. These concern men who were judged to be free of cardiovascular disease at the entry examinations. If men with entry cardiovascular disease are not excluded, the picture is essentially the same. All of the correlations are negative, that is, age-specific mortality decreases with increasing relative weight and fatness, but none of the coefficients is statistically significantly different from zero. So the large differences in ten-year mortality among the cohorts cannot be explained by the differences in relative weight and fatness.

Figures 10.1 through 10.4 show that the differences among the cohorts in the rates of total and of coronary mortality are not accounted for by differences in body mass index or sum of the skinfolds. These measures of relative weight and fatness also fail to account for the differences among the cohorts in the incidence of coronary heart disease. Table 10.1 summarizes the correlations of the body mass index and skinfold sums with the incidence of coronary heart disease, including nonfatal incidence, in all cohorts, except the American railroad men whose nonfatal coronary incidence in the last five years of follow-up is unknown and, for sum of skinfolds, the men of Tanushimaru because that measurement was not made at entry. With the exception of the correlation of soft CHD with sum of the skinfolds

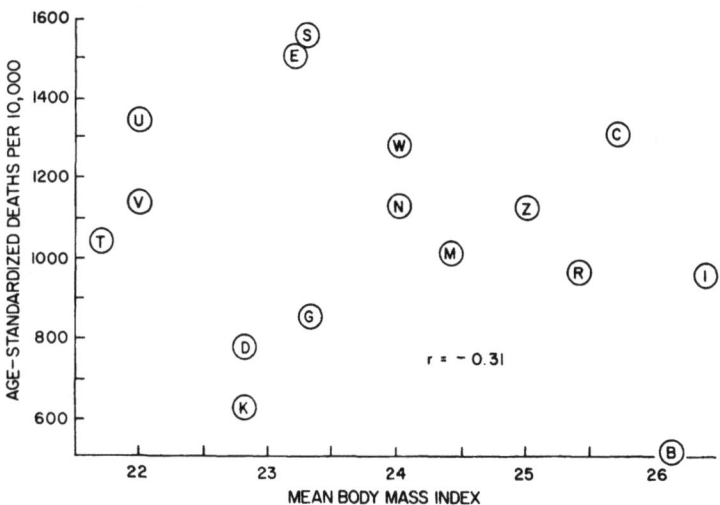

Figure 10.1. Age-standardized ten-year all-causes death rates of the cohorts versus their mean body mass index at entry. B = Belgrade; C = Crevalcore; D = Dalmatia; E = east Finland, G = Corfu; I = Italian railroad; K = Crete; M = Montegiorgio; N = Zutphen; R = U.S. railroad; S = Slavonia; T = Tanushimaru; U = Ushibuka; V = Velika Krsna; W = west Finland; Z = Zrenjanin. All men free of cardiovascular disease at entry.

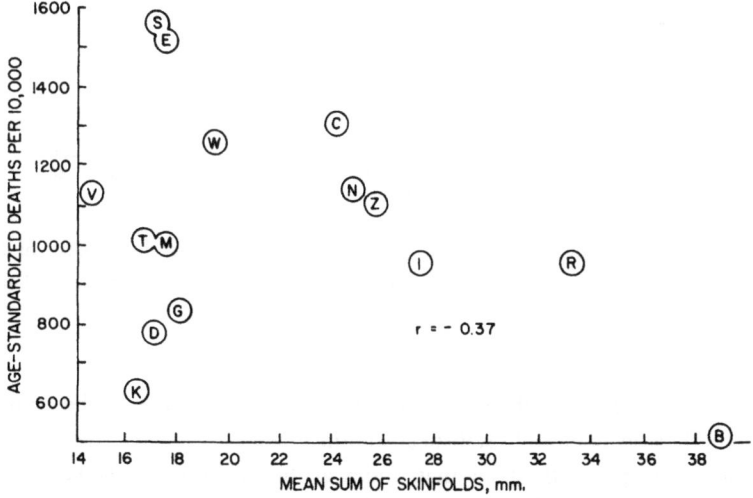

Figure 10.2. Age-standardized ten-year all-causes death rates of the cohorts versus their mean sum of skinfold thickness at entry. Cohorts as in figure 10.1.

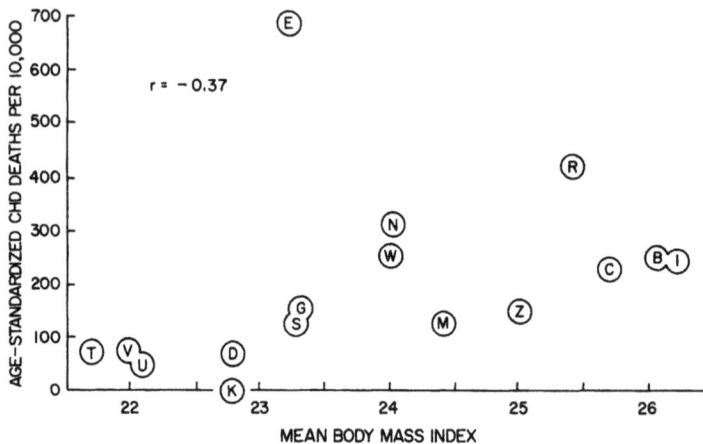

Figure 10.3. Age-standardized ten-year coronary heart disease death rates of the cohorts versus their mean relative body weight at entry. Cohorts as in figure 10.1.

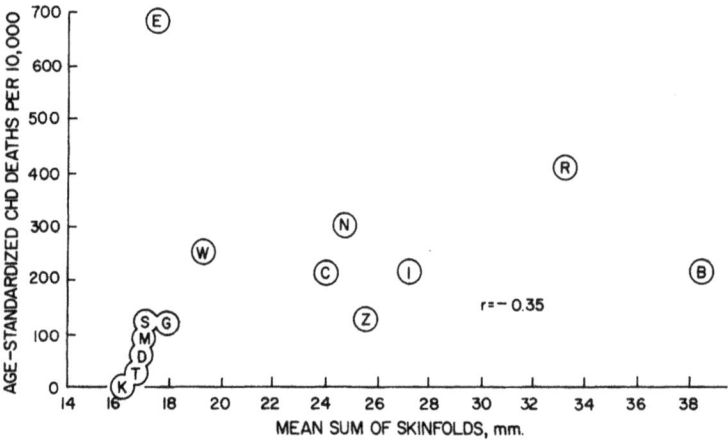

Figure 10.4. Age-standardized ten-year coronary heart disease death rates of the cohorts versus their mean sum of skinfold thickness at entry. Cohorts as in figure 10.1.

where $r = -0.01$, all of the correlations are positive, but none of the correlation coefficients is close to statistical significance.

Though we prefer the body mass index as the measure of relative weight, for men aged 40–59 the relative weight calculated as a percentage of the average weight for men of the same height and age in United States life insurance tables is very highly correlated with the body mass index, with a cor-

Table 10.1. Correlation coefficient (r) of age-standardized ten-year incidence rate of coronary heart disease with mean body mass index (fifteen cohorts) and with mean skinfold thickness (fourteen cohorts) (men without cardiovascular disease at entry).[a]

CHD	r with BMI	CHD	r with skinfold
Hard	0.22	Hard	0.08
Any	0.40	Any	0.15
Soft	0.24	Soft	−0.01

a. With fifteen pairs of values, $r = 0.48$ is the smallest value to assure, with 95% probability, that r is not actually zero.

Table 10.2. Correlation (r) between body mass index and relative body weight (expressed as percentage of the average weight at that height in U.S. insurance tables for men aged 40 through 59) and coefficients in the least-squares regression of BMI on RBW ($BMI = a + b\, RBW$).

Cohort	r	a	SE	b	SE
U.S. railroad	0.993	0.195	(0.084)	0.243	(0.001)
East Finland	0.991	−0.063	(0.109)	0.245	(0.001)
Crevalcore	0.991	0.466	(0.108)	0.242	(0.001)

relation coefficient of $r = 0.99$ or higher in all cohorts. Table 10.2 gives three typical examples and the regression coefficients. From the latter it is evident that the relative body weight can be estimated from the body mass index divided by 0.24 with no more than a trivial error.

The demonstration that the differences in ten-year incidence among the cohorts are not explained in any part by the differences among the cohorts in average body mass index, relative body weight, or body fatness (sum of skinfold thicknesses) does not, of course, dispose of those measures of relative weight or obesity as possible risk factors within the cohorts. But before considering the relations between incidence rate and those weight and fatness indicators within the cohorts, it is important to examine some correlations. Table 10.3 shows correlation coefficients of body mass index with each of eight characteristics in each of the sixteen cohorts.

In examining the coefficients in table 10.3, it should be recalled that the numbers are large—500 or more in each cohort—so values of $r = 0.09$ or greater reach $p = 0.05$.

Except for west Finland and Corfu, BMI is negatively correlated with age, but the coefficient is very small. The high correlation of BMI with the sum

Table 10.3. Correlation between body mass index and other characteristics at entry.

Cohort	Age	Skinf.	Lat/lin[a]	S BP	D BP	Chol.	Pulse	Smoking
U.S. railroad	−0.02	0.75	0.43	0.23	0.27	0.09	0.05	−0.10
Dalmatia	−0.08	0.82	—	0.38	0.30	0.24	0.05	−0.20
Slavonia	−0.07	0.83	0.35	0.34	0.39	0.26	0.10	−0.38
Tanushimaru	−0.09	0.54	—	0.05	0.04	0.03	0.08	−0.04
East Finland	−0.04	0.77	0.32	0.11	0.21	0.10	0.16	−0.21
West Finland	0.00	0.80	0.40	0.21	0.28	0.13	0.20	−0.26
Ushibuka	−0.03	—	—	0.17	0.19	0.09	−0.07	−0.08
Crevalcore	−0.01	0.71	0.47	0.20	0.22	0.21	0.12	−0.21
Montegiorgio	0.01	0.80	0.39	0.21	0.27	0.33	0.17	−0.23
Zutphen	−0.08	0.70	0.61	0.32	0.36	0.21	0.08	−0.09
Crete	−0.05	0.79	0.40	0.27	0.33	0.28	0.09	−0.20
Corfu	0.01	0.84	0.44	0.29	0.35	0.28	0.23	−0.25
Rome railroad	−0.08	0.77	0.49	0.26	0.34	0.09	0.10	−0.25
Velika Krsna	0.06	0.76	0.29	0.06	0.10	0.21	0.05	−0.15
Zrenjanin	−0.06	0.87	—	0.23	0.32	0.26	—	−0.27
Belgrade	−0.06	0.77	—	0.12	0.21	0.13	—	−0.16
Mean	−0.04	0.77	0.42	0.21	0.26	0.19	0.10	−0.19
SE	0.01	0.02	0.02	0.02	0.02	0.02	0.02	0.02

a. Standing height divided by the sum of the biacromial and bicristal diameters.

of the skinfolds is not unexpected, but note that on the average BMI accounts for only about half of the variance in skinfold thickness. The highly significant correlation between BMI and the index of laterality/linearity is interesting though, again, not unexpected. Men with relatively wide skeletal form tend to be relatively heavy for their height, again emphasizing that relative weight is not simply a measure of obesity. The correlation between BMI and blood pressure confirms other surveys and common opinion, but it should be observed that, on the average, the body mass index accounts for only 4 percent of the systolic and 5 percent of the diastolic blood pressure variance. Serum cholesterol concentration is also positively correlated with the body mass index in all of the cohorts, but on the average, BMI accounts for only 4 percent of the cholesterol variance. The resting pulse rate is also positively correlated with the body mass index in all of the cohorts save the men of Ushibuka; that correlation accounts for 1 percent of the average variance of the resting pulse rate. Finally, the habit of smoking cigarettes is negatively correlated with the body mass index; body mass index, or relative weight, tends to decrease with cigarette smoking in all the cohorts. The net

Overweight and Obesity | 169

result of the correlation analysis is that three characteristics that are positive risk factors, arterial blood pressure, serum cholesterol, and resting pulse rate, are positively correlated with relative body weight, whereas age and cigarette smoking, also positive risk factors, are negatively correlated with BMI. A suitable multivariate analysis is required to evaluate the independent contribution of relative weight to risk. However, with three positive and two negative correlations with BMI among five characteristics that are positive risk factors, it would seem that the results of univariate analysis of incidence as related to relative weight would not be grossly misleading.

Ten-year Death Rate

All men in the study were classified at entry into deciles, specific for five-year age class and cohort, of relative body weight and the sum of the skinfold thicknesses. The distribution into those decile classes of the men who died in the succeeding ten years examines the relationship between mortality and the measures of overweight and obesity without making any assumptions about the nature of the distributions. In the absence of a relationship the deaths would not significantly differ from a random distribution among the ten classes.

Figure 10.5 shows the findings for all-causes deaths among the American railroad men who were free of signs of CHD at entry. Among the men in the top 20 percent of the fatness distribution 51 died, and among those in

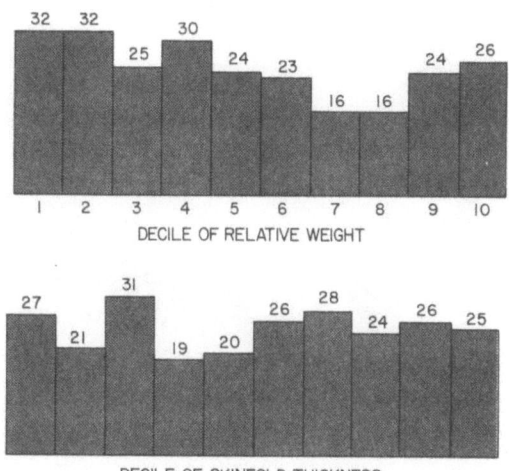

Figure 10.5. Distribution of all-causes ten-year deaths into the age- and cohort-specific entry decile classes of relative body weight and of skinfold thickness for American railroad men. All men free of coronary heart disease at entry.

the bottom 20 percent 48 died. Mortality in regard to relative body weight does not show such close correspondence with chance expectation; there was a tendency for the men at the upper end of distribution to have a reduced mortality. If relative weight had no effect, the chance expectation would be 124 deaths in both the upper and the lower halves of the distribution. Actually there were 105 deaths among the relatively heavier men, and 143 among the lighter men (chi-square = 5.82). Such a distribution would occur by chance in only about 2 in 100 trials.

Figure 10.6 is the corresponding picture for deaths from coronary heart disease. The relatively fatter men are indicated as having an excessive coronary death rate. In the upper half of the distribution of the sum of the skinfolds there were 69 coronary deaths compared but only 44 in the lower half of the distribution (chi-square = 5.53). Only about 1 in 50 trials would be so distributed by chance. On the other hand, relative body weight shows some tendency in the opposite direction, 52 coronary deaths in the upper half of the distribution, 61 in the lower half (chi-square = 0.72).

Figure 10.7 summarizes ten-year mortality in Croatia (Dalmatia and Slavonia). No analysis of probability is needed to conclude that mortality was inversely related to both relative body weight and body fatness. Compared with the men in the top 20 percent of the relative weight distribution, those in the bottom 20 percent had a death rate 3.5 times greater. Compared with

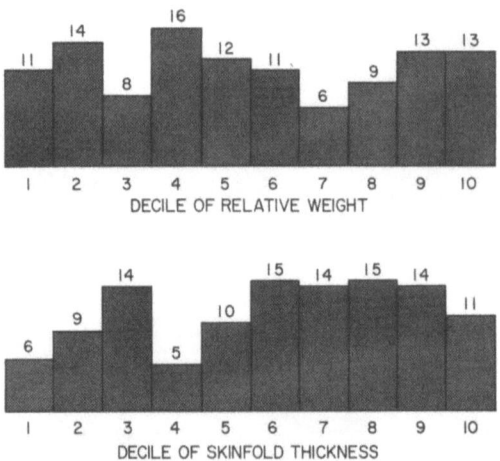

Figure 10.6. Distribution of ten-year coronary heart disease deaths into the age- and cohort-specific entry decile classes of relative body weight and of skinfold thickness for American railroad men. All men free of coronary heart disease at entry.

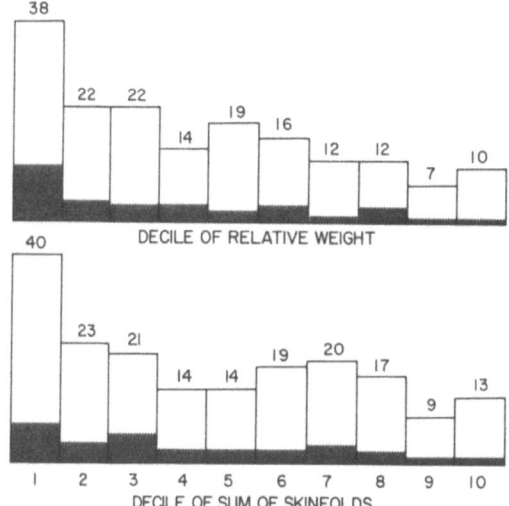

Figure 10.7. Distribution of all-causes ten-year deaths into the age- and cohort-specific entry decile classes of relative body weight and of skinfold thickness for Croatia (Dalmatia and Slavonia). All men free of coronary heart disease at entry. Shaded areas represent deaths from infectious disease.

the fatter men, the thinner Croatians had a similarly bad experience. It should be recalled, of course, that these Croatians generally tended to be lighter and much thinner than the Americans of the same age and height. Coronary deaths in Croatia were too few (21) to merit separate analysis; they will be included in an analysis of all Yugoslavs combined.

Figure 10.8 summarizes the distributions of the ten-year deaths in Finland from all causes. The men at the upper ends of the distributions of relative weight and of fatness had a favorable death rate compared with the lighter and thinner men. In the upper 20 percent of the relative weight distributions, 40 men died compared with 63 deaths among the same number of men at risk in the bottom 20 percent (chi-square = 6.10, $p = 0.014$). The penalty associated with being thin was even greater, 77 deaths for the bottom 20 percent in fatness versus 39 for the top 20 percent (chi-square = 15.13, indicating only about 1 chance in 10,000 for chance explanation).

Deaths in Finland attributed to coronary heart disease were seemingly independent of relative weight and body fatness; this is shown in figure 10.9. There were 46 CHD deaths in the upper half of the relative weight distribution, and 34 in the lower half (chi-square = 2.06, $p = 0.15$). In regard to skinfold thickness the split between upper and lower halves of the distribution was even closer, 40 versus 42.

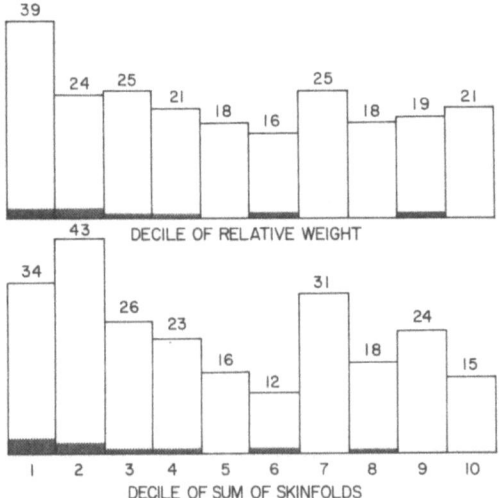

Figure 10.8. Distribution of all-causes ten-year deaths into the age- and cohort-specific entry decile classes of relative body weight and of skinfold thickness for east and west Finland. All men free of coronary heart disease at entry. Shaded areas represent deaths from infectious disease.

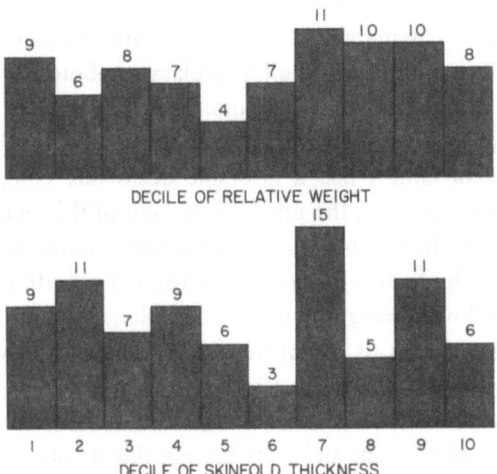

Figure 10.9. Distribution of ten-year coronary heart disease deaths into the age- and cohort-specific entry decile classes of relative body weight and of skinfold thickness for east and west Finland. All men free of coronary heart disease at entry.

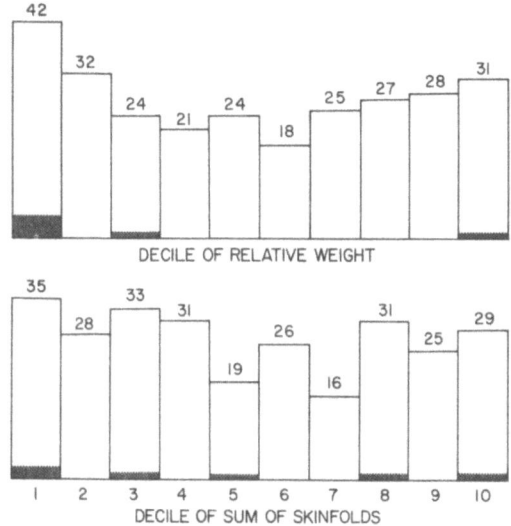

Figure 10.10. Distribution of all-causes ten-year deaths into the age- and cohort-specific entry decile classes of relative body weight and of skinfold thickness for Italy (Crevalcore, Montegiorgio, and Rome railroad). All men free of coronary heart disease at entry. Shaded areas represent deaths from infectious disease.

Figure 10.10 summarizes the ten-year all-causes death experience of the Italians. The highest mortality rate was observed in the men in the lowest 10 percent of the distributions of relative weight and of fatness, and the lowest death rates tended to be in the middle of the distributions; these trends are statistically rather impressive. In the distribution of relative body weight, the top and bottom quintiles accounted for 133 deaths while the other 60 percent included only 139 deaths; chi-square for this distribution = 8.97, indicating a probability of less than 2 in 1,000 for chance explanation. Chance could much more easily account for the observed distribution of the deaths in the deciles of skinfolds thickness.

Among the Italians free of coronary heart disease at entry, 49 died from that disease in ten years, 30 being in the top half of the relative weight distribution; with chi-square = 2.52, that distribution would be expected in about 1 our of 9 trials. In regard to entry body fatness the distribution of the deaths from coronary heart disease above and below the median was 28 and 21, respectively; chi-square = 1.02, and this distribution has about 1 out of 3 chances for occuring if there were no relation between body fatness and CHD death. For graphical display of the distribution into ten decile classes the Italians and the Greek men in this study are combined.

Figure 10.11 shows the distributions of ten-year all-causes deaths of the

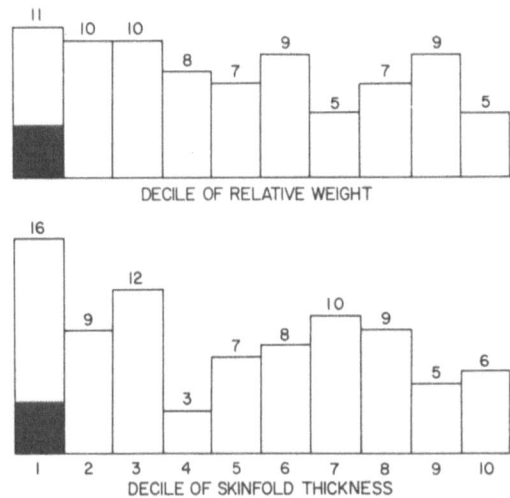

Figure 10.11. Distribution of all-causes ten-year deaths into the age- and cohort-specific entry decile classes of relative body weight and of skinfold thickness for Greece (Crete and Corfu). All men free of coronary heart disease at entry. Shaded areas represent deaths from infectious disease.

Greek men of Crete and Corfu. The apparent tendency of the death rate to be inversely related to relative body weight is not statistically convincing. For example, chi-square = 1.5 for the numbers observed above and below the median; and with 31 deaths in the bottom three deciles versus 50 in the other seven deciles chi-square = 2.72; those values have probability about 0.2 and 0.1, respectively. In the distribution of skinfold thickness the thinner Greeks had a higher death rate than can easily be attributed to chance. There were 37 deaths in the bottom 30 percent of the distribution, 55 in the upper 70 percent; chi-square test of the numbers observed and expected in the bottom 30 and the upper 70 percent of the distribution gives 10.22, a probability of chance explanation of less than 1 in 1,000.

Only 9 Greeks, initially CHD-free, died from that disease in ten years. The Greeks have been combined with the Italians for the examination of the relation of death from coronary heart disease to relative weight and to body fatness shown in figure 10.12. The tendency for the relatively heavier and fatter men to be more prone to death from coronary heart disease is evident. Among men in the upper half of the relative weight distribution, 37 died from CHD, and in the lower half 20 died from CHD (chi-square = 4.48, $p = 0.03$. The experience of the fatter men was also strongly in favor of a positive relation between fatness and risk of coronary death. In the top 20 percent of the skinfold distribution 20 men died from CHD; the expected

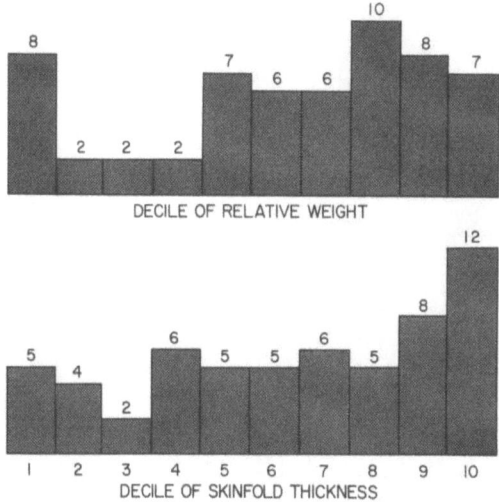

Figure 10.12. Distribution of ten-year coronary heart disease deaths into the age- and cohort-specific entry decile classes of relative body weight and of skinfold thickness for Italy and Greece (all five cohorts). All men free of coronary heart disease at entry.

number in the absence of a true relationship would be only 11.6; for the observed distribution of deaths between the top 20 percent and the other 80 percent of the men at risk, chi-square = 7.73, which would occur by chance in only about 5 out of a 1,000 trials.

The three Serbian cohorts, Velika Krsna, Zrenjanin, and Belgrade, have been combined for the distributions of ten-year all-causes deaths in the deciles of relative body weight and of sum of skinfolds (figure 10.13). The all-causes death rate is inversely related to both relative weight and body fatness. The death rate of the men in the top 20 percent of relative weight suffered less than half the death rate in the bottom 20 percent. The inverse relationship of death rate to body fatness is less marked but still statistically important; comparison of the deaths in the lower versus the upper halves of the distribution of the sum of the skinfold thicknesses gives chi-square = 4.88 and $p = 0.03$.

All five cohorts of men in Yugoslavia were combined for an examination of the distribution of deaths from coronary heart disease into the age- and cohort- specific deciles of relative weight and skinfold thickness (figure 10.14). The analysis fails to indicate any relationship of coronary heart death rate to either relative weight or body fatness.

Among 845 men of Zutphen judged free of coronary heart disease at the entry examination, 101 died from all causes in the ten-year follow-up. The distributions of those men into the decile classes of relative weight and of

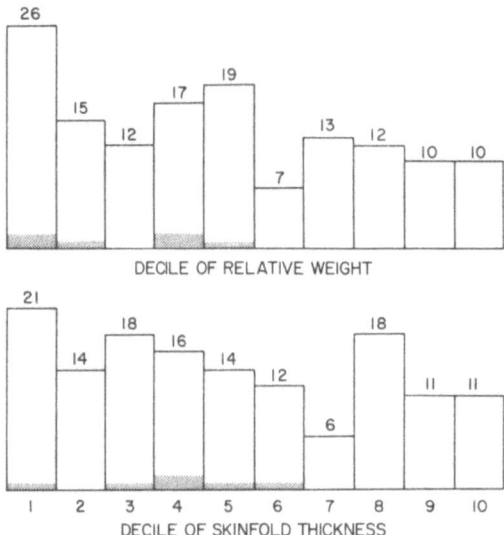

Figure 10.13. Distribution of all-causes ten-year deaths into the age- and cohort-specific entry decile classes of relative body weight and of skinfold thickness for Serbia (Velika Krsna, Zrenjanin, Belgrade). All men free of coronary heart disease at entry. Shaded areas represent deaths from infectious diseases.

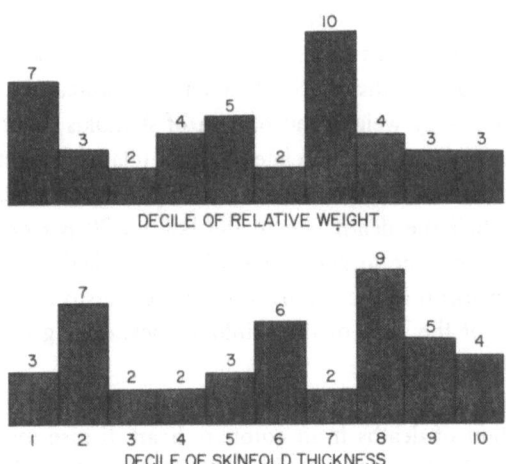

Figure 10.14. Distribution of ten-year deaths from coronary heart disease into the age- and cohort-specific entry decile classes of relative body weight and of skinfold thickness for Yugoslavia (Croatia and Serbia). All men free of coronary heart disease at entry.

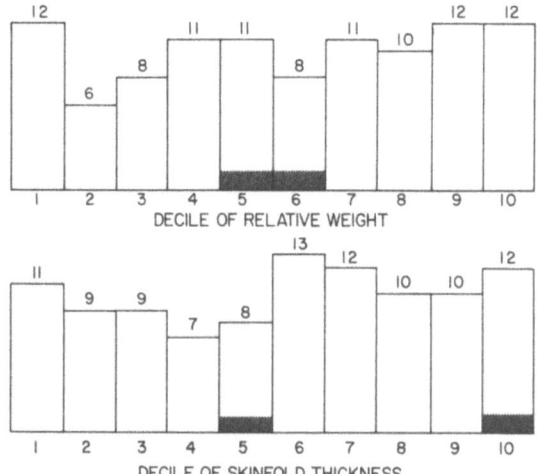

Figure 10.15. Distribution of ten-year all-causes deaths into the age- and cohort-specific entry decile classes of relative body weight and of skinfold thickness for Zutphen. All men free of coronary heart disease at entry. Shaded areas represent two deaths from infectious disease.

skinfold thickness at the time of the entry examination are shown in figure 10.15. The data show no relationship between weight or fatness and subsequent all-causes mortality. On the other hand, the data for those deaths caused by coronary heart disease, summarized in figure 10.16, indicate that the death rate from that cause is directly related to increasing relative weight and body fatness. There were 22 deaths in the upper half of the relative weight distribution and 9 in the lower half, a ratio of 2.44 (chi-square = 5.65, $p = 0.02$). The discrepancy between the upper and lower halves of the skinfolds distribution is even greater, 24 versus 7 (chi-square = 9.67), a distribution that would occur by chance in only about 2 out of 1,000 trials.

The relationship of ten-year all-causes death rate to relative body weight at entry in Japan is summarized in figure 10.17. There seems to be a definite trend for the death rate to be inversely related to relative body weight. Among the 299 men in the lower 30 percent of the distribution of relative weight, 48 died in ten years, and 71 of the other men died. This distribution yields chi-square = 7.02, $p = 0.008$. If deaths from infectious diseases are omitted chi-square = 4.15, $p = 0.042$.

Skinfold thickness was not measured at entry at Ushibuka. The distribution of the ten-year deaths at Tanushimaru in the decile classes of skinfold thickness indicated some trend for more of the thinner than the fatter men

178 | Seven Countries

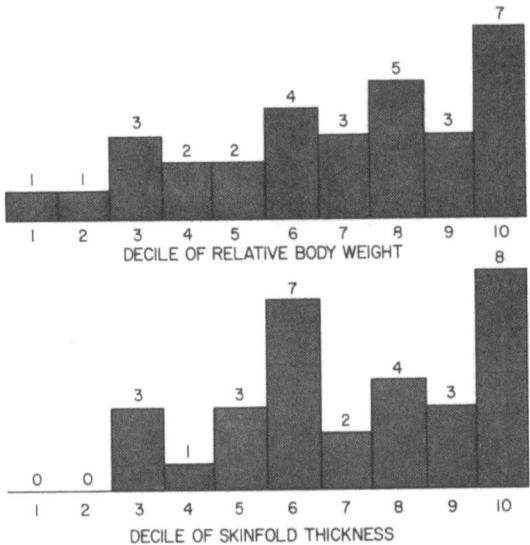

Figure 10.16. Distribution of ten-year deaths from coronary heart disease into the age- and cohort-specific entry decile classes of relative body weight and skinfold thickness for Zutphen. All men free of coronary heart disease at entry.

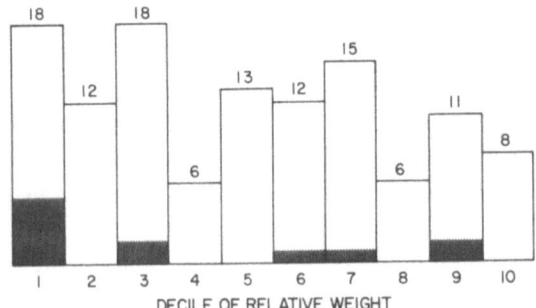

Figure 10.17. Distribution of ten-year all-causes deaths into the age- and cohort-specific entry decile classes of relative body weight for Japan (Tanushimaru and Ushibuka). All men free of coronary heart disease at entry. Shaded areas represent deaths from infectious diseases.

to die, but the trend is not statistically significant. Among men in the lower half of the distribution there were 30 deaths; in the upper half, 24.

During ten years of follow-up in Japan only 8 deaths were attributed to coronary heart disease, a number too small to warrant detailed analysis of any relationship to the entry characteristics of the men. For what it is worth it may be noted that 5 of those men were in the lower half of the distribution of relative weight, that is, the relatively underweight men. At the entry examination no evidence of coronary heart disease was found in any of the 8 men who subsequently died from the disease.

Infectious diseases. Out of a total of 1,512 deaths in ten years from all causes in this study, 74 were attributed to infectious diseases, 62 of them from tuberculosis. It is very probable that these men had acquired tuberculosis long before they entered this study, so the question arises as to whether the disease influenced their relative weight and body fatness as recorded at entry. In figures 10.7, 10.8, 10.9, 10.10, 10.11, 10.13, 10.15, 10.17, showing the distribution of all-causes deaths into the decile classes of relative weight and of skinfold thickness, deaths from infectious diseases are indicated by shaded portions of the columns. There is a distinct tendency for the deaths from infectious diseases to be concentrated in the lower decile classes, the lighter and thinner men. This explains some but not all of the tendency for the all-causes death rate to be inversely related to relative weight and to body fatness. Note that in the cohort of American railroad men, no deaths were attributed to infectious disease, but as noted earlier (see figure 10.5), there was a statistically significant trend for the relatively heavier men to have a lower ten-year death rate than the lighter men.

Curvilinear relationship. The current analysis of relationships within cohorts between mortality and relative weight or body fatness has involved no assumptions about the character of the relationships. On the other hand, in many reports about relative weight and obesity, it is implicitly assumed that any relationships to mortality are linear. However, in the five-year data from the Seven Countries Study, curvilinear U-shaped relations were suggested for Finland, rural Italy, and Zutphen (Keys 1970, p. 61, 73, 87). The ten-year follow-up continues to show such a trend for Italy (figure 10.10) and less clearly for Finland and Zutphen. Further analysis of this trend in the ten-year data requires a multivariate approach because intercorrelated variables are involved, so this subject is treated in more detail in chapter 15. It is enough to state here that for all-causes deaths a U-shaped distribution with body mass index clearly holds for the men in southern Europe, even when other characteristics of the men at entry are controlled. The tendency is similar but less marked for the men of northern Europe. For the American railroad men there is a suggestion that all-causes deaths have a curvilinear relationship to body mass index. For none of the cohorts or groups of cohorts is there an indication of a curvilinear relationship for coronary heart disease.

180 | Seven Countries

Incidence Rate

In the present study deaths from coronary heart disease represented only about one-fourth of all incidence of this disease during ten years among men who showed no evidence of the disease at the entry examinations.

Figure 10.18 shows the distribution into deciles of relative body weight at entry of the 305 Finns who became ten-year incidence cases. There is no statistically significant trend for the incidence of any of the diagnostic categories of coronary heart disease, or all of them combined, to be related to the age- and cohort-specific decile class of relative body weight. Among men below the median relative weight, 69 became cases of hard CHD and 573 exhibited no signs of any kind of CHD, and above the median the corresponding numbers are 82 and 554, so chi-square is only 1.39 ($p = 0.24$). All other comparisons result in still smaller values for chi-square.

Figure 10.19 shows the corresponding data with respect to the distribution of these Finns into decile classes of the sum of the skinfolds. Here again there is no suggestion that the incidence is in any way related to the entry characteristic skinfold thickness, taken to be a measure of body fatness or obesity. None of the chi-square values for the distribution of any of the categories of CHD is as large as 1.6.

The distribution in regard to relative weight decile classes of the men who developed CHD in Croatia in ten years is shown in figure 10.20. Hard CHD conforms to chance expectation in regard to the distribution of relative body weight; there are 13 men in each half of the distribution. For angina pectoris only, however, the distribution is 3 versus 10 (chi-square = 4.07, $p = 0.04$). For all cases of CHD combined, the distribution shows 27 cases and 620 noncases below the median and 41 and 591 above the median, so

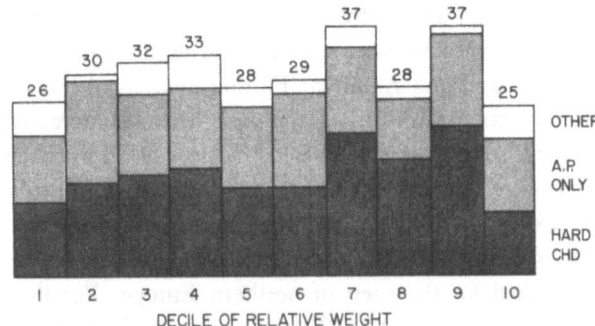

Figure 10.18. Distribution of ten-year incidence of coronary heart disease, by diagnostic category, into the age- and cohort-specific entry decile classes of relative body weight for east and west Finland. All men free of coronary heart disease at entry.

Overweight and Obesity | 181

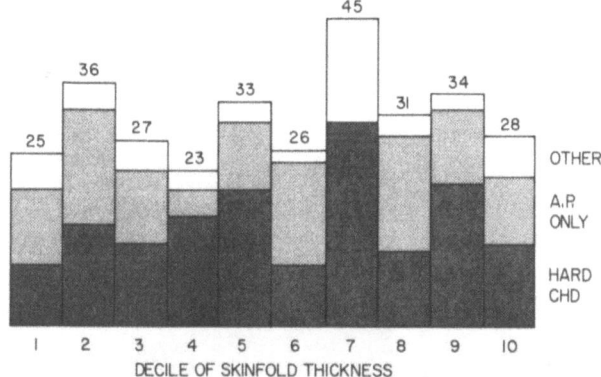

Figure 10.19. Distribution of ten-year incidence of coronary heart disease, by diagnostic category, into the age- and cohort-specific entry decile classes of skinfold thickness. All men free of coronary heart disease at entry.

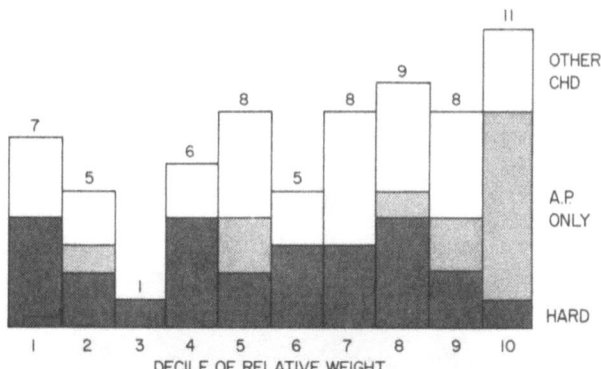

Figure 10.20. Distribution of ten-year coronary heart disease, by diagnostic category, into the age- and cohort-specific entry decile classes of relative body weight for Croatia (Dalmatia and Slavonia). All men free of coronary heart disease at entry.

chi-square = 3.40 and $p = 0.065$, and statistical significance cannot be claimed.

In regard to the distribution into the entry decile classes of the sum of the skinfolds, the ten-year data from Croatia more strongly indicate a relationship with angina pectoris only and with the total of all CHD incidence. The numbers above and below the median give chi-square = 6.43 and $p = 0.01$ for angina and chi-square = 6.15 and $p = 0.013$ for total CHD. Hard CHD incidence seems to be unrelated to the entry sum of the skinfolds.

182 | Seven Countries

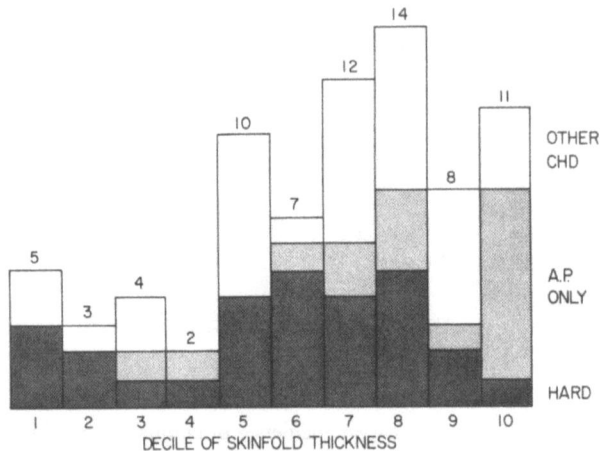

Figure 10.21. Distribution of ten-year coronary heart disease, by diagnostic category, into the age- and cohort-specific entry decile classes of skinfold thickness for Croatia (Dalmatia and Slavonia). All men free of coronary heart disease at entry.

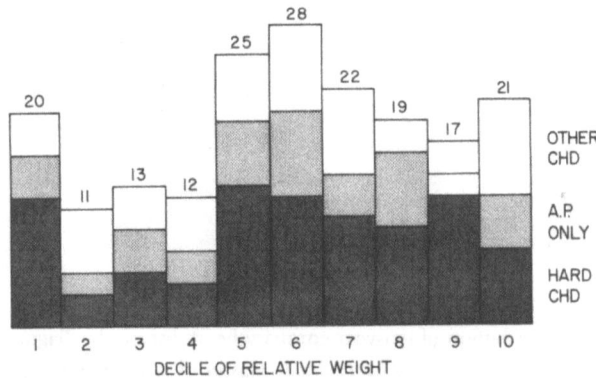

Figure 10.22. Distribution of ten-year incidence of coronary heart disease, by diagnostic category, into the age- and cohort-specific entry decile classes of relative body weight for Italy (Crevalcore, Montegiorgio, and Rome railroad). All men free of coronary heart disease at entry.

In the data for the Italians, shown in figure 10.22, there is no indication that entry relative weight was related to the ten-year CHD incidence among those free of the disease at entry when hard CHD, angina pectoris alone, and other CHD are considered separately. Combining all diagnostic categories, the distribution below and above the median was 81 cases and 1,050 noncases versus 107 and 1,009, yielding chi-square $= 4.44$, $p = 0.035$.

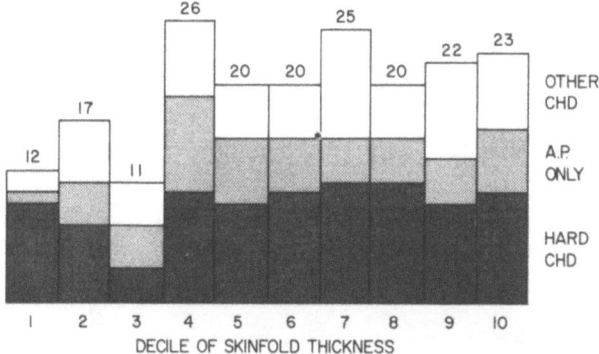

Figure 10.23. Distribution of ten-year coronary heart disease, by diagnostic category, into the age- and cohort-specific entry decile classes of skinfold thickness for Italy. All men free of coronary heart disease at entry.

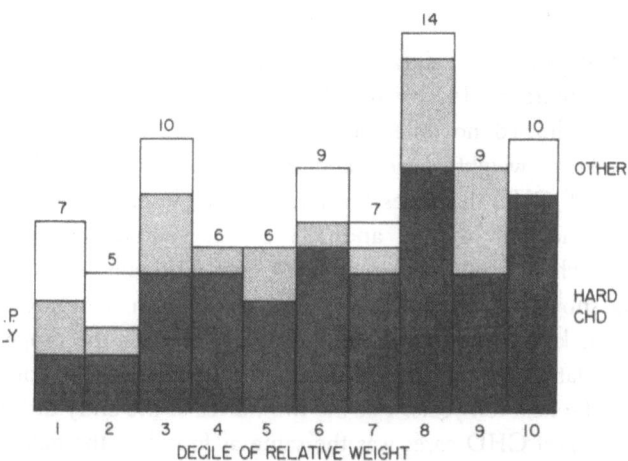

Figure 10.24. Distribution of ten-year incidence of coronary heart disease, by diagnostic category, into the age- and cohort-specific entry decile classes of relative body weight for Zutphen. All men free of coronary heart disease at entry.

In regard to the distribution into the entry skinfold decile classes, shown in figure 10.23, none of the above- and below-median comparisons gave a value of chi-square lower than 2.28, a probability of at least 7.5 percent chance distribution.

The corresponding analysis of the ten-year findings with the men of Zutphen is shown in figures 10.24 and 10.25. Hard CHD incidence tended to rise with increasing relative body weight; below the median, there were 18

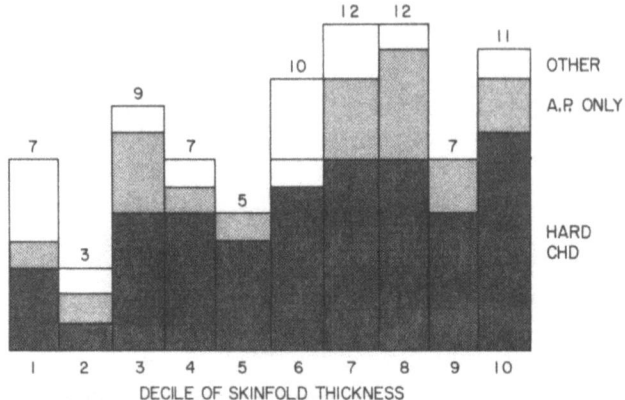

Figure 10.25. Distribution of ten-year incidence of coronary heart disease, by diagnostic category, into the age- and cohort-specific entry decile classes of skinfold thickness for Zutphen. All men free of coronary heart disease at entry.

cases and 357 noncases; above the median, the numbers were 33 and 333, giving chi-square = 5.14, $p = 0.023$. However, angina pectoris and other CHD cases showed no difference in numbers in the above- and below-median relative weight classes, and the comparison in regard to the incidence of all CHD diagnoses combined shows 34 cases and 357 noncases below the median, and 49 and 333 above, yielding chi-square = 3.44, $p = 0.064$, which would be interpreted conventionally as nonsignificant. The data shown in figure 10.25 for the distribution in regard to skinfold thickness make a somewhat more convincing case for the proposition that the relative fatness at entry was important for the incidence of coronary heart disease in the next ten years. For the two halves of the entry distribution the number of hard CHD cases was the same as found in the data for relative weight, but the distribution of cases of angina only was 7 and 12; for any CHD 31 and 52 (chi-square = 5.95, $p = 0.015$).

The experience of the Greeks of Crete and Corfu is shown in figure 10.26. As noted earlier, the incidence of coronary heart disease in the Greek cohorts was low, and the ten-year total of any CHD diagnosis was only 39 cases; 1,069 men never showed evidence of the disease. In regard to relative body weight, above- and below-median comparisons of numbers of men, CHD-free at entry, who eventually were given diagnoses of hard CHD gives 8 and 8, and for any CHD incidence, 19 and 20. In the distribution into the entry decile classes of skinfold thickness the above- and below-median classes give 7 and 9 for hard CHD; 21 and 17 for any diagnosis of coronary heart disease. These numbers give no suggestion that the incidence of

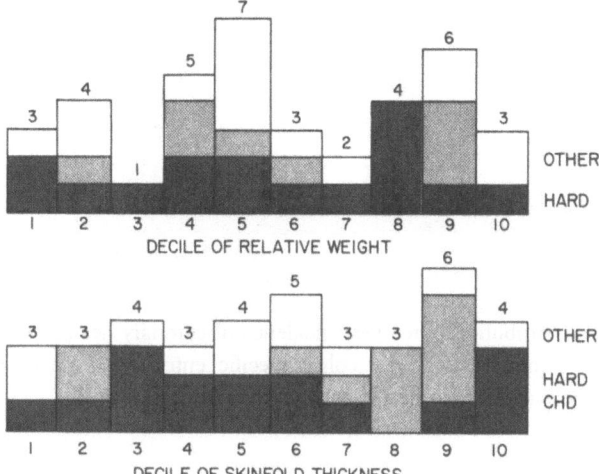

Figure 10.26. Distribution of ten-year incidence of coronary heart disease, by diagnostic category, into the age- and cohort-specific entry decile classes of relative body weight and of skinfold thickness for Greece (Crete and Corfu). All men free of coronary heart disease at entry.

coronary heart disease was related in any way to either relative weight or body fatness in the Greek men.

The corresponding ten-year follow-up data for the men in Serbia—Velika Krsna, Zrenjanin, and Belgrade—are given in figures 10.27 and 10.28. The tendency for the incidence of coronary heart disease to increase with increasing relative weight and increasing fatness is confirmed by chi-square

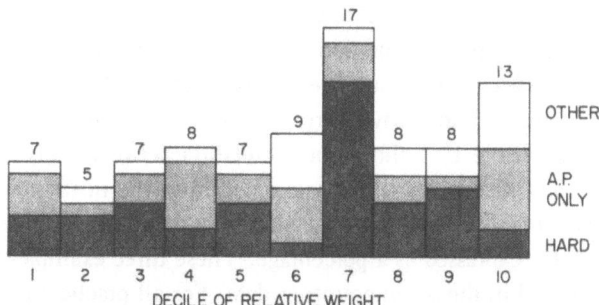

Figure 10.27. Distribution of ten-year incidence of coronary heart disease, by diagnostic category, into the age- and cohort-specific entry decile classes of relative weight for Serbia (Velika Krsna, Zrenjanin, and Belgrade). All men free of coronary heart disease at entry.

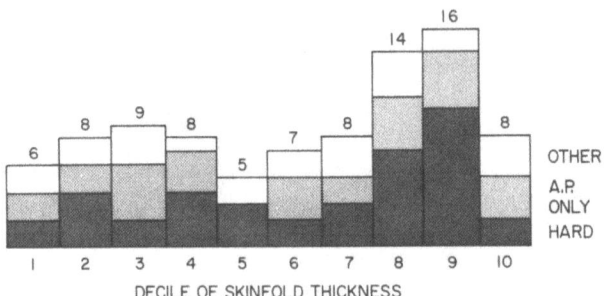

Figure 10.28. Distribution of ten-year incidence of coronary heart disease, by diagnostic category, into the age- and cohort-specific entry decile classes of skinfold thickness for Serbia. All men free of coronary heart disease at entry.

test for the total of all CHD cases combined in the distribution of the entry decile classes of relative weight. Below the entry median there are 34 cases and 685 noncases; above the median, 55 and 658 giving chi-square = 5.47, $p = 0.019$. Analysis of the data in regard to the distribution into the entry decile classes of the sum of the skinfold thickness does not show such an impressive difference from chance expectation. In the above- versus below-median comparison there are 24 versus 15 cases of hard CHD, but chi-square is only 2.14, $p = 0.14$. All CHD cases in the above-median class for skinfolds number 53 as compared with 36 in the below-median class; the result is chi-square = 3.26, $p = 0.07$.

Correlation with Other Variables

In our material body mass index is very highly correlated with the relative body weight as calculated from insurance company actuarial tables for the average weight of American men of given height and age. For the age range of the men at the entry examination, there is very little age trend in either the body mass index or the insurance company tables of average weight for height. So no more than a trivial error would result from disregard of age over that range. Table 10.1 shows the correlation between body mass index and relative body weight, the latter calculated from the insurance company height and weight tables, and the regression of body mass index on that relative body weight, expressed as a percentage. These three examples typify the relationship found in the seven countries data. For all practical purposes the body mass index for men aged 40 through 59 can be estimated from the relative body weight by multiplying the latter by 0.24. Conversely, relative body weight can be estimated from body mass index by multiplying the latter by 4.1.

It is interesting to check this simple method of estimating relative body weight with data from cohorts other than the American railroad, Crevalcore, and east Finland. Referring to figure 10.1, it may be noted that the mean body mass index ranges from 21.8 for Tanushimaru and 22.1 for Velika Krsna to 26.3 for the men of the Italian railroad. Multiplying by 4.1 gives estimated relative body weight values of 89, 91, and 108, respectively. The corresponding means of the recorded relative body weight are 90, 92, and 108.

Table 10.2 gives the product-moment coefficient of correlation between body mass index and eight other characteristics recorded at the entry examinations of the men in the sixteen cohorts. As noted earlier, table 10.1 shows that there is no appreciable correlation between BMI and age. The correlation between BMI and the sum of skinfold thickness is high, $r = 77$, on the average, but 40 percent of the variance of body fatness is still not explained by the body mass index. BMI is correlated with the index of laterality/linearity with a high degree of significance. In other words, the body mass index tends to reflect the shape of the skeleton. Although not surprising, this fact is commonly neglected in the effort to charge all overweight to obesity.

In all of the cohorts there is a statistically significant correlation between blood pressure, both systolic and diastolic, and BMI, but from the seven countries data it appears that some 94 percent of blood pressure variance remains unexplained by variations in body mass index. Serum cholesterol shows even less correlation than blood pressure with BMI. All except one of the Japanese cohorts show a small positive correlation between resting pulse rate and BMI. Finally, in all cohorts there was a significant negative correlation between BMI and cigarette smoking; smokers tend to have lower body weights than nonsmokers of the same height and age.

Other Studies

Death rate. Other studies are of two kinds, those of the American life insurance industry and those in which subject selection is free of the economic pressures that operate to make rated insurance policy holders a highly selected sample. By *rated* is meant persons who pay substantial extra premiums because they are grossly overweight. Such persons make up a tiny fraction of policy holders, perhaps 2 percent, but in the population at large persons of that degree of overweight are estimated to be around 7 percent (Keys 1955a,b), so the crucial question concerns the character of the sample of overweight persons who are willing to pay such a high price for life insurance.

The Metropolitan Life Insurance Company reported that the death rate from coronary heart disease of policy holders paying extra premiums because they were 20 percent or more above the average weight of all insurance applicants of the same height was 42 percent greater than that of men in their standard risk category (Dublin and Marks 1958). Such an outcome may justify the extra premiums demanded from such overweight applicants, but there is no evidence that the general population of overweight persons has a similar death rate. A long-accepted maxim in the insurance industry is that the insurance applicant "selects against the company," and the underwriter must protect the company in setting the premium rates. There is an interesting parallel in the history of life insurance rates for women. Formerly, women were required to pay larger premiums than men of the same age, and the few women policy holders proved to have a mortality that justified the high premiums charged. But the development of family policies brought many more women into the insured class, and the mortality experience of insured women dramatically changed; women proved to be better risks than men.

At the start of this chapter other serious defects in the American life insurance data and their analyses were mentioned. Still, for many years there was no challenge to the dictum of the American insurance industry about a simple direct relationship between relative weight and death rate. Insurance companies in other countries simply accepted the figures from the American actuaries; they either adjusted their rates accordingly or took the socialist view that life insurance should be a greater equalizer with no extra premium to anyone not obviously ill. Even in the United States the life insurance rating structure has given scant attention to the thesis of a simple direct relation to mortality to relative weight. In a review of the practice of the companies in 1958, Wilson (1958) stated that "all lives not more than 30 percent underweight and not more than 20 percent overweight are generally accepted at standard rates, on the theory that the broad group should yield 100 percent mortality." Today, many companies apply standard risk rates to persons as much as 25 percent or anything under 30 percent above average weight for height.

Questions about the teaching of the American life insurance industry were first directed to death from coronary heart disease. Yater et al. (1948) reported on 866 United States Army men under 40 years of age who died from coronary heart disease; autopsy data were at hand for more than half the cases. The distribution of relative body weight was substantially identical to that for soldiers of the same age who were killed in military accidents in the same period. Much publicity was given to a preliminary report on 80 of those soldiers dead of coronary heart disease whose average body weight at death was greater than that of men of the same height just entering the service at that time (French and Dock 1944). It turned out that the soldiers who died from heart attacks had gained weight since entering the service but no more so than the Army men who stayed well (Yater et al. 1948). The final report received no publicity.

Prospective research studies outside the life insurance industry are generally free from the insurance company defects of biased samples and inadequate entry examination data, but until lately they have reported little on mortality; the focus has been on the incidence of coronary heart disease and deaths were few. From Framingham it was reported that sudden death was unduly common among the 18 percent of the most overweight men but for the other 82 percent of the men there was no sign of a relationship between relative weight and sudden death (Kannel et al. 1967). The Framingham experience with all-causes deaths reported by Shurtleff (1974) shows a marked negative relation between mortality and relative weight, but the persons at risk are only specified as being alive at the last examination before death. A recent publication from Framingham shows an inverse relation between death rate and the incidence of cardiovascular disease but a positive regression of the incidence of cardiovascular disease on relative weight (Gordon and Kannel 1976). Framingham data will be examined further in the light of multivariate analysis in chapter 15.

A ten-year follow-up of almost all San Francisco longshoremen showed that mortality was directly related to age, blood pressure, and the use of cigarettes, but there was "no indication of a steady gradient between mortality and degree of overweight in this population" (Borhani, Hechter, and Breslow 1963). This somewhat oblique statement seems to reflect hesitancy to challenge the view popularized by insurance companies. Put more simply, the data show no significant relation between death rate and relative body weight.

In 1963 one-third of all men in Gothenburg, Sweden, born in 1913 were invited at random for medical examination and 88 percent accepted. After ten years of follow-up "the measures of obesity, skinfold thickness and relative weight showed no relation with the endpoints" (Tibblin, Wilhelmsen, and Werkö 1975); the end points were all-causes death, coronary heart death, incidence of coronary heart disease. The data from thirteen years of follow-up when 80 men had died were analyzed in more detail (Larsson 1978). The mean body mass index of the men who died was 24.3 (SE = 0.42) and 24.8 (SE = 0.12) of those who survived. Relative weight and obesity were not significant risk factors for any end point, including incidence of coronary heart disease. A major follow-up study in Stockholm similarly failed to find that relative body weight was a risk factor (Carlson and Böttiger 1972; Böttiger and Carlson 1973).

Ten years of follow-up of middle-aged men employed by the Chicago

Peoples Gas Company indicated that men in the upper half of the relative weight distribution were less apt to die prematurely than men in the lower half (Berkson et al. 1970). A more elaborate analysis utilized the fourteen-year experience of those men (Dyer et al. 1975). The men classified by body mass index into five groups of similar size were compared in regard to fourteen-year mortality from all causes, from cardiovascular-renal diseases, and from coronary heart disease. The 245 men with the highest body mass index did not differ significantly from the rest of the men in death rate from any of the classes of death cause.

The 243 gas company men in the lowest class of body mass index had the most unfavorable rates for all three classes of death, but the difference between their death rate and that of the other 990 men is statistically significant only for all-causes deaths ($t = 3.85$). On the other hand, the 228 men in the fourth body mass index class, who would be described as moderately overweight in the scale of the distribution of all men in the study, were outstanding in having the lowest death rate. Their fourteen-year all-causes death rate was 127.2 per 1,000; that of the other 1,005 men in the study was 215.9, 70 percent higher. The difference in these rates, 88.7 per 1,000, has a standard error of 29.3 ($t = 3.03$). That group of moderately overweight men was also favored in respect to deaths from coronary heart disease, having a rate of 48.2 per 1,000, only 63 percent of the rate of 76.6 for the rest of the men, but with $t = 1.50$ the difference is not significant.

The extensive application of the multiple logistic equation to the Chicago material by Dyer et al. will be discussed in chapter 15. Dyer et al. (1975) concluded: "The weights corresponding to the lowest mortality are found to be about 25–35 percent above the ideal published by the Metropolitan Life Insurance Company. Thus, for this cohort moderate overweight appears to be a sign of good health. Those individuals with the highest risk are those near the so-called ideal weight and those who are markedly obese, say with a relative weight above 150 or 160." The findings in the Seven Counties Study are in general agreement with that conclusion.

Only one large epidemiological series has indicated that body fatness is a risk factor for death. Fifteen years after a tuberculosis survey covering some 25,000 persons of both sexes, blacks and whites, ages 15 and over, estimates of body fatness were made from the fluorograms of the chest and a search was made for death records of the subjects (Comstock, Kendrick, and Livesay 1966). It was concluded that mortality was associated with fatness, but the analysis did not distinguish within the broad age groups 15–34, 35–54, 55 and over, thereby disregarding the fact that on the average body fatness increases markedly over the years from puberty to middle age and that age is the most important of all risk factors. In the report it was also claimed that death from coronary heart disease was also related to fatness, but it was admitted that the numbers were small. It is significant that for the persons aged 55 or more the data indicate decreasing mortality both from all causes and from coronary heart disease with increasing fatness.

The findings in a follow-up of hypertensive men classified in respect to relative weight are interesting. Dimond (1963) reported on 527 railway operating employees who developed hypertension between 1925 and 1942 and were followed to 1962. During the follow-up period 318 of these men died, 131 of the deaths being attributed to acute myocardial infarction and another 35 to myocardial failure. "Clinical obesity in this hypertensive group was associated with a significantly increased frequency of diabetes but was not related to the development of coronary heart disease, cerebral vascular accident, or to longevity" (p. 150). Sokolow and Perloff (1961) reported that hypertensive patients who are obese have a better prognosis than hypertensive patients otherwise comparable; they offered no explanation for the difference.

There are some suggestions that duration of life after a heart attack may be influenced by relative weight. In the combined material of the Framingham and Albany studies it appeared that among 234 men who died from coronary heart disease the 109 men who died suddenly tended, on the average, to be relatively heavier than the men whose deaths were not so abrupt (Doyle et al. 1976). There were some discrepancies between the two studies in this regard, and it should be noted that the data in the report do not show that relatively overweight men are unduly prone to die from this disease; they simply indicate that among men who die from this disease the overweight men tend to die more quickly. On the other hand, among 240 patients with acute myocardial infarction admitted to a hospital in Nashville, Tennessee, the thirty-day survival among the patients recorded as obese on admission was better than that of the patients judged to be normal in fatness, and the patients classified as being thin had the worst experience (Billings et al. 1949). These two reports are not necessarily discordant; the Albany-Framingham study concerned sudden death, in most cases before hospital admission was possible, whereas all of the Nashville patients survived long enough for hospital admission.

Incidence rate. The foregoing discussion on other studies focused on mortality, but the incidence rate of all coronary heart disease is much greater than the rate of death from that disease. In the present study 40 percent of the men who developed the disease in ten years died from that cause. In less prolonged studies the proportion of fatal to nonfatal cases is smaller. After five years of follow-up in the present study the coronary deaths represented only 20.6 percent of all men who were given diagnoses of the disease in that period (see Keys 1970, p. 188).

Many epidemiological studies have combined fatal and nonfatal cases in reporting on the incidence of coronary heart disease, an understandable expedient when numbers are small. However, the relationship of incidence to various previous characteristics is not necessarily the same for all manifestations of the disease. Angina pectoris may well be more closely associated with overweight than other categories of the disease. It stands to reason that with the same degree of limitation of the coronary circulation, physical exertion that involves movement of the mass of the body should more easily provoke angina in the overweight than in lighter persons.

The pioneering prospective studies that popularized the risk factor concept began with the conviction that besides discovering new risk factors they would document the importance of overweight as taught by the insurance industry. The attitude was apparent in the emphasis on relative weight in the first symposium in 1956 (Measuring the risk of coronary heart disease in adult population groups, 1957 *Am. J. Public Health* vol. 47, part 2). Overweight was stressed, in reporting the early experience of the Framingham study (Dawber, Moore, and Mann 1957), and later reports from that study continued the emphasis (Kannel et al. 1961; Dawber, Kannel, and Lyell 1963; Dawber and McNamara 1967). It was even stated: "We might expect a 20 percent reduction in weight in the obese to result in a 40 percent reduction in the chances of CHD" (Kannel and Gordon 1974). A more critical approach, with larger numbers of cases and appropriate multivariate methods, sharply downgraded the factor of overweight as risk at Framingham: "It would appear that physique in terms of relative weight or its equivalent might be accorded a relatively minor role in the etiology of coronary heart disease despite the striking relationship noted in the insurance data" (Gordon and Kannel 1973). As will be shown in chapter 15, further critical analysis of Framingham data showed that relative weight was not significant for coronary death or myocardial infarction.

In the prospective study of civil servants in Los Angeles relative weight did not appear to be related to the incidence of coronary heart disease in the first ten years of follow-up (Chapman and Massey 1964). After five more years of follow-up unifactor analysis indicated only a relatively insignificant relation of relative weight to incidence, but from a multifactor discriminant function analysis it was thought that ponderal index was significant for myocardial infarction for men starting at ages 30 to 39 but not for other ages (Chapman et al. 1971). There were only sixteen cases in the age group 30–39. Moreover, when there are multiple opportunities for chance to play a role, as here where several age groups were treated as independent samples, allowance for the fact should be made in the evaluation of probability; a finding of a result expected by chance 5 percent of the time is not very convincing when it occurs in only 1 of 4 trials.

In the Western Collaborative Group Study, 257 men developed coronary heart disease by the end of follow-up at 8.5 years, and their mean relative weight was greater than that of the men who stayed well (Rosenman et al. 1975). Nothing was reported about relative weight as a risk factor independent of other variables.

Japanese men living in Japan, in Hawaii, and in California were studied in a prospective study and followed for an average of five years (Robertson et al. 1977). It was concluded that relative weight was a risk factor for the men in Hawaii but not for those in Japan. Relative weight was expressed as departure from "standards" developed from a special study in Honolulu (Gordon, Kagan, and Rhoads 1975).

In Sweden rather elaborate follow-up studies failed to incriminate overweight or obesity as risk factors for the development of coronary heart disease in middle-aged men in Stockholm (Carlson and Böttiger 1972: Böttiger and Carlson 1973) and in Gothenburg (Larsson 1978). Several reviews have concluded that overweight and obesity could not be labeled as important risk factors for coronary heart disease (Heyden 1975; Mann 1974). The need for multivariate analysis is evident in many examples. For example, in Evans County, Georgia, the incidence of coronary heart disease among men in sedentary occupations was significantly higher than among men in jobs requiring physical effort, but there were also other important differences between the two categories of men; the sedentary men smoked more and had higher incomes and socioeconomic status.

Summary

Relative body weight and obesity (sum of skinfold thickness) varied widely among and within cohorts. The highest average relative weight was in Belgrade and in the Italian railroad, 108 percent of the average for American men of like age applying for life insurance, and the average for the Japanese men was only 86 percent on the same scale. The median sum of the skinfolds was highest at Belgrade with 39 mm, and the United States railroad men were next with 33 mm.

The differences among the cohorts in ten-year death rates and in incidence of coronary heart disease were not significantly related to differences in average relative weight or obesity.

Within none of the areas of this study was relative overweight or obesity associated with extra risk of all-causes death. Among the American railroad men the ten-year mortality semed to be independent of relative fatness, but a U-shaped relationship with relative weight was suggested. The lowest age-specific death rate was in the men in the seventh and eighth decile classes of relative weight.

In Finland, Croatia, Italy, Greece, Serbia, and Japan, the all-causes death rate tended to be inversely related to relative body weight and to relative fatness. At Zutphen the ten-year all-causes death rate was not significantly related to either relative weight or fatness.

For men with no evidence of coronary heart disease at entry, the ten-year death rate from that disease was not significantly related to either relative weight or body fatness in the United States, Finland, Italy, or Yugoslavia. At Zutphen, 11 of 31 men who died from coronary heart disease were in the top 20 percent of the distribution of body fatness at entry. In Greece, only 9 men, free of coronary heart disease at entry, died from the disease in ten years. In Japan, also, the number of coronary deaths (7) was too few for useful analysis.

The ten-year incidence of coronary heart disease, including nonfatal cases, involved 305 Finns with no evidence of the disease at entry. No category of coronary heart disease, nor all combined, was related to either relative weight or obesity. The ten-year incidence of coronary heart disease in Croatia and Italy was similarly not significantly related to either relative weight or obesity.

In Serbia, 89 men, CHD-free at entry, developed the disease in ten years. Fifty-five of the cases were in the upper half of the distribution of relative weight at entry, but that disproportion depended entirely on an excess of cases in the seventh decile class of relative weight. In Japan only 19 men suffered myocardial infarction or died from coronary heart disease in ten years. There was no indication that the incidence of coronary heart disease was related to relative weight or fatness in Japan.

For the American railroad men there are no data on the incidence of nonfatal coronary heart disease in the second five years of follow-up, but in the first five years the incidence of coronary heart disease with any diagnosis was directly related to relative body weight and to obesity. That relationship depended on diagnoses of uncomplicated angina pectoris and other soft diagnoses. The incidence of hard CHD was not related to relative weight or body fatness.

In none of the areas of this study was overweight or obesity a major risk factor for death or the incidence of coronary heart disease. In most of the areas the probability of death in ten years appeared to be least for the men somewhat over the average in relative weight or fatness. Findings in other prospective studies support the conclusion that overweight and obesity are much less serious risk factors than popularly supposed and suggested by the older reports from the life insurance industry.

11 | Physical Activity

All men in this study were classified at entry according to their habitual physical activity. Class 1 men were sedentary, engaging in little exercise; class 2 men were moderately active during a substantial part of the day; and class 3 men performed hard physical work much of the time. Classification was based on the responses to questions about the occupation and usual activities, including part-time jobs and notable nonoccupational exercise. In addition, the American railroad men answered a detailed questionnaire about leisure time and recreational activity, but only their occupational activity is considered here.

The sampling design for the American and Italian railroad men sought to provide random samples of men contrasting in physical activity by the nature of their jobs. In both countries railroad men are remarkably stable in their occupations, and the work in those occupations is defined in detail. For the great majority of the men in the other fourteen cohorts the classification by activity also turned out to be determined by their occupation. Most men reported some nonoccupational activity—work around the home, maintaining a small garden, walking or cycling to work, occasional hunting—but this rarely involved strenuous exercise or many hours a week. Vigorous exercise for its own sake was extremely uncommon, and most of the men were not concerned about physical fitness. Sports were universally popular—as something to follow as spectators, commonly on the radio or television.

Some American men reported bowling as a recreation, but such vigorous exercise as jogging or tennis had not begun to be popular when this study started. In Finland, Sunday cross-country skiing was fairly common among men in all occupations, but it was generally done at an easy pace, often as a family outing, a bit more energetic but otherwise something like the family walk after Sunday dinner in more southerly parts of Europe. Except for the Finnish and American cohorts, the idea of exercise for its own sake was considered a little mad by men beyond the age of 40; that view prevails today in many rural areas.

In the final classification, allowance was made, when warranted, for exercise beyond that required by the occupation, but this affected very few men. Occasionally, men in relatively sedentary occupations reported secondary work, mostly seasonal, that merited upgrading from class 1 to class 2. Downgrading was justified for a few men who had long done heavy work but in recent years were pleased to "take it easy." It should be noted again that our analyses concern only men with no evidence of cardiovascular disease at entry, men who were not limited in activity by health.

Activity class 1 embraces accountants, artists, barbers, bartenders, clerks, dentists, druggists, engineers, lawyers, managers, officials, pastors, physicians, priests, proprietors, salesmen, shoemakers, tailors, taxi drivers, teachers, watchmen, and writers. In class 1 are most of the American railroad men—executives, clerks, dispatchers—and the Italian railroad station masters and clerks. Activity class 2 applies to bakers, butchers, carpenters, drivers who load and unload their vehicle, electricians, mechanics, plumbers, shepherds, many small shopkeepers and peddlers, and tile setters. Activity class 3, embracing a majority of the men in Europe and Japan, included blacksmiths, almost all of the farmers, fishermen (a small group in Dalmatia and most of the men in Ushibuka, Japan), common laborers, masons, plasterers, quarriers, road builders (old-style methods), and railroad maintenance men in Italy. None of the American railroad men in this study were in class 3. The list of occupations into which the men were classified has been published (Keys et al. 1967, pp. 350–354); occupations were used as a guide and were not the only criterion for classification by physical activity.

Table 11.1 shows, for men without cardiovascular disease at entry, the percentages in the three activity classes in each cohort. Class 1 contained from 3.9 percent of the men at Tanushimaru to 99.4 percent at Belgrade; class 3 ranged from 0 percent at Belgrade and United States railroad to 80 percent in west Finland. In some cohorts small numbers in class 1 mean that incidence rates in that class have large standard errors; combinations of cohorts allow more meaningful comparisons between activity classes. Accordingly, east and west Finland are combined as Finland; Crevalcore and Montegiorgio, as rural Italy; Crete and Corfu, as Greece; the two Japanese cohorts, as Japan; and all the Yugoslav cohorts except Belgrade as Yugoslavia.

Table 11.1. Distribution by physical activity class at entry in men free of cardiovascular disease (activity class 1 = sedentary; 2 = moderate activity; 3 = heavy work, very active).

Cohort	Activity class (%)			Cohort	Activity class (%)		
	1	2	3		1	2	3
U.S. railroad[a]	49.7	35.3	0	Montegiorgio	5.8	25.8	68.4
Dalmatia	7.9	11.6	80.5	Zutphen	23.7	65.7	10.6
Slavonia	17.1	9.2	73.7	Crete	6.6	30.9	62.5
Tanushimaru	3.9	36.6	59.5	Corfu	31.0	37.8	31.2
East Finland	9.6	12.6	73.8	Rome railroad	22.0	40.4	37.6
West Finland	7.5	12.5	80.0	Velika Krsna	8.5	24.5	67.0
Ushibuka	7.6	17.1	75.3	Zrenjanin	35.2	35.2	29.6
Crevalcore	10.5	18.8	70.7	Belgrade	99.4	0.6	0

a. 15.1 percent not readily classifiable between activity classes 1 and 2.

Correlation with Other Variables

Before assessing the possible relationship of physical activity to the subsequent experience, we shall examine some characteristics of the men in the different classes of physical activity who showed no evidence of cardiovascular disease at entry. Age is important because, as noted in chapter 6, the average experience in this study is that a difference of a single year of age is associated with a 9 percent difference in the all-causes death rate. The age effect is about half as great for the incidence of coronary heart disease.

In ten of the sixteen cohorts there was no significant difference in age between the activity classes, but in four the average age decreased significantly with increasing activity. The difference in average age in activity class 1 minus the most active men was 1.8 years for Montegiorgio, 2.7 years for both the American railroad and the Ushibuka men, 5.0 years for the Serbians at Velika Krsna. The average expectation is that these differences should be associated with a difference in all-causes death rate of 16 percent for Montegiorgio, 24 percent for the American and Ushibuka men, 45 percent for the Serbians at Velika Krsna. In contrast, at Zutphen the least active group averaged 1.5 years younger than the men in the very active class. Because all but three men in the Belgrade cohort were classified as sedentary, no examination of the age relationship is possible.

Accordingly, for five cohorts age could be a confounding variable in comparisons of incidence rates in the physical activity classes. For this reason here and in other chapters the rates are age standardized. In all multivariate analyses (chapter 15), age, in single years, is one of the independent variables.

In seven cohorts, men in the three activity classes did not differ significantly in average resting blood pressure at entry: east Finland, west Finland, Tanushimaru, Ushibuka, Zutphen, Rome railroad, Zrenjanin. At Belgrade, again, no comparisons are possible. In all of the remaining eight cohorts the mean blood pressure was lowest in the men with the most physical activity. In some cases, notably the American railroad and Velika Krsna, some part of the blood pressure relationship may be attributed to the relationship of activity to age. The differences in mean systolic blood pressure, millimeters of mercury, for most active men minus least active men are as follows: Dalmatia, -7.3; Slavonia, -2.2; Corfu, -7.4; Crete, -3.2; Crevalcore, -5.8; Montegiorgio, -6.1; Velika Krsna, -6.4; American railroad, -2.2. Not all of these differences are statistically significant.

Serum cholesterol concentration did not vary with physical activity in west Finland, Tanushimaru, Ushibuka, or American railroad men. In east Finland the mean value for serum cholesterol was 6.5 mg/dl higher in class 3 than in class 1, but the difference is not statistically significant. In all other cohorts the men in activity class 3 had the lowest average cholesterol values, the difference from the sedentary men ranging from 4.3 mg/dl (Montegiorgio) to 17.5 (Dalmatia). Considering all fifteen cohorts in which comparison is possible, the average cholesterol value was 7.2 mg/dl lower in the more active than in the sedentary men in the same cohort ($SE = 2.3$).

It is not possible to conclude that these data indicate a cholesterol-lowering effect of physical activity. Five of the fifteen cohorts do not show lower cholesterol values in the most active men, and in the other cohorts the most active men generally had the lowest incomes and therefore the smallest leeway to maintain a rich diet. But whatever may be the explanation of the tendency toward lower cholesterol levels in the most active men, the fact remains that they tended to have the least unfavorable cholesterol concentrations.

In all cohorts the average resting pulse rate was inversely related to the activity class and was lowest in the most active men. The average difference between the most active men and their sedentary fellows was 5.03 beats per minute ($SD = 2.99$, $SE = 0.77$, $t = 6.53$). Typical means for activity classes 1, 2, and 3, respectively, are 74.8, 67.2, and 66.5 beats per minute for west Finland; 80.6, 77.3, and 75.8 for Dalmatia. In the American railroad cohort the average for the clerks and executives was 72.6 and for the switchmen 70.4; standard errors are 0.37 and 0.42, respectively, and $t = 3.90$.

At the entry examinations the vital capacity, the maximum forced expiratory volume, was measured in only about half of the men in the United States railroad and in none of the men in Dalmatia, Slavonia, Tanushimaru, Ushibuka, Zutphen, or the Rome railroad. For the seven cohorts with acceptable measurements at entry, the vital capacity averages for classes 1, 2, and 3, respectively, were 2.34, 2.40, and 2.44 liters/m of height. Except for the men of Crete, the mean values of the most active men (class 3) were higher than those of the sedentary men in the same cohort. Though in most of the cohorts the higher values for the most active men are statistically significant, the differences are really very small, only an average of 4.6 percent.

Ten-year Death Rate

Before analyzing relationships within cohorts the first question is whether differences in the incidence of death and coronary heart disease in the follow-up are related to the differences shown in table 11.1. Are the proportions of less active to more active men in the cohorts reflected in the ten-year death and CHD incidence rates? Figure 11.1 compares the percentages of sedentary men in the cohort groups with their ten-year age-standardized death rates from all causes. There is a distinct tendency for mortality to fall with increasing percentage of relatively sedentary men in the group. The Belgrade group is important in this regard, but even omitting Belgrade the

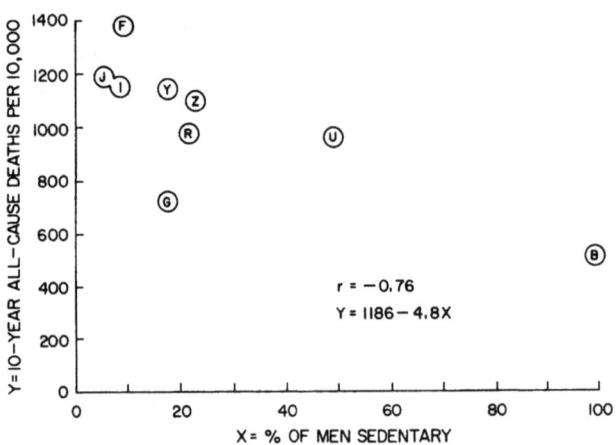

Figure 11.1. Ten-year all-causes age-standardized death rates of population samples versus percentage of sedentary men in those samples. All men aged 40–59 and free of cardiovascular disease at entry. B = Belgrade; F = Finland; G = Greece; I = rural Italy; J = Japan; R = Rome railroad; U = American railroad; Y = Yugoslavia except Belgrade; Z = Zutphen.

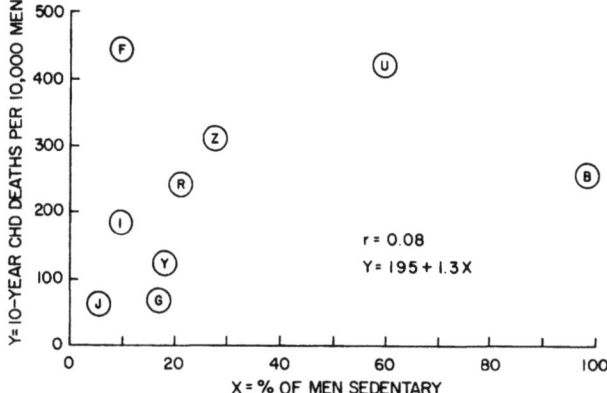

Figure 11.2. Ten-year coronary heart disease age-standardized death rates of population samples versus percentage of sedentary men in those samples. All men aged 40–59 and free of evidence of cardiovascular disease at the start of follow-up. Groups as in figure 11.1.

correlation is interesting, $r = -0.41$. This must not be overinterpreted; the conclusion is simply that the differences among the groups in mortality are in no way explained by the differences in physical activity, unless it is proposed that being sedentary is associated with better health.

Figure 11.2 shows that the differences among the groups in CHD death rate are unrelated to the representation of sedentary men in those groups. The incidence rates of hard CHD (infarct or coronary death) and any CHD (any diagnosis of coronary heart disease) are examined in figures 11.3 and 11.4. For neither end point is there any indication that the proportion of sedentary men in the population makes any difference to the average risk of developing coronary heart disease in that population. For all of these comparisons the limitations of justifiable conclusions are the same; consideration of the frequency of inactivity in these groups does not help to understand why they differ as they do in the incidence of this disease. But this negative finding says nothing about the possible importance of differences of physical activity within groups. That question is examined below.

American Railroad Men. Of the American railroad men 15.1 percent were not readily classifiable as activity class 1 or 2. Although called clerks by the union and the employer, on closer scrutiny they were not ordinary sedentary clerks; they worked in warehouses and other places where they were less sedentary. At entry the nonsedentary clerks and miscellaneous men did not differ significantly from the men in purely sedentary jobs in any of

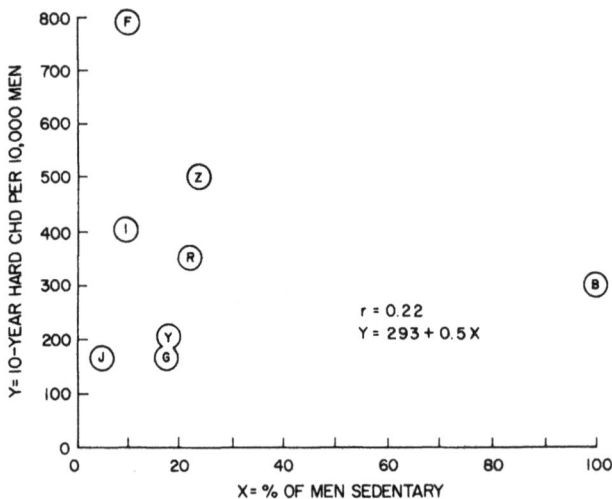

Figure 11.3. Ten-year age-standardized incidence of hard CHD (myocardial infarction or death from coronary heart disease) in population samples versus percentage of sedentary men in those samples. All men aged 40–59 and free of cardiovascular disease at entry. Groups as in figure 11.1.

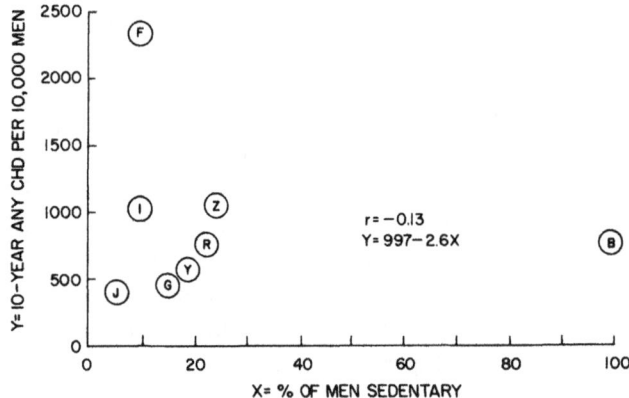

Figure 11.4. Ten-year age-standardized incidence of any CHD (any diagnosis of coronary heart disease) in population samples versus percentage of sedentary men in those samples. All men aged 40–59 and free of cardiovascular disease at the start of follow-up. Groups as in figure 11.1.

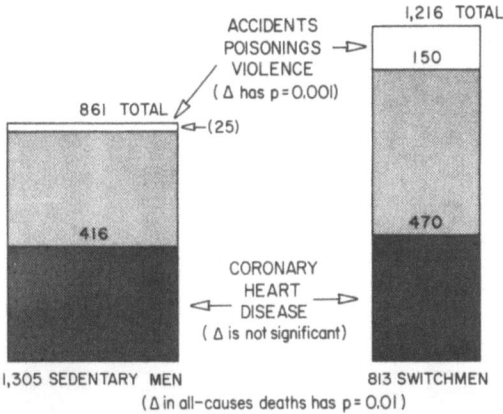

Figure 11.5. For American railroad men, ten-year age-standardized deaths per 10,000 at risk classified by habitual physical activity in their occupation. All men free of evidence of cardiovascular disease at entry. Width of the bars is proportional to the number at risk.

the suggested risk factors or in the five-year incidence of death and coronary heart disease (Taylor, Blackburn, and Keys 1970), and they did not differ significantly in the ten-year experience. Accordingly, the analysis of the ten-year experience of the railroad cohort compares these men, labeled class 1, with the more active switchmen, class 2.

Figure 11.5 summarizes the findings for men free from cardiovascular disease at entry. The age-standardized all-causes death rate of activity class 1 was only 71 percent that of the more active men, the switchmen; that difference would be expected by chance in fewer than 1 in 100 trials. An important part of this unfavorable experience of the more active men was a highly significant difference ($p < 0.001$) in deaths caused by accidents, poisonings, and violence. Excluding those deaths the difference in mortality in the two activity classes is not significant ($p = 0.18$). The switchmen also had a higher rate of death from coronary heart disease, but the difference does not approach significance; it would be expected to occur by chance alone in 45 percent of trials.

Finland. The relationship in Finland between physical activity and all-causes mortality in the ten-year follow-up, shown in figure 11.6, is in great contrast to the findings in the American railroad cohort. In Finland the all-causes death rate of the sedentary men was 62 percent greater than that of the moderately active men (class 2), 2.33 times that of the very active men who made up over three-fourths of the entire study population in

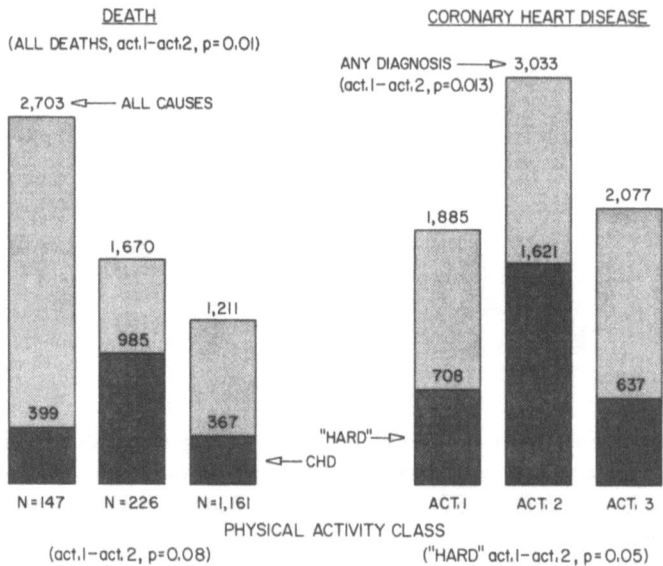

Figure 11.6. For Finland, ten-year age-standardized incidence of death and of coronary heart disease per 10,000 at risk classified by habitual physical activity. All men free of cardiovascular disease at entry.

Finland. The bad experience of the sedentary men is statistically highly significant even when compared only with the moderately active men ($p = 0.008$).

The finding of a large progressive negative gradient of death rate from class 1 to class 3 is important, but this concerns all-causes deaths and does not necessarily support the thesis that inactivity causes or promotes coronary heart disease. For coronary deaths there is no difference between activity classes 1 and 3, but class 2 men had a rate 2.5 times that of class 1 men and 2.7 times that of class 3 men.

The special vulnerability to coronary heart disease of the moderately active Finns is confirmed by the data on hard and any CHD incidence. The incidence rate of hard CHD in the moderately active men was 2.3 times that of the sedentary men and 2.5 times that of the very active men. For the incidence of any CHD the corresponding multiples are 1.6 and 1.5; these differences, like those for hard CHD, are statistically highly significant, but there are no significant differences in either hard or any CHD between the sedentary and the most active men.

As stated earlier, the mean values for entry risk factors in the men in the three activity classes were not significantly different in east or in west Finland. When east and west Finland are combined, there is still no suggestion that the moderately active Finns differed from the men in classes 1 and 3 in age or smoking habits. However, the mean systolic pressure in class 2 was 2.2 mm higher than in classes 1 and 3 (SE = 1.4). Mean serum cholesterol in class 2 was 5.54 mg/dl higher than in the other activity classes, but because SE = 3.97, this is not significant. These small differences could not explain more than a tiny fraction of the indicated higher susceptibility of the class 2 men to coronary heart disease.

The main peculiarity in the all-causes death rates in the three activity classes can be attributed to a greatly excessive death rate from causes other than coronary heart disease in class 1. The numbers of coronary and other deaths in class 1 are 7 and 37; the corresponding numbers for class 2 are 18 and 13, and the result is chi-square = 14.54. The peculiarity could also be attributed to a remarkable predilection of the men in activity class 2 to die from coronary rather than other causes; their high susceptibility to coronary heart disease is evident in the right side of figure 11.6.

These findings provoked a review of all death records of the Finns in activity classes 1 and 2. This confirmed the coronary deaths and the fact that deaths from heart disease other than coronary were very few (4 in activity class 1, 3 in class 2). The question that remains is why the sedentary Finns were excessively prone to die from causes other than coronary heart disease; neoplasms account for around half of the excess. Why the moderately active Finns were so susceptible to coronary heart disease is even more mysterious.

Rural Italy. After five years of follow-up the incidence rate of myocardial infarction in rural Italy (Crevalcore and Montegiorgio) was highest in the sedentary men, lowest in the very active men, and intermediate in the men with moderate physical activity. However, there were few cases, and the differences were not statistically significant (Menotti et al. 1969). The ten-year experience of these men, summarized in figure 11.7, is confirmatory.

The all-causes death rate in the sedentary men was 53 percent higher than in the moderately active men, 81 percent higher than in the very active men, and those differences are statistically significant ($t = 1.96$ and 3.12, respectively). The coronary death rate of the sedentary men was 2.58 times that of the moderately active men, 3.57 times that of the very active men with t values of 1.92 and 3.12, respectively. Neither for all-causes or coronary deaths are the differences between activity classes 2 and 3 statistically significant ($t = 1.03$ and 0.75).

The activity classes are compared in regard to the incidence of coronary heart disease on the right side of figure 11.7. Here again the disadvantage of the less active men is evident; in the sedentary men the incidence rate of hard CHD was 60 percent higher than in the moderately active group, 2.5

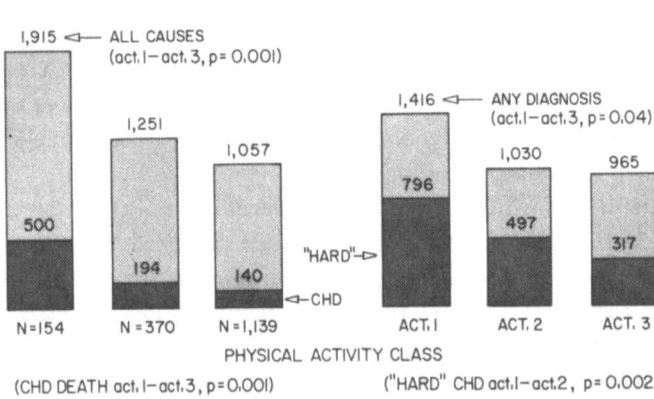

Figure 11.7. For rural Italy (Crevalcore and Montegiorgio), ten-year age-standardized incidence of death and of coronary heart disease per 10,000 at risk. All men free of cardiovascular disease at entry.

times higher than in the very active men, the latter difference having $p = 0.002$. For the incidence of any CHD the differences are in the same direction but smaller. Any incidence was 47 percent higher in the sedentary rural Italians than in the most active men in their cohorts; that $p = 0.04$ means such a difference could occur by chance in about 1 out of 25 trials.

This experience indicates that in rural Italy physical inactivity is a risk factor for coronary heart disease; the risk of developing the disease is inversely related to the habitual level of physical activity. Earlier we noted that the sedentary rural Italians tended to have higher blood pressures and serum cholesterol concentrations than their more active fellows. In rural Italy the sedentary men also tended to have a faster resting pulse rate and to more often be heavy smokers than their more active fellows. The men in activity classes 2 and 3 did not differ significantly in their ten-year experience so they are combined for comparison with class 1. The mean differences for class 1 minus classes 2 and 3 (142 and 1,416 men, respectively) are as follows: systolic BP, 5.86 mm Hg (SE = 1.818, $t = 3.22$); cholesterol, 3.61 mg/dl (SE = 3.60, $t = 1.00$); resting pulse, 6.78 beats per minute (SE = 1.12, $t = 6.05$). Comparison of the numbers of heavy smokers (twenty or more cigarettes daily) also indicates that men in class 1 are more at risk than the men in classes 1 and 2 (chi-square = 1.32). Though these comparisons show the sedentary men at a disadvantage and the differences in blood pressure and pulse rate are highly significant, it is doubtful that the differences in coronary incidence can be fully explained in this way. Finally, we note that the differences in coronary death rates do not account for more than a part of the total difference in all-causes death rates. The noncoronary deaths for classes 1, 2, and 3, respectively, are 1,415, 1,057 and 917. The death rate for the sedentary men is significantly higher ($p = 0.03$) than that of the most active men. There is no significant difference between classes 1 and 2 ($p = 0.19$) or between classes 2 and 3 ($p = 0.41$).

Rome Railroad. The Rome railroad men were classified by physical activity according to occupation, as was done with their American counterparts; about one-third of the cohort was made up of men habitually doing heavy manual work. The ten-year experience of the Rome railroad men who showed no evidence of cardiovascular disease at entry is summarized in figure 11.8.

In spite of the impressive differences in the height of the bars for all-causes death rate, the differences between activity classes are not statistically significant. The largest difference, that between classes 1 and 3, has $p = 0.07$, which means that the observed difference could be expected by chance in about 1 out of 14 trials. For coronary heart death, however, the difference between classes 1 and 3 has a value of $p = 0.02$, whereas the difference between classes 1 and 2 has $p = 0.06$.

Evaluation of the incidence of nonfatal coronary heart disease in the Ital-

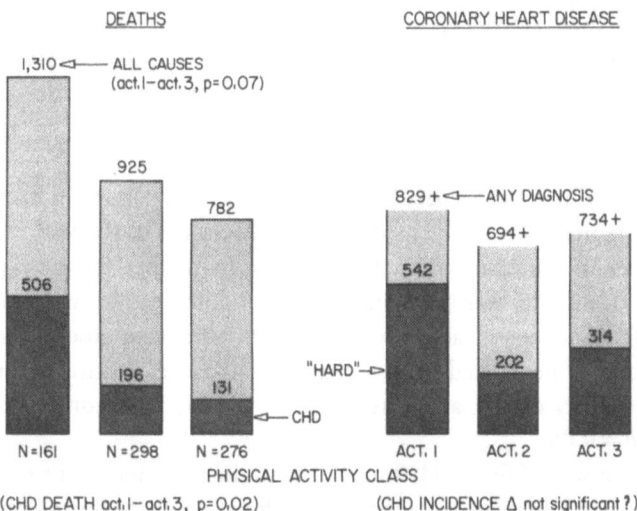

Figure 11.8. For Rome railroad men, ten-year age-standardized incidence of death and of coronary heart disease per 10,000 classified by habitual physical activity. All men free of cardiovascular disease at entry.

ian railroad cohort is limited by the fact that a substantial number of the men were not reexamined on the tenth anniversary of entrance. The right side of figure 11.8 is based on the incomplete sample reexamined plus the death and disability records of the Italian State Railroad, which, like the Railroad Retirement Board in the United States, seldom misses deaths or major illness and disability for the simple reason that those events allow claims for payments by the worker or his heirs. The rates for hard CHD should not be seriously in error, but it is possible that an appreciable number of soft diagnoses of coronary heart disease escaped notice. Such as they are, the rates for any CHD do not indicate a real difference between the activity classes, but the rate of hard CHD in class 1 is close to being significantly higher than the rate in class 2, $p = 0.06$. The difference between classes 1 and 3 does not approach significance. The conclusion is that the data available from the Rome railroad men do not indicate any significant difference between the activity classes in any form of coronary heart disease other than coronary death.

Menotti et al. (1969) analyzed the death records over four years of 105,595 employees of the Italian State Railroad who were 40 to 59 years old at the start. Among the men in jobs requiring the lowest physical activity, the death rate from coronary heart disease was significantly higher than for the men classed as moderately or very active; there was no difference between the latter two classes. On the other hand, the men in activity class 3 had the highest all-causes death rate. Other relevant characteristics of the men in the three activity classes are not reported but it may be remarked that the men doing the heaviest work are, as elsewhere, at the bottom of the socioeconomic scale with attendant limitations in expenditures for expensive foods and cigarettes.

Zutphen. Zutphen was peculiar among the sixteen cohorts in that the majority of the men were in the moderate activity class. The ten-year experience at Zutphen is summarized in figure 11.9. In neither the all-causes nor coronary death rates was there any significant difference between the sedentary and the moderately active men, but both rates were much lower in the small group of men rated most active. For all-causes deaths the difference between activity class 1 and class 3 has $p = 0.001$; for coronary deaths the value is $p = 0.06$.

The right side of figure 11.9 shows the findings for incidence of coronary heart disease. The differences in the rates for the activity classes are not statistically significant. For hard CHD the largest difference between activity classes is that between 2 and 3, which has $p = 0.10$. So at Zutphen the most active men seemed to be favored in the all-causes death rate, but the

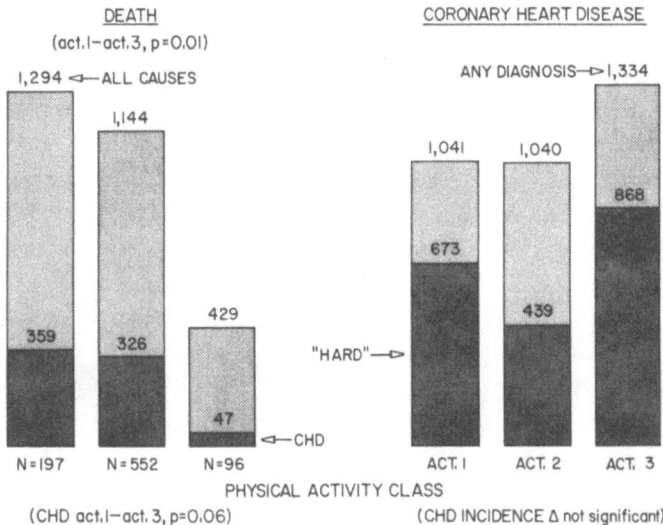

Figure 11.9. For Zutphen, ten-year age-standardized incidence of death and of coronary heart disease per 10,000 classified by habitual physical activity. All men free of cardiovascular disease at entry.

numbers are too small for conclusions about activity and coronary death. For the incidence of coronary heart disease there is no indication of a relationship to physical activity.

Yugoslavia. Substantially all of the Belgrade men were sedentary, and that cohort had a more favorable ten-year experience than the other Yugoslavs. The present analysis considers Dalmatia, Slavonia, Velika Krsna, and Zrenjanin as Yugoslavia. The ten-year experience of the men classified by physical activity is summarized in figure 11.10. There were no significant differences in all-causes deaths or in coronary deaths between the sedentary and the most active groups. However, the moderately active men suffered no coronary deaths, and that peculiarity makes a significant difference compared with class 1 ($p = 0.004$) and with class 3 ($p = 0.02$).

The favorable experience of the moderately active (class 2) men in Yugoslavia is also shown in the incidence rates of both hard and any CHD. When class 2 is compared with classes 1 and 3 in the incidence of hard CHD, the differences in rates have $p = 0.007$ and $p = 0.01$, respectively; the difference between the sedentary and the most active men is not significant. In the incidence of any CHD the rate for the sedentary men is significantly higher than for the moderately active ($p = 0.008$) as well as for the most active men ($p = 0.006$). Explanation of these data from Yugoslavia is obscure;

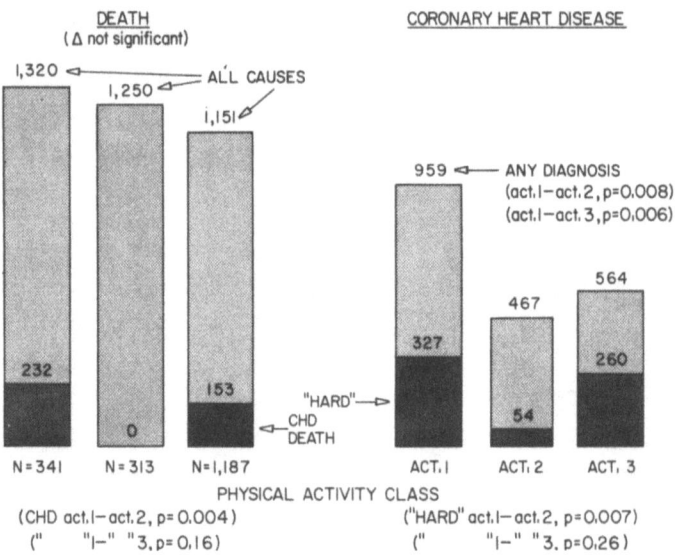

Figure 11.10. For Yugoslavia except Belgrade, ten-year age-standardized incidence of death and of coronary heart disease per 10,000 at risk classified by habitual physical activity. All men free of cardiovascular disease at entry.

the data do not indicate that the incidence of coronary heart disease has a simple relationship with physical activity.

Greece. Although the low death and very low coronary incidence rates of the men of Crete and Corfu have much epidemiological interest, the incidence cases are so few that it is difficult to establish significant differences between activity classes. The data are given in figure 11.11. In all-causes deaths the sedentary men had the poorest experience. The differences between them and the men in classes 2 and 3 have $t = 1.78$ and 1.93, respectively; when classes 2 and 3 are combined the difference has $t = 2.03$ ($p = 0.02$).

Coronary deaths in the Crete and Corfu cohorts were too few to allow firm conclusions. The incidence of coronary heart disease, indicated on the right side of figure 11.11, did not differ significantly among the activity classes.

Japan. Because Japan had only 57 sedentary men free of cardiovascular disease at entry, in the analysis of the relationship between ten-year experience and physical activity it was necessary to combine activity classes 1 and 2 to have suitable numbers for comparison with class 3. The results are

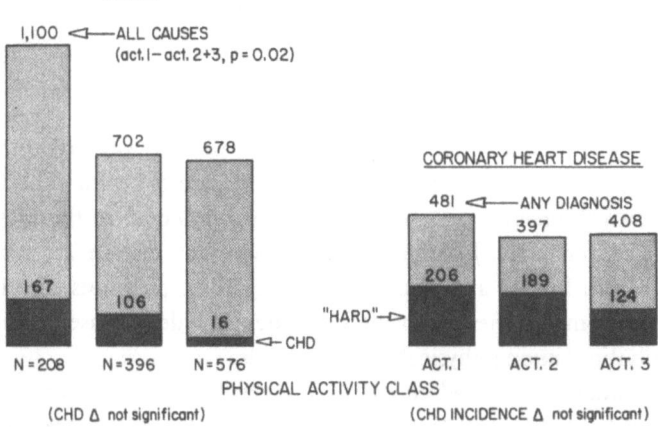

Figure 11.11. For Greece (Crete and Corfu), ten-year age-standardized incidence of death and of coronary heart disease per 10,000 classified by habitual physical activity. All men free of evidence of cardiovascular disease at entry.

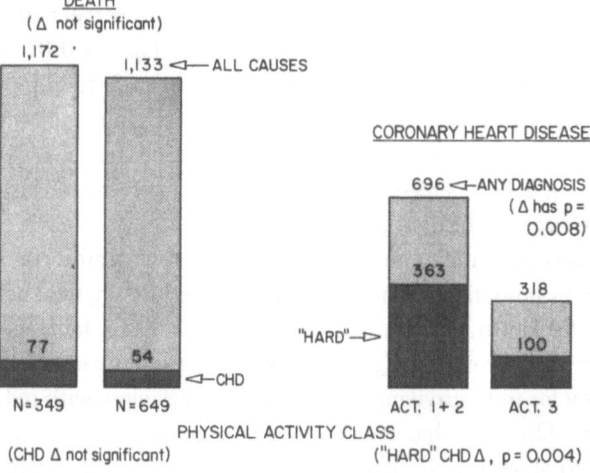

Figure 11.12. For Japan, ten-year age-standardized incidence of death and of coronary heart disease per 10,000 classified by habitual physical activity. All men free of evidence of cardiovascular disease at entry.

given in figure 11.12. Neither all-causes nor coronary deaths give any indication of a significant difference. For the incidence rate of coronary heart disease, summarized on the right side of the figure, the data indicate highly significant differences between the less active and the most active men. A comparison of cases to noncases results in chi-square values of 8.50 for hard CHD and 6.95 for any CHD.

Prevalence versus Incidence Rates

At the entry examinations, a not-surprising finding was that some men were restricted in their physical activity by their state of health. This was obvious from volunteered statements and was documented in the prevalence findings (see chapter 3). Men with cardiovascular disease at entry were excluded from further analyses, except in regard to prognosis, but it is instructive to compare them with the subsequent incidence cases in regard to the distribution among physical activity classes.

In the American railroad cohort 11.7 percent of the sedentary men had cardiovascular disease at entry, and 7.1 percent of the more active men were so afflicted; the difference has chi-square = 10.2, indicating around 1 in 1,000 of chance explanation. In contrast, in the follow-up of the men starting free of cardiovascular disease, the sedentary men showed no disadvantage compared with their more active colleagues. Among 8,154 European men cardiovascular disease was diagnosed at entry in 6.97 percent of the class 1 men, 4.77 percent of class 2 men and 3.57 percent of the class 3 men. The difference between class 1 and class 2 has $p = 0.01$; for the difference between classes 1 and 3, p is less than 0.000005. In comparison, the incidence of any CHD in the next ten years in that same combined population of European men but excluding the prevalence men was 10.7 percent in activity class 1, 9.8 percent in class 2, and 10.7 percent in class 3; the differences are not statistically significant.

The prevalence of major abnormalities in the electrocardiograms recorded at the entry examinations of our subjects classified by physical activity is reported in Blackburn, Parlin, and Keys (1967). Their table G11, which shows the frequency of large Q waves (old myocardial infarction), illustrated the tendency for men surviving heart attacks to seek work with reduced physical activity. This table has recently been "adapted" and misrepresented as purporting to show the ill effect on the heart of physical inactivity (Mann 1977). In our report on the electrocardiograms at entry, it was also shown that the percentage of men with large Q waves who had stopped smoking was almost twice that of heavy smokers; using Mann's logic this would indicate that stopping smoking greatly increases the risk of having a heart attack!

Other Studies

The theory that physical inactivity is an important risk factor for coronary heart disease gained prominence from a report on mortality of busmen and postal employees in London (Morris et al. 1953). The bus drivers, whose work is sedentary, were more prone to coronary death than the conductors who spent much time standing and now and then climbed the steps of the double-decker buses to collect fares. Similarly, London postal clerks were more frequently coronary victims than the letter carriers; a study of death records of postal employees in Washington, D. C., indicated a like difference between clerks and carriers (Kahn 1963). Job selection and job changes pose serious questions in these and other studies comparing men in different occupations, but in any case the contrasts in physical activity are similar to those between classes 1 and 2 in the present study, that is, a difference between men who are mainly sedentary and men whose work involves low-level exercise.

From a review of the literature, Leon and Blackburn (1977) state, "it appeared that a sedentary individual might have to increase his activity by no more than 100 kilocalories per day to be placed in a more favorable intermediate activity group" (p. 571) in regard to the risk of coronary heart disease. Such a difference is certainly much less than the average difference between activity classes 1 and 2 and the two classes of busmen and postal employees in London. For the American railroad men measurements of oxygen consumption and time-motion studies in representative job activities indicate an average difference between activity classes 1 and 2 of 500 to 600 kcal per day (Blackburn et al. 1965; Taylor 1978). This may be a fair estimate of the average difference between classes 1 and 2 in the other cohorts with a similar additional difference between the men in classes 2 and 3. Dietary studies in Italy indicate an average of 3,078 kcal per day for men in industry compared with a figure of 3,692 for farmers; in terms of physical activity these men belong in classes 2 and 3, respectively.

Lately it has been proposed that anaerobic work, exercise that involves the accumulation of an oxygen debt and provokes puffing and panting is the "protective" kind of activity (Morris et al. 1973). Much of the propaganda for jogging and tennis is based on the idea that exercise must involve anaerobic work to be beneficial to the cardiocirculatory system. Exercise to the point of getting out of breath is speculated to provoke an increase in the size of the coronary vascular bed, thereby lessening the chance of coronary insufficiency in the future. Without debating that argument it must be pointed out that bus conductors and letter carriers never get the least out of breath on the job, so such advantage as they may enjoy in regard to the risk of heart attack cannot be explained in this way. Nor can it be suggested that the supposed immunity of the Masai in Africa is due to anaerobic work; walking with their cattle does not involve anaerobic work. Actually, it is not possible to credit anaerobic exercise for the reported relative protection from heart attacks of the more active men in any of the positive reports on occupation summarized by Leon and Blackburn (1977).

Scarcely any ordinary occupation ever demands exertion that provokes breathlessness in healthy persons. The farmer cultivating his fields by hoe and handheld plough, the mason moving, cutting, and setting stone, the lumberjack felling trees by axe and saw—all do very hard work using large muscle masses, but they never get out of breath except in rare crises of accident. They do their work at a pace that can be kept up hour after hour, all day long, never puffing and panting, never developing a notable tachycardia. Their work involves none of the anaerobic cardiorespiratory training lately advocated in the hope of preventing coronary heart disease.

The findings in the present study can offer nothing to the debate about the possible value of anaerobic exercise. Furthermore, like practically all other epidemiological studies on men habitually at different levels of physical activity, the groups contrasting in activity are not identical in other characteristics, and even elaborate attempts at multivariate analysis can only hope to balance out a few known or suspected risk factors. Accordingly, inferences and conclusions from the findings in regard to physical activity must be strictly limited. The fact that no relationships emerge consistently in the sixteen cohorts is enough to give pause to drawing conclusions.

The data from Finland illustrate the necessity for careful analysis with precise definition of the hypothesis under test. Since Morris's report on the London busmen, the popular hypothesis has been that physical inactivity promotes coronary heart disease; so far as it has not been proposed that heavy physical labor for most of the working day is required for protection. But if, in fact, the latter were the hypothesis under test, the data from Finland could be presented so as to seem strongly confirmatory. If we disregard the fact that the men in classes 1 and 2 are very different both in physical activity and in the ten-year experience, we may combine them because they did not do heavy work most of the time as did the men in class 3. The 10-year incidence rates for the men not engaged in heavy labor (classes 1 and 2) and the men in class 3 are, respectively, with standard errors in parentheses: all-causes deaths 2,077 (210) and 1,211 (98); coronary deaths 754 (137) and 378 (55); hard CHD 1,261 (171) and 637 (72). The respective t values for the differences are 4.17, 3.10, 3.88, indicating that such differences would very rarely occur by chance.

The analysis of the ten-year data on the Finns by Punsar and Karvonen (1976) emphasizes how wrong it would be to use the foregoing example in support of the theory that heavy exercise protects against coronary heart disease. They divided our activity class 3 into two classes to provide a fourth class of 427 lumberjacks who were more active than the other men of activity class 3. The analysis led to the conclusion that "vigorous physical activity at work was not associated with a reduction in the risk of developing CHD."

Elsewhere we and others have pointed out the severe limitations of permissible conclusions about the health effects of exercise from findings on population samples (Keys 1970, 1975, pp.1153–161; Taylor et al. 1966; Taylor, Buskirk, and Remington 1973; Montoye 1975). Confounding factors confuse relationships between physical activity and other risk factors (Montoye et al. 1976). Several examples of the latter difficulty emerged from continuing studies on the London busmen (Morris, Heady, and Raffle 1956; Kagan 1960). Although the inclusion of other risk factors in multivariate analyses is helpful, as will be seen in chapter 15, some problems remain.

Summary

The sampling of the railroad men in the United States and in Italy was designed to provide groups contrasting in physical activity. In the other cohorts the effort was made to enroll all men aged 40–59 in the designated area, regardless of activity.

At entry men were classified by habitual physical activity: class 1, primarily sedentary; class 2, moderate activity during a substantial part of most days; class 3, hard physical work. Classification of the American and Italian railroad men was based on their long-time jobs. Men in the other cohorts were asked about their activities on and off the job, but occupational work usually determined the activity classification because prolonged, frequent or heavy nonoccupational activity exercise was rare. None of the American or Belgrade men and only 11 percent of the Zutphen men were in activity class 3. About a third of the men of Corfu, the Italian railroad, and Zrenjanin (Serbia) were in class 3. Most men in the other ten cohorts were in class 3.

In ten cohorts, activity level did not differ with age; in four cohorts activity level tended to be higher in younger men, but at Zutphen the most active men tended to be older.

In eight cohorts the mean blood pressure decreased with increasing activity; in the other cohorts blood pressure was not related to activity. Except in the United States, Finland, and Japan, serum cholesterol concentration tended to decrease with activity. In all cohorts the resting pulse rate tended to be lowest in the most active men. The vital capacity was trivially larger in the most active men. In general, smoking habits differed little among activity classes except in the American railroad men where the more active switchmen tended to be the heavier smokers.

The differences in the distributions by physical activity of the cohorts do not help to explain the cohort differences in the incidence of coronary heart disease. A tendency for the all-causes death rate to fall with the percentage of sedentary men in the group depended mainly on the very low death rate of the sedentary Belgrade professors. The incidence rate of coronary heart disease was unrelated to the physical activity characteristics of the groups.

Among the American railroad men, the ten-year death rate of the sedentary men was lower than that of the more active switchmen, but the difference reflects an excessive accident death rate of the switchmen. The coronary death rate was not different in the two activity classes of railroad men.

In Finland, the all-causes death rate of the sedentary men was excessive because of an undue frequency of death from neoplasms. In coronary deaths there was no difference between Finns in class 1 and in class 3, but the rate of the moderately active men (class 2) was over twice that of the other men. The incidence rate of coronary heart disease in the moderately active Finns was also much higher than in the other two activity classes.

In rural Italy, both all-causes and coronary death rates tended to be inversely related to habitual activity, and the incidence of coronary heart disease was significantly elevated among the sedentary men. For the Rome railroad men, too, both all-causes and coronary death rates were inversely related to habitual physical activity.

At Zutphen, the small group of most active men had the lowest death rates for both all-causes and coronary death, but there was no difference in mortality between the larger groups of sedentary and of moderately active men. The Dutchmen classified by activity did not differ significantly in the incidence rate of coronary heart disease.

In Yugoslavia, class 1 and class 3 men did not differ in ten-year all-causes or coronary death rates or in the incidence rate of coronary heart disease. The experience of men in activity class 2, however, was significantly more favorable.

In Greece, the sedentary men had the highest all-causes death rate, but the men in class 2 did not differ from those in class 3 in that respect. Coronary deaths in Greece were too few for analysis, but in the incidence of coronary heart disease there were no significant differences among the activity classes.

Because only 57 Japanese men free of cardiovascular disease were sedentary, activity classes 1 and 2 were combined for comparison with the most active men. These activity groupings did not differ in ten-year all-causes death rates, but the more active men had a significantly lower incidence of coronary heart disease.

The findings in regard to the ten-year experience of men differing in habitual activity at entry clearly do not support the theory of a simple direct relationship between physical inactivity and the development of coronary heart disease or the risk of early death. The varying experience of the several groups suggests that where physical activity seems to be important this may be because of interrelations with other more primary risk factors. In any case these data do not bear on the recently popular idea that periodic anaerobic exercise will give protection against development of coronary heart disease. None of the occupations represented in this study involve anaerobic work and substantially none of the men ever engaged in anaerobic exercise other than in very rare emergencies.

12 | Resting Pulse Rate

The resting pulse rate as a risk factor for mortality of middle-aged men was reported on the basis of a ten-year follow-up of men, initially aged 40–59, employed by the Peoples Gas Company, Chicago (Berkson et al. 1970). Rates of 80 or more beats per minute were found to have an ominous significance in regard to the death rate in the next ten years from all causes, cardiovascular-renal diseases, coronary heart disease, and sudden death.

As in the Chicago study, the resting pulse rate was estimated from the electrocardiogram recorded at the entrance examination. That method has the obvious disadvantage that for each man the estimation is based on a relatively short time period, and in many cases it may be a poor indication of the true resting average for the individual. This disadvantage was extreme for the Japanese men because the electrocardiographic examination at entry was made by an experienced cardiologist who based his diagnoses on what he saw on the oscilloscope and the records of only one or two complexes from each lead. Later, when interest in the pulse rate developed from the report by Berkson et al. (1970), its estimation for entry at Tanushimaru and Ushibuka was necessarily based on that material. This chapter will make only limited use of the entry pulse rate data from Japan.

Insofar as the recorded electrocardiograms are random samples for each man, their brevity should introduce no bias, but the pulse rates for the individuals will involve substantial random errors. It follows, of course, that the strength of relationships of pulse rate to other variables, including the follow-up experience, must be underestimated. The effect of dilution with random "noise" will reduce the apparent importance of the pulse rate as a risk factor but should not produce spurious relationships or distort the group averages. The estimated standard errors of the means may be somewhat larger than would be found with longer sampling of the individual rates, but for the cohort averages the estimated standard errors of the mean are only of the order of half a beat per minute. However, comparisons among the cohort means have other limitations.

Differences among Cohorts

Although the electrocardiograms were recorded under substantially constant conditions, it was not possible to assure that the conditions were identical from one region to another. For all cohorts, certain stipulations were constant: no vigorous exercise or major meal within several hours of the recording, no smoking or stimulating beverages just before starting through the routine of registration and examination, recording of the electrocardiograms at the end of the sequence of answering questionnaires, anthropometry, respiratory function tests, medical history, physical examination, and at least some minutes of recumbent repose. But some conditions of relevance to the heart rate that were practically constant within each cohort varied among cohorts: the size, noise level, and temperature of the examining rooms, the professional status, sex, and age of the persons recording the electrocardiograms, distance from the home, and transportation to the examination place. Possibly of relevance too is the fact that the season for the entry examinations varied from spring in rural Italy to fall in Finland, Greece, and Yugoslavia except at Belgrade where the examinations were made during the winter.

Among the sixteen cohorts the mean resting pulse rate varied from 60.1 beats per minute at Tanushimaru to 77.3 at Belgrade, but no great emphasis should be put on those differences in view of the variability of conditions noted above. In any case figure 12.1 shows that consideration of the mean pulse rates of the cohorts does not help explain the differences in death rates among the cohorts. Figure 12.1 concerns all-causes deaths; the picture for deaths from coronary heart disease is so nearly identical that a separate graph is not warranted; the coefficient of correlation between resting pulse rate and the coronary death rate is $r = 0.08$. Similarly, there is no relationship between the mean pulse rate and the ten-year incidence of coronary heart disease (figure 12.2; $r = 0.015$).

The failure of the resting pulse rate to throw any light on the differences among the cohorts in death and coronary incidence rates has no necessary implication about the importance of the pulse rate as a risk factor for individuals within the cohorts. In fact, univariate analysis shows the resting pulse rate to be an important risk factor for all-causes deaths in the following ten years, though it is of less interest for the risk of developing coronary heart disease. However, the correlation between the resting pulse rate and other risk factors must be considered.

Correlation with Other Variables

Table 12.1 gives, for several groups of men, the coefficient of correlation between resting pulse rate and some other characteristics at entry. In no cohort or group is there any significant correlation between resting pulse rate and age. The correlation between pulse rate and cigarette smoking is positive and highly significant ($p < 0.01$) for the American railroad men and for the group of all cohorts in southern Europe, but not for rural Italy, Serbia, Greece, or Finland. No ready explanation is at hand for these discrepancies concerning smoking. Table 12.1 shows that the resting pulse rate consistently has a relatively strong correlation with blood pressure and physical activity (negative) and a consistent but less strong correlation with serum cholesterol and with vital capacity (negative). These interrelationships with other characteristics give warning that final evaluation of the resting pulse rate as an independent risk factor must await detailed multivariate analysis (see chapter 15). However, the lack of correlation of the pulse rate with age provides some justification for the univariate analysis in the present chapter.

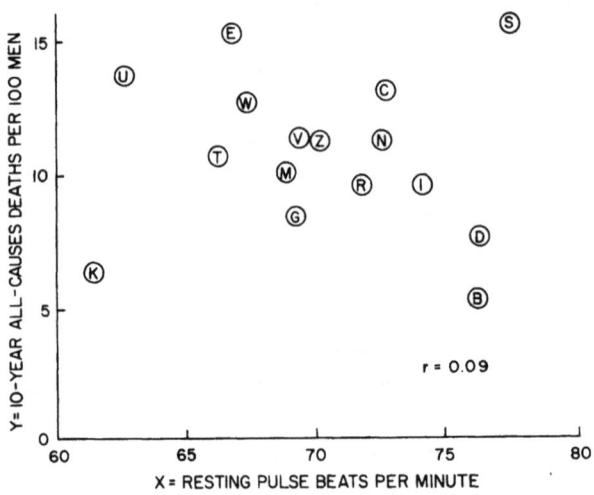

Figure 12.1. Mean resting pulse rates of the cohorts at entry versus the age-standardized ten-year all-causes death rates of the cohorts. B = Belgrade; C = Crevalcore; D = Dalmatia; E = east Finland; G = Corfu; I = Rome railroad; K = Crete; M = Montegiorgio; N = Zutphen; R = American railroad; S = Slavonia; T = Tanushimaru; U = Ushibuka; V = Velika Krsna; W = west Finland; Z = Zrenjanin. All men free of cardiovascular disease at entry.

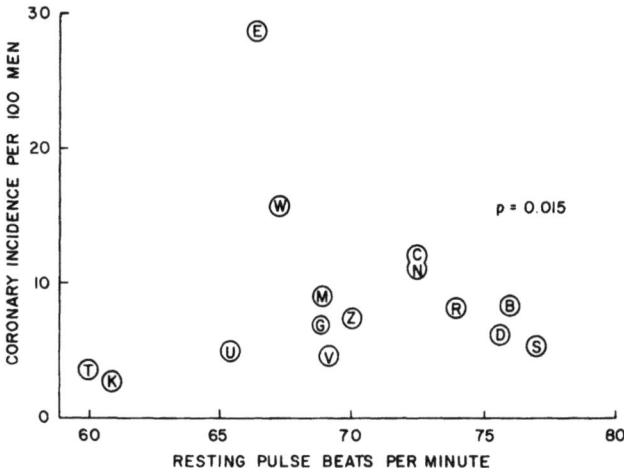

Figure 12.2. Mean resting pulse rates of the cohorts at entry versus the ten-year age-standardized incidence rates of coronary heart disease of the cohorts. Cohorts as in figure 12.1.

The negative correlation of resting pulse rate with habitual physical activity is striking, though perhaps not unexpected in view of the well-known fact that physical training tends to lower the pulse rate at rest as well as in exercise. Table 12.2 gives the mean resting pulse rate of the men in each of the sixteen cohorts classified by habitual physical activity. The regularity of the inverse relationship is notable.

Table 12.1. Correlation of resting pulse rate with other variables recorded at entry in men free of cardiovascular disease.

	Age	S BP	Chol.	Smoking	Vital cap.	Activity
U.S. railroad	0.06	0.31	0.07	0.13	−0.10	−0.07
Finland	−0.06	0.16	0.04	−0.01	−0.07	−0.17
Rural Italy	0.02	0.32	0.11	−0.01	−0.15	−0.21
Serbia	0.08	0.19	0.21	0.05	−0.13	−0.17
Greece	−0.06	0.28	0.17	−0.06	−0.08	−0.24
Southern Europe[a]	0.02	0.13	0.16	0.12	−0.11	−0.05

a. Dalmatia, Slavonia, Rome railroad.

Table 12.2. Resting pulse rate at entry by class of physical activity in men free of cardiovascular disease.

Cohort	All classes N	All classes Mean (SE)	Class 1 N	Class 1 Mean (SE)	Class 2 N	Class 2 Mean (SE)	Class 3 N	Class 3 Mean (SE)
U.S. railroad	2,280	71.7 (12.2)	1,476	71.8 (12.2)	804	70.4 (12.0)	—	—
Dalmatia	640	76.3 (17.0)	49	80.6 (16.7)	74	77.3 (17.3)	517	75.8 (16.9)
Slavonia	650	77.3 (13.6)	111	79.8 (13.7)	60	82.4 (14.9)	479	76.1 (13.2)
Tanushimara [a]	335	60.1 (10.4)	14	66.9 (10.5)	130	60.8 (10.0)	211	59.3 (10.5)
East Finland	695	66.5 (12.7)	67	74.4 (14.2)	115	67.8 (11.5)	513	65.2 (12.4)
West Finland	765	67.2 (12.2)	57	74.8 (16.0)	96	67.2 (12.4)	612	66.5 (11.5)
Ushibuka [a]	421	65.5 (11.2)	32	70.0 (11.3)	72	68.5 (11.9)	317	64.4 (10.8)
Crevalcore	884	72.5 (12.9)	93	77.9 (14.5)	166	75.7 (12.5)	625	70.8 (12.3)
Montegiorgio	674	68.8 (12.3)	39	75.8 (18.2)	174	72.2 (13.4)	461	67.0 (10.6)
Zutphen	781	72.6 (12.6)	185	72.8 (12.5)	513	73.1 (12.7)	83	68.9 (11.4)
Crete	611	61.4 (11.2)	40	64.9 (10.8)	189	63.0 (11.0)	382	60.2 (11.2)
Corfu	510	68.2 (12.8)	158	70.6 (14.1)	193	68.0 (12.1)	159	66.2 (11.9)
Rome railroad	715	74.1 (13.7)	157	75.8 (13.6)	289	73.3 (14.2)	269	73.9 (13.1)
Velika Krsna	489	69.2 (11.2)	32	70.4 (10.9)	101	70.7 (12.1)	276	68.5 (10.9)
Zrenjanin	435	70.0 (11.3)	153	70.3 (10.4)	153	69.8 (11.5)	129	69.9 (12.3)
Belgrade	501	76.2 (11.4)	498	76.3 (11.4)	3	63.3 (10.1)	—	—

a. Excludes men with ECGs unsatisfactory for pulse rate estimation.

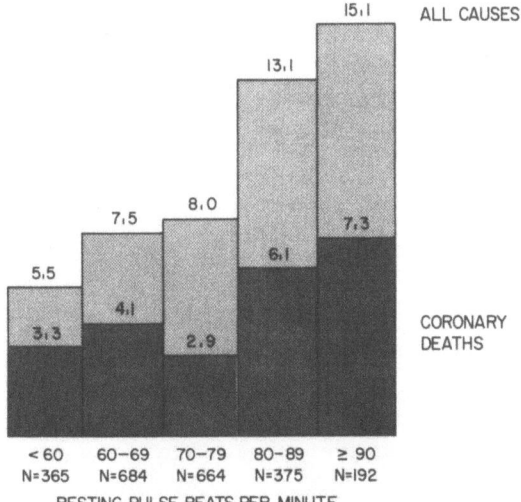

Figure 12.3. For American railroad men, ten-year deaths per 100 from all causes and from coronary heart disease of men classified by resting pulse rate at entry and free of cardiovascular disease at that time.

Ten-year Death Rate

The relationship of pulse rate at entry to deaths in the succeeding ten years among American railroad men is shown in figure 12.3. The all-causes death rate of the men with pulse rates of 90 or more is almost three times that of the men with rates less than 60, but with only 192 men at risk in the 90 or above class the rate of 15.1 has SE = 2.58. The 567 men with pulse rates of 80 or more had 13.8 deaths per 100, SE = 1.45; that rate is 2.8 times the death rate of the 1,049 men with pulse rate under 70. The risk of coronary death was less strikingly related to the pulse rate, but it is statistically significant; the difference in this respect between the men with pulse rates of 80 or more and those with rates under 70 has $p = 0.03$.

The corresponding picture for the men of northern Europe (east and west Finland and Zutphen) is given in figure 12.4. Though both all-causes and coronary death rates tend to rise with increasing resting pulse rate, the slope is much less than for the American men. Comparing, for all deaths, the men with rates of 80 or more with those with rates less than 70, chi-square = 2.00 and $p = 0.16$. For coronary deaths the corresponding chi-square = 3.38 and $p. = 0.07$.

Figure 12.5 summarizes the data from the five cohorts in Italy and Greece, indicating that the resting pulse rate is a highly significant risk factor for death. The all-causes death rate of the men with pulse rates of 90 or

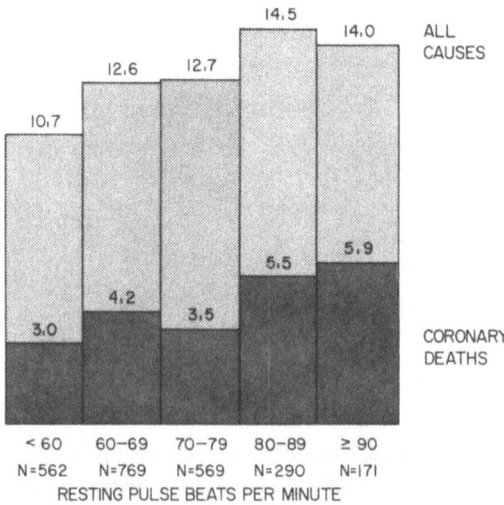

Figure 12.4. For northern Europe (east and west Finland, Zutphen), ten-year deaths per 100 from all causes and from coronary heart disease of men classified by resting pulse rate at entry and free of cardiovascular disease at that time.

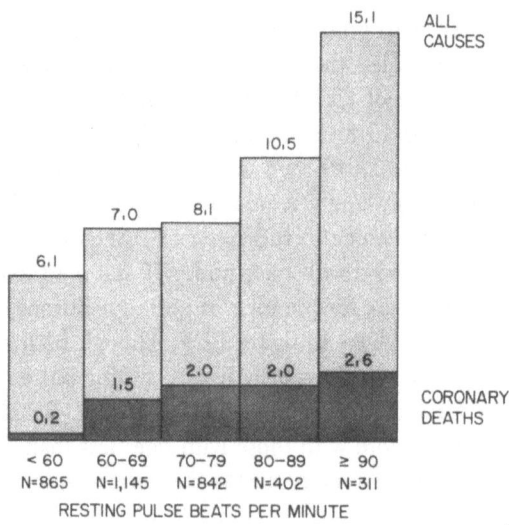

Figure 12.5. For Italy and Greece (five cohorts), ten-year deaths per 100 from all causes and from coronary heart disease of men classified by resting pulse rate at entry and free of cardiovascular disease at that time.

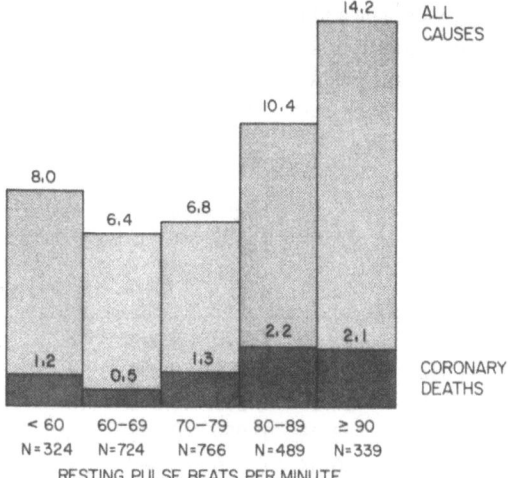

Figure 12.6. For Yugoslavia (five cohorts), ten-year deaths per 100 from all causes and from coronary heart disease of men classified by resting pulse rate at entry and free of cardiovascular disease at that time.

more was 2.5 times greater than that of the men with pulse rates under 60. The total number of deaths from coronary heart disease is too small for comparison with those cutting points, but the death rates of the men with pulse rates of 80 or more and of men with rates under 70 are 2.24 and 0.95, respectively (chi-square = 7.00, $p < 0.01$).

The data on resting pulse rate as a risk factor for ten-year death in the five cohorts of men in Yugoslavia are summarized in figure 12.6. When the men with pulse rates of 80 or more are compared with those with rates under 70, the result for all-causes deaths has chi-square = 14.08 and for coronary heart disease deaths chi-square = 4.38; the latter figure indicates that the difference in death rate might occur by chance in about 1 out of 30 trials.

The histograms shown in figures 12.3 through 12.6 suggest a linear relationship between the resting pulse rate and the death rate for the 10-year follow-up so the data were examined with the regression equation, $y = a + bx$, where x is the pulse rate in beats per minute and y is assigned 0 for survival, 1 for death. Table 12.3 gives the solutions for the regression equation and also the standard error of the slope, t, and the percentage of men at entry with resting pulse rates of 60 and 80 that would be predicted to be dead in ten years. Except for the men of Zutphen and Serbia, the t values indicate high probability that the death rate is positively related to the pulse rate.

Table 12.3. Resting pulse rate and ten-year death rate in men free of cardiovascular disease at entry (least-squares solutions for $y = a + bx$, where y = ten-year deaths per 100 men, x = pulse rate; predicted dead are deaths per 100 estimated from the regression solution for men with entry pulse rates of 60 and of 80; SE_b = standard error of the slope, b; $t = b/SE_b$.

Area	Death cause	Regression				Predicted dead	
		a	b	SE_b	t	Pulse 60	Pulse 80
U.S. railroad	All	−7.66	0.230	0.048	4.8	6.1	10.7
	CHD	−1.63	0.081	0.034	2.4	3.2	4.9
Croatia	All	−10.65	0.258	0.052	5.0	2.3	10.0
	CHD	−3.23	0.059	0.021	2.8	0.3	1.5
Finland	All	0.63	0.156	0.067	2.3	10.0	13.1
	CHD	−3.72	0.122	0.044	2.8	3.6	6.0
Serbia	All	6.97	0	0.059	0	7.0	7.0
	CHD	−0.31	0.023	0.026	0.9	1.1	1.5
Italy and Greece	All	−4.32	0.185	0.035	5.3	6.8	10.5
	CHD	−2.69	0.060	0.015	4.0	0.9	2.1
Zutphen	All	7.28	0.045	0.085	0.5	10.0	10.9
	CHD	2.09	0.018	0.050	0.4	3.2	3.5

Several of the histograms suggest that the death rate may be a curvilinear function of the resting pulse rate. The question was examined with the quadratic model, $y = a + bx + cx^2$. In none of the cohorts did the quadratic model yield a better fit to the data than the linear model.

In table 12.3 the slope of the regression of all-causes deaths on pulse rate is greater than the slope of the regression of coronary deaths on the pulse rate in all cases except Serbia, where neither slope is statistically significant. This suggests that the resting pulse rate is a more important risk factor for noncoronary than for coronary death. The question was examined further by calculating the regression of noncoronary death on the pulse rate and comparing the result with the coronary heart disease regression data given in table 12.3. For the American railroad men the slope for noncoronary death is 1.85 times steeper than the slope for coronary death. The corresponding ratio of noncoronary to coronary to coronary death slope is 3.41 for Croatia, 2.07 for Italy and Greece, and only 0.33 for Finland. Weighted by the number of men at risk, the average slope of the regression of noncoronary death on pulse rate is 1.92 times greater than the slope of coronary death. For both Zutphen and Serbia none of the slopes of death rate on resting pulse rate is statistically significant. It appears, therefore, that where the pulse rate is a major factor for death it tends to be considerably more important for noncoronary than for coronary death.

Incidence Rate of Coronary Heart Disease

The ten-year follow-up showed that the resting pulse rate is an important risk factor for all-causes deaths in ten years but less consequential for death from coronary heart disease. The incidence of coronary heart disease, including nonfatal cases, presented a very different picture of pulse rate as a risk factor. For the American railroad men there are no data on the ten-year incidence of nonfatal coronary heart disease. The findings for the Finns are summarized in figure 12.7. With 165 cases of coronary death or nonfatal myocardial infarction (hard CHD) among 1,492 Finns with no evidence of cardiovascular disease at entry there was no significant trend for the incidence rate to be related to the resting pulse rate. For 328 men given any diagnosis of coronary heart disease, there was also no indication of any relation to the resting pulse rate.

Figure 12.8 presents the corresponding data for 832 men at Zutphen free of evidence of cardiovascular disease at entry. For neither hard CHD (45 cases) nor any CHD (90 cases) is there any indication of a relation to the resting pulse rate.

The men in southern Europe, in contrast, showed a consistent rise in the incidence of coronary heart disease with either hard or any CHD as the cri-

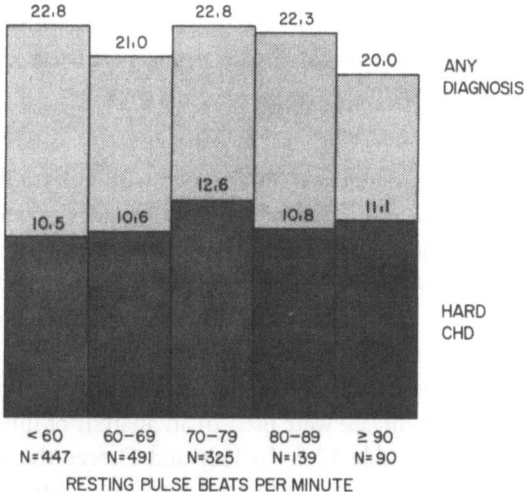

Figure 12.7. For Finland, ten-year incidence of coronary heart disease per 100 men classified by entry resting pulse rate and free of cardiovascular disease at that time.

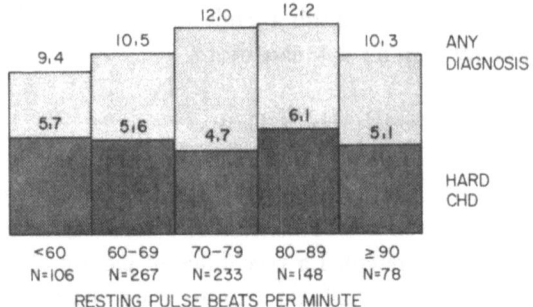

Figure 12.8. For Zutphen, ten-year incidence of coronary heart disease per 100 men classified by resting pulse rate at entry and free of cardiovascular disease at that time.

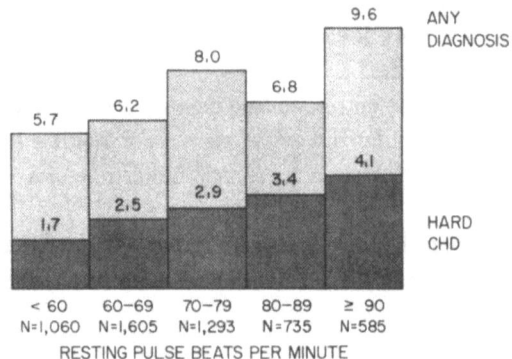

Figure 12.9. For southern Europe (Italy, Greece, Yugoslavia), ten-year incidence of coronary heart disease per 100 men classified by resting pulse rate at entry and free of cardiovascular disease at that time.

terion (figure 12.9). The incidence rate for men with entry pulse rates of 80 or more was roughly twice that for men with pulse rates under 60 per minute. However, the trend for any CHD to rise with increasing pulse rate is entirely accounted for by hard CHD; for the 224 men given soft diagnoses of coronary heart disease, there was no tendency for the incidence rate to be related to the entry resting pulse rate.

As in the case of the mortality data, the findings in regard to the incidence of coronary heart disease were used in an analysis of linear regression. The results are given in table 12.4. In Italy and Greece the incidence rate of hard CHD was significantly related to the entry pulse rate. In Croatia and in Finland the incidence rate of hard CHD was related to the resting pulse rate at a probability level close to the conventional $p = 0.05$ taken to indicate

Table 12.4. Resting pulse rate and ten-year incidence rate of coronary heart disease in men free of cardiovascular disease (least-squares solutions for $y = a + bx$, where y = ten-year incidence, x = pulse rate; predicted cases are cases per 100 estimated from the regression solution for men with resting pulse rates of 60 and of 80; SE_b = standard error of the slope; $t = b/SE_b$).

Area	CHD	Regression				Predicted cases	
		a	b	SE_b	t	Pulse 60	Pulse 80
Croatia	Hard	−1.43	0.051	0.028	1.82	1.63	2.65
	Other	2.30	0.016	0.033	0.48	3.26	3.58
Finland	Hard	8.20	0.043	0.023	1.87	10.78	11.64
	Other	12.43	−0.023	0.065	−0.35	11.05	10.59
Zutphen	Hard	7.15	−0.002	0.071	−0.03	7.03	6.99
	Other	2.30	0.023	0.055	0.43	3.68	4.14
Italy and Greece	Hard	−1.23	0.071	0.024	2.96	3.03	4.45
	Other	0.50	0.050	0.024	2.08	3.50	4.50
Serbia	Hard	−1.22	0.051	0.038	1.50	2.20	3.34
	Other	3.45	<0.001	0.042	—	3.45	3.45

statistical significance; in Serbia the trend was similar but might be expected to occur by chance in perhaps one out of seven trials. Except in Italy and Greece the incidence of other CHD was not related to the resting pulse rate. When it is remarked that Table 12.4 covers five population groups, the fact that other CHD incidence appeared to be related to the resting pulse rate in one of those groups with a value of $p = 0.05$ would seem to have little significance.

We have remarked about the limitations of the entry pulse rate data from the Japanese cohorts. Still, there is no reason to suggest the data are biased; the problem is that random "noise" from moment-to-moment intra-individual variability will tend to obscure relationships. There is also a question as to whether the time calibration of the electrocardiographic records was the same as in the other records where, in general, a time calibration was included in the permanent file. The measurement of the complexes in the central laboratory in Minnesota indicated pulse rates under 50 beats per minute in 5.8 percent of the men of Ushibuka and 13.7 percent of the men of Tanushimaru. The average for all of the other cohorts was 2.7 percent with such low pulse rates.

Nevertheless, as figure 12.10 shows, the all-causes death rate of the men in Japan was related to the resting pulse rate. The 190 men with pulse rates

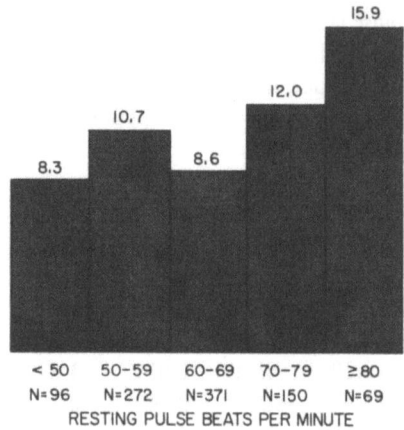

Figure 12.10. For Japan (Tanushimaru and Ushibuka), ten-year deaths per 100 from all causes among men classified by resting pulse rate at entry and free of cardiovascular disease at that time.

of 80 or more had a death rate 41 percent higher than that of the 808 men with rates less than 80. The chi-square test gives 4.41 for the comparison and $p = 0.036$ for chance explanation. The Japanese data do not indicate any relationship between pulse rate and the incidence of coronary heart disease, but the number of cases of the disease is too small to warrant conclusions.

Other Studies

In the original report from Chicago on the resting pulse rate as a risk factor, only rates of 80 or more beats per minute were identified as portending an increased risk of death in ten years. In the gas company study 18.5 percent of the 1,329 men had such high pulse rates; below that level there was no apparent trend for mortality rate to be related to the pulse rate. The idea of a threshold for risk seems to have arisen from the finding that, whereas the death rate of the 480 men with entry pulse rates of 70 through 79 was 98.2, the 445 men with rates from 60 through 69 had a higher rate, 108.5 per 1,000 men. However, the 95 percent confidence limits of these rates are 7.6, 12.5, and 8.0, 13.7, respectively, so it could easily be that with larger numbers a continuous trend for mortality to rise with pulse rate would emerge. The larger material of the present study shows no sign of a threshold; the data are well fitted by straight lines; regressions are shown in figure 12.11.

Data on the relationship of the resting heart rate to the subsequent incidence of coronary heart disease in the Framingham study show no sign of

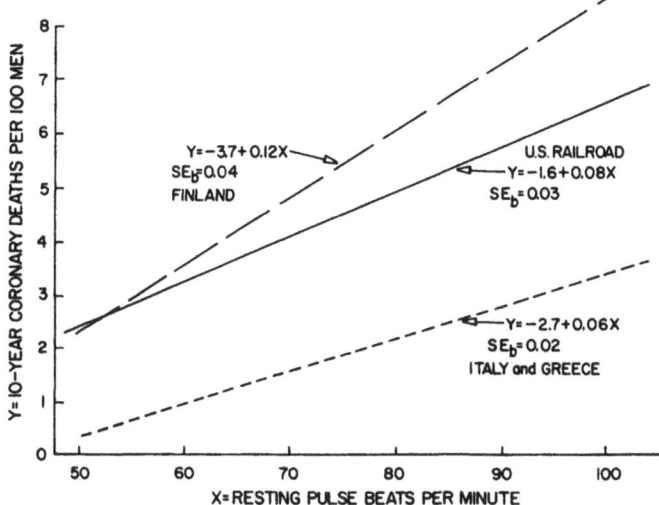

Figure 12.11. Linear regressions of ten-year death rate from coronary heart disease on resting pulse rate at entry for men without cardiovascular disease at entry in Finland, the United States railroad, and in Italy and Greece (five cohorts).

a threshold, and in the detailed analysis of the Framingham data Shurtleff (1974) selected a linear model. In the Seven Countries Study the data on the relationship of the incidence of coronary heart disease to entry resting pulse rate also show no sign of a threshold. The regressions for northern and southern Europe with hard CHD as the end point are depicted in figure 12.12. Note that the slope in both cases is small but steeper for southern Europe than for northern Europe. For any CHD the corresponding regressions are given in figure 12.13. We have no explanation for the curious difference in the slopes in figure 12.13 except to point out that in the category of any CHD angina pectoris accounts for a substantial proportion of all the diagnoses, and angina pectoris does not necessarily represent the same physical condition in the several cohorts.

Comparison of the data reported from Framingham with those obtained in the Seven Countries Study is complicated by the fact that the Framingham data on the incidence of coronary heart disease concern men initially free of coronary heart disease but not necessarily free of cardiovascular disease as specified for the analysis of the seven countries data. For all-causes deaths the reported data from Framingham concern men only specified to have been alive at the last examination preceding death. It should be noted, also, that the Framingham study covers a much smaller number of men in the age range of concern than the Seven Countries Study—1,379

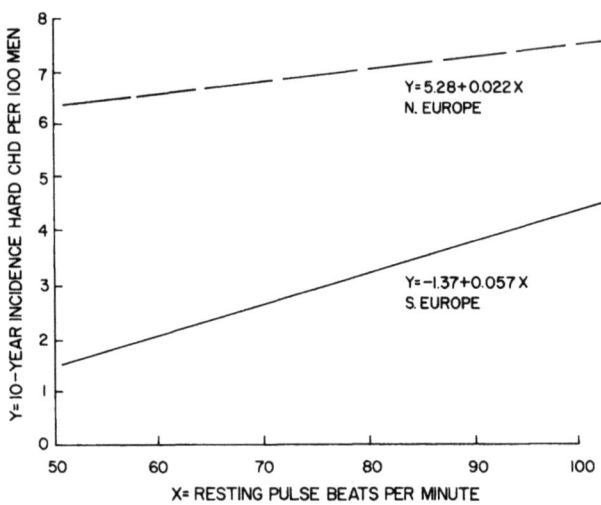

Figure 12.12. Regression of ten-year incidence of hard coronary heart disease on resting pulse rate at entry, men starting free of cardiovascular disease. N. Europe = Finland and Zutphen; S. Europe = Italy, Greece, and Yugoslavia.

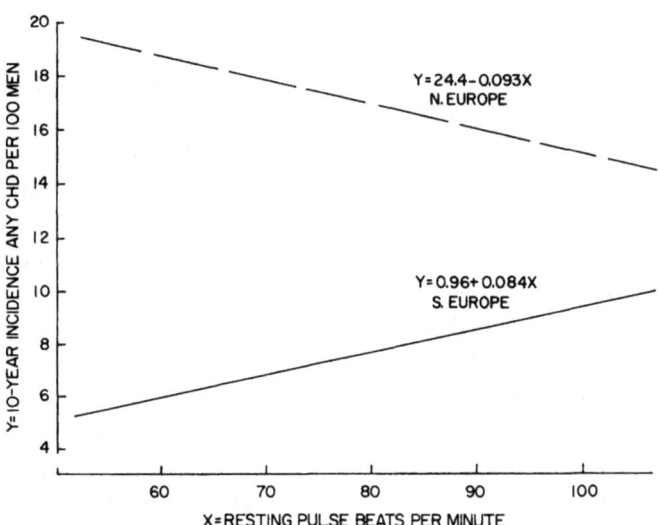

Figure 12.13. Regression of ten-year incidence of any diagnosis of coronary heart disease on resting pulse rate at entry, men starting free of cardiovascular disease. N. Europe = Finland and Zutphen; S. Europe = Italy, Greece, and Yugoslavia.

versus 12,763 men in the sixteen cohorts of the Seven Countries Study—but the follow-up reported by Shurtleff (1974) extended over eighteen years with biennial reexaminations. Because the men reentered the group at risk at each biennial examination, most of the men were counted many times. That methodological device differed greatly from the simple method used here.

In spite of these differences some comments are in order. The Framingham report indicates that the resting pulse rate is a significant risk factor for men, but not for women, for any CHD when other risk factors are ignored. But even for men the slope of the incidence on pulse rate is not steep. When the risk of the men with pulse rate 80 is compared with that of the men with pulse rate 60, the coefficients of the logistic function indicate a risk ratio of 1.11 for men aged 45–54, 1.29 for ages 55–64. In the Framingham study the resting pulse rate was not a significant factor for myocardial infarction but appeared to be consequential for death from coronary heart disease; calculation indicates that men with a pulse rate of 80 had about twice the risk of men with pulse rate 60. Another feature of interest in the Framingham data is that the importance of the resting pulse rate tended to decline with age. For CHD death the risk ratio for pulse 80 versus pulse rate 60 was 2.09 for ages 45–54, 2.00 for ages 55–64, 1.29 for ages 65–76. Finally, in the multivariate analysis of the Framingham data, the resting pulse rate had no statistical significance as an independent risk factor for the development of any CHD or for myocardial infarction but was significant ($t = 2.97$) for death from coronary heart disease.

In the analysis of the ten-year experience of the seven countries in this chapter, in which other risk factors are not considered, the importance of the resting pulse rate was greatest for death from all causes, less for coronary heart disease death, very little for the incidence of nonfatal CHD. Coronary heart disease diagnosed only on the basis of soft criteria was substantially unrelated to the resting pulse rate.

Summary

The resting pulse rate was calculated from the electrocardiogram recorded at the entry examination. The rate proved to be independent of age and had no consistent correlation with smoking habit. It had low-order direct correlations with blood pressure and the serum cholesterol concentration and negative correlation with the vital capacity. In all cohorts the men most active physically had the slowest average resting pulse rate.

In all areas, among men with no cardiovascular disease at entry, the ten-year death rate tended to be linearly related to the entry pulse rate. In the American railroad men and the men in northern and southern Europe, 20 to 25 percent had resting pulse rates of 80 or more beats per minute. Those men with the faster pulse rates had ten-year death rates roughly double the rate of the other men in the same cohort for both coronary and for other causes of death. In Japan, too, the all-causes death rate of men free of cardiovascular disease at entry was linearly related to the pulse rate.

The ten-year incidence of coronary heart disease was not significantly related to the resting pulse rate in Finland or in Zutphen. In southern Europe the incidence of coronary disease tended to be linearly related to the pulse rate but the relationship was more important for the incidence of hard CHD (myocardial infarction or coronary death) than for other diagnoses. Men in the top 20 percent of the pulse rate distribution in southern Europe had an incidence of hard CHD 44 percent higher than the rest of the men, but they did not differ in the incidence rate of other diagnoses of the disease, including angina pectoris.

13 | Respiratory Function

Interest in the vital capacity as a possible risk factor for coronary heart disease was stimulated by a report from the Framingham study indicating an inverse relationship between the vital capacity and subsequent incidence of coronary heart disease (Dawber, Kannel, and Friedman 1966). Five-year follow-up data from the Seven Countries Study did not agree, and we pointed out that the Framingham conclusion was unwarranted because age and body size, items strongly correlated with vital capacity, had been ignored (Keys et al. 1972a).

Recently analyses of data in the files of the Kaiser-Permanente Hospitals in California reportedly confirmed "the original finding from the Framingham Study that the total vital capacity is a predictor of clinical coronary heart disease" (Friedman, Klatsky, and Siegelaub 1976). The Kaiser-Permanente study was a retrospective case-control comparison. Both cases and controls had had a health checkup at about the same time and were matched in sex and race and "as closely as possible" in age, blood pressure, serum cholesterol, and other possibly relevant characteristics. The persons who later suffered myocardial infarction or sudden cardiac death averaged 59 years of age at the health checkup prior to the event, which occurred, on the average, about eighteen months later.

Among the Kaiser-Permanente subjects roughly 20 percent were women and 10 percent were "nonwhite." Another notable difference from the Seven Countries Study is the age at entry, old people in contrast to middle-aged men, and a much shorter follow-up period. Even if a retrospective case-control study was equivalent to a prospective study starting with healthy persons, it is questionable that the Kaiser-Permanente study could be considered comparable to the present study.

The Kaiser-Permanente study emphasized that it confirmed the Framingham report but the fact is that more careful analysis of Framingham data did not agree with the original published conclusion (Shurtleff 1974). For Framingham men the univariate logistic coefficient for vital capacity, ignoring age and other variables, is statistically significant for the incidence of coronary heart disease but not for death from that cause. When age was controlled the vital capacity was not significant for any coronary event category. The multivariate analysis even more clearly indicated no significance for the vital capacity as a risk factor for Framingham men, though it seemed to be consequential for women. The question remains, however, what the case would be if persons with cardiovascular disease were excluded. The Framingham subjects were only stipulated to have been free of coronary heart disease at entry. In the Seven Countries Study 254 men were excluded from the analysis because of coronary heart disease at entry; with the stipulation that any cardiovascular disease at entry is cause for exclusion, another 403 men were eliminated. A sample free of coronary heart disease will include many subjects with cardiovascular disease.

Measurements

Measurements of respiratory function were included in the entry examinations for ten of the cohorts in this study, but in the American railroad cohort only 40 percent of the men took the tests. The vital capacity (maximum expiratory volume) was recorded for all ten cohorts; the forced expiratory volume at ¾ second (FEV ¾) was also measured in eight of those cohorts. At the five-year reexaminations the respiratory measurements were repeated in the same ten cohorts, and measurements were made in three more cohorts, Dalmatia, Slavonia, and Zutphen.

It was not possible to provide the same kind of spirometers for all regions, but in general the same spirometers were used for the cohorts within each region. The same spirometer was used in east and west Finland, another spirometer was used both in Crete and Corfu, and so on. A spirometer with high airflow resistance was used at the entry examinations at Crevalcore and Montegiorgio; a more suitable instrument was provided for the later reexaminations of the men in those cohorts. Accordingly, it is not warranted to emphasize comparisons among cohorts in regard to respiratory function. However comparisons among men within cohorts are perfectly valid.

Relation to Height and Age

In reporting on the five-year experience of the Seven Countries Study, we emphasized the necessity of allowing for both body size and age in any consideration of the vital capacity. Table 13.1 summarizes the multiple regression analysis, $y = a - b \text{(age)} + c \text{(height)}$, where y is the total vital capacity.

Table 13.1. Multiple regression of vital capacity y (deciliters) on age x (years) and height z (centimeters): $y = a + bx + cz$ (all men free of cardiovascular disease; R = multiple correlation coefficient).

Cohort	N	a	b	SE	c	SE	R
U.S. railroad	1,134	−35.6	−0.42	0.03	0.57	0.03	0.59
Dalmatia[a]	536	−47.5	−0.23	0.06	0.60	0.04	0.56
Slavonia[a]	514	−12.1	−0.43	0.05	0.46	0.05	0.51
East Finland	584	−30.9	−0.38	0.05	0.57	0.04	0.57
West Finland	654	−29.0	−0.33	0.04	0.54	0.04	0.54
Crevalcore	605	−51.1	−0.23	0.04	0.54	0.04	0.60
Montegiorgio	602	−30.2	−0.40	0.05	0.54	0.04	0.58
Crete	545	−31.3	−0.26	0.04	0.50	0.03	0.53
Corfu	422	−35.1	−0.28	0.05	0.52	0.04	0.54
Velika Krsna	452	−22.8	−0.45	0.06	0.52	0.06	0.51
Zrenjanin	466	−26.2	−0.34	0.05	0.51	0.04	0.59
Belgrade	445	−39.1	−0.28	0.05	0.56	0.05	0.54

a. Measured at the five-year reexamination.

In every cohort the regression coefficients for both age (negative) and height are highly significant, and the coefficient of multiple correlation ranges from 0.5 to 0.6, which means that over 25 percent of the total variation in the vital capacity is accounted for by age and height alone.

Among men aged 40 through 59, height is only slightly related to age. In terms of correlation between height and age at the entry examination, the coefficient ranged from $r = -0.02$ at Belgrade to $r = -0.21$ at Corfu, and the mean for all cohorts was $r = -0.11$. At the five-year reexamination of the same men, the average height was 0.2 cm less than at entry.

In contrast to height, the vital capacity decreased substantially over the years of follow-up and reexaminations: The average decrease in five years was 251 ml, or 5.9 percent of the vital capacity at entry. This decrease of vital capacity with age is important because age itself is the most powerful of the risk factors.

Figure 13.1 shows the regression of vital capacity on age of 1,238 men in Finaland at entry, after five years, and finally at the ten-year reexamination. Although the three regressions are very similar, the slope increased over time. The difference between the slopes at entry and after ten years has $t = 1.94$.

Figure 13.2 shows the regression of vital capacity on age for 822 men in Greece (Crete and Corfu) at entry and on the same men ten years later. The

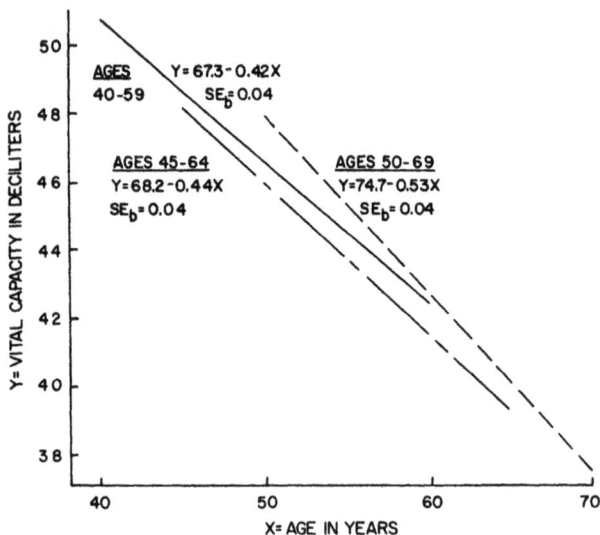

Figure 13.1. Regression of vital capacity on age, data on the same 1,238 men in Finland at entry, five years and ten years later. All men free of cardiovascular disease at entry.

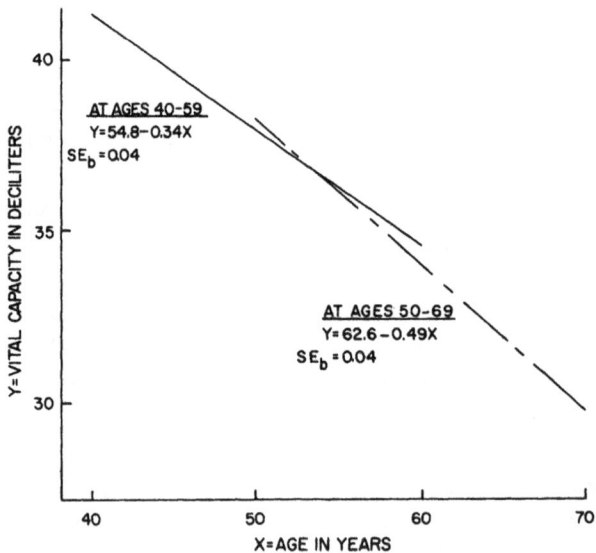

Figure 13.2. Regression of vital capacity on age, data on the same 833 men in Greece at entry and again ten years later. All men free of cardiovascular disease at entry.

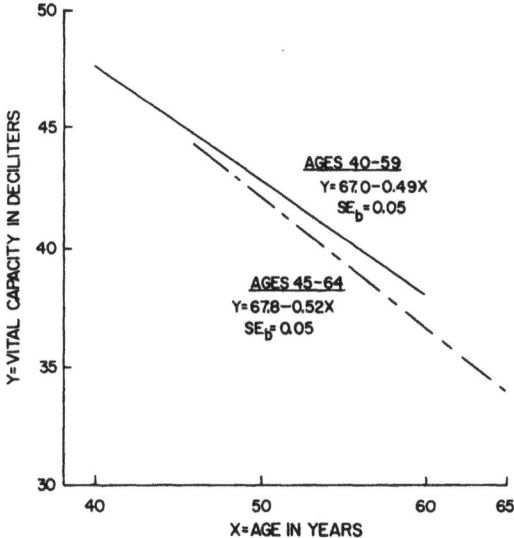

Figure 13.3. Regression of vital capacity on age, data on the same 1,571 American railroad men at entry and again five years later. All men free of cardiovascular disease at entry.

slope is substantially greater after ten years, and the difference from the slope at entry has $t = 2.65$.

The corresponding picture for 571 United States railroad men at entry and again after five years is given in figure 13.3. Again the slope is steeper at the older age, but in contrast to the findings in Finland and in Greece, the difference is not statistically significant. Finally, figure 13.4 shows the regression of vital capacity on age for 1,139 men in Serbia recorded on two occasions five years apart. The slope shows a trivial decrease after five years.

Ten-year Death Rate

The most elementary way of examining the role of vital capacity as a risk factor is to compare the entry vital capacity of the men differing in health status after ten years of follow-up. However, allowance must be made for the fact that, in all cohorts, the average entry age of the men who died or developed coronary heart disease was older than that of the men who stayed well. Allowance for that age difference can be made from the regression of vital capacity on age for the men in each group calculated from their entry data. Those regressions, together with the corresponding regressions of the forced expiratory volume at 0.75 second (FEV ¾) on age, are shown in table 13.2. Before using the data in table 13.2 for adjusting the mean entry vital capac-

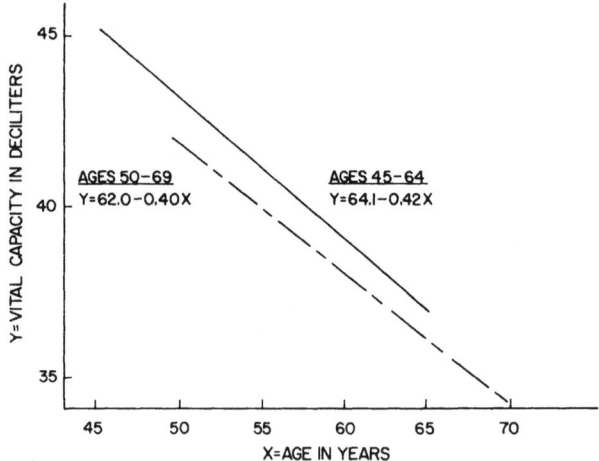

Figure 13.4. Regression of vital capacity on age, data on the same 1,139 men in Serbia at entry and again five years later. All men free of cardiovascular disease at entry.

ity values to constant age, it may be remarked that the regressions, and the correlations, are very much alike in all five areas.

The use of the regressions in table 13.2 for the adjustment of mean vital capacity to constant entry age of the men in different categories according to ten-year outcome is illustrated with the data from the men in Finland who stayed well and those who died from coronary heart disease. At entry their mean ages were 48.96 and 51.14 years and their mean vital capacities were 27.54 and 26.22 deciliters per meter height. From table 13.2 the slope of vital capacity was −0.248 per year of age, and corrected to mean age 50 years at entry, the values are 27.28 and 26.50, respectively. The difference at age 50 is 0.78 dl/m with a standard error of the difference of 0.46 and

Table 13.2. Regression of respiratory function, y, on age, x, at entry in men free of cardiovascular disease (vital capacity and FEV ¾ in deciliters per meter height; least-squares solutions of $y = a + bx$).

Group	N	Vital capacity			FEV ¾		
		a	b	r	a	b	r
Finland	1,448	38.80	−0.248	−0.313	29.61	−0.222	−0.327
U.S. railroad	1,033	36.80	−0.288	−0.365	28.61	−0.250	−0.402
Rural Italy	1,531	33.58	−0.244	−0.300	23.11	−0.184	−0.290
Greece	1,125	32.79	−0.205	−0.333	25.51	−0.202	−0.362
Serbia	1,424	34.72	−0.221	−0.330	27.67	−0.233	−0.391

$t = 1.52$. Table 13.3 summarizes the data calculated in this way for the five areas and the four end points (two for the American railroad men).

Table 13.3 indicates that, after adjusting for age and body size, the vital capacity was a highly significant risk factor for all-causes deaths except for the Greeks where the difference between those who died and those who

Table 13.3. Vital capacity (deciliters per meter height) at entry of men classified by ten-year health status, all free of cardiovascular disease at entry ($\bar{y}$ = vital capacity at entry; y' = vital capacity adjusted to age 50 by the regression in table 13.2; age = mean at entry; difference = y' for no CHD minus y' for men with specified incidence).

Ten-year status by group	N	Age	$\bar{y}$	y'	Difference Mean	SE	t
Finland							
No CHD	827	48.96	27.54	27.28			
CHD deaths	64	51.14	26.22	26.50	0.78	0.46	1.52
Hard CHD	157	51.45	26.59	26.95	0.33	0.31	1.06
Any CHD	316	50.57	26.82	26.96	0.32	0.24	1.33
All-causes deaths	159	51.93	25.61	26.09	1.19	0.32	3.72
U.S. railroad							
No CHD	932	49.23	24.41	24.19			
CHD deaths	53	51.53	22.62	23.06	1.13	0.56	2.02
All-causes deaths	101	52.39	21.87	22.56	1.63	0.42	3.88
Rural Italy							
No CHD	1,207	49.33	23.29	23.13			
CHD deaths	27	52.41	21.05	21.64	1.49	0.62	2.41
Hard CHD	74	51.30	21.77	22.09	1.04	0.39	2.70
Any CHD	159	50.93	22.50	22.73	0.40	0.28	1.45
All-causes deaths	158	52.54	21.30	21.93	1.21	0.27	4.41
Greece							
No CHD	864	49.34	22.96	22.55			
CHD deaths	8	51.25	21.33	21.59	0.96	1.05	0.92
Hard CHD	21	50.76	21.60	21.67	0.88	0.65	1.35
Any CHD	50	51.66	21.91	22.25	0.30	0.43	0.69
All-causes deaths	61	53.33	21.36	22.04	0.51	0.40	1.26
Serbia							
No CHD	1,191	48.62	24.16	23.86			
CHD deaths	18	52.39	23.20	23.73	0.13	0.90	0.14
Hard CHD	37	50.74	23.58	23.74	0.12	0.63	0.19
Any CHD	89	50.50	23.57	23.63	0.18	0.42	0.43
All-causes deaths	101	52.39	21.87	22.40	1.46	0.40	3.66

stayed well could arise by chance in about 1 out of 9 trails. For hard CHD or death from coronary heart disease the vital capacity is indicated to be a significant risk factor for the American railroad men and the Italians but not for the Finns or the Serbians. If all diagnoses of coronary heart disease are accepted, vital capacity was not significant for any of the areas.

Table 13.4. Forced expiratory volume, FEV ¾, deciliters per meter height, at entry of men classified by ten-year health status, all free of cardiovascular disease at entry ($\bar{y}$ = FEV ¾ at entry; y' = FEV ¾ adjusted to age 50 by the regression in table 13.2; age = mean at entry; difference = y' for no CHD minus y' for men with specified incidence; see table 13.3 for numbers and mean ages).

Ten-year status by group	$\bar{y}$	y'	SE	t
Finland				
No CHD	19.03	18.80	0.11	—
CHD deaths	16.98	17.23	0.56	3.35
Hard CHD	17.64	17.96	0.32	2.71
Any CHD	17.96	18.09	0.21	3.09
All-causes deaths	16.24	16.69	0.36	6.71
U.S. railroad				
No CHD	16.57	16.38	0.11	—
CHD deaths	14.63	15.01	0.44	2.80
All-causes deaths	14.28	14.88	0.38	4.08
Rural Italy				
No CHD	14.23	14.07	0.08	—
CHD deaths	12.06	12.55	0.67	2.53
Hard CHD	12.45	12.69	0.41	3.72
Any CHD	13.97	14.14	0.29	−0.27
All-causes deaths	12.10	12.57	0.28	5.71
Greece				
No CHD	15.53	15.40	0.10	—
CHD deaths	15.58	15.83	1.16	−0.39
Hard CHD	14.94	15.09	0.63	0.45
Any CHD	15.45	15.79	0.33	−0.87
All-causes deaths	14.31	14.98	0.45	1.02
Serbia				
No CHD	16.50	16.17	0.09	—
CHD deaths	15.55	16.17	0.76	0
Hard CHD	16.13	16.30	0.64	−0.23
Any CHD	15.67	15.79	0.38	1.04
All-causes deaths	14.10	14.66	0.43	4.32

Table 13.4 summarizes the corresponding analysis of the data on the FEV ¾ at entry classifying, again, the men according to their ten-year health status. It appears that the forced expiratory volume at 0.75 second is a more significant risk factor than the simple vital capacity, at least for the Finns, Italians, and Americans.

Correlations with Other Variables

Evaluation of vital capacity and the timed forced expiratory volume as possible risk factors requires examination of interrelationships of those respiratory function measures with other characteristics of the persons under study (table 13.5). The forced expiratory volume at ¾ second is highly correlated with the vital capacity, but about half the variance of the one measure of respiratory function remains unaccounted for by the other. Thus it is possible that vital capacity and the timed expiratory volume are relatively independent risk factors.

Table 13.5 shows that adjustment only for age is not enough for the evaluation of vital capacity as a possible independent risk factor. In all of the population samples, vital capacity is inversely related to blood pressure, resting pulse rate, and serum cholesterol concentration, three variables that are in themselves important risk factors. Except in Serbia, the vital capacity is positively correlated with habitual physical activity. This means that the vital capacity is so correlated with other variables, in themselves risk factors, that evaluation of the significance of the ventilatory function as an independent risk factor requires appropriate multivariate analysis. Obviously, the vital capacity cannot be blamed for differences in age, but questions may be asked

Table 13.5. Correlation of vital capacity and confidence limits with other characteristics of men free of cardiovascular disease (vital capacity and FEV ¾ in deciliters per meter height).

Group	N	FEV ¾	Age	S BP	Pulse	Activity	Chol.
Finland	1,431	0.75	−0.31	−0.11	−0.07	0.10	−0.03
U.S. railroad	1,011	0.77	−0.37	−0.10	−0.11	0.09	−0.02
Rural Italy	1,565	0.62	−0.30	−0.20	−0.19	0.11	−0.08
Greece	1,088	0.75	−0.33	−0.15	−0.08	0.10	−0.01
Serbia	1,361	0.76	−0.33	−0.17	−0.08	−0.06	−0.04
Total[a]	6,456	0.724	−0.325	−0.150	−0.109	0.067	−0.033
Lower 95% CL		0.712	−0.346	−0.174	−0.173	0.057	−0.057
Upper 95% CL		0.735	−0.302	−0.126	−0.125	0.105	−0.009

a. Mean weighted by N of each group.

about possible cause and effect in regard to the other variables. From table 13.3 it is clear that the differences in mean vital capacity between the men who stayed well and those who died or developed coronary heart disease are small. Even in the case of all-causes death, where the difference is largest and statistically most significant, the difference between mean age- and height-standardized vital capacity of the men who died and those who stayed well is only 9 percent. It seems most unlikely that such a trivial difference could cause important differences in the blood pressure, resting pulse rate, habitual physical activity, and serum cholesterol concentration. The proposition that high blood pressure, fast pulse rate, and low physical activity result in a reduced level of pulmonary function appears more reasonable if, indeed, the relationships are cause and effect.

Because in all cohorts there is a highly significant correlation between age and blood pressure, it is useful to calculate the partial correlation between the respiratory function measurements and blood pressure, with age held constant. The result is summarized in table 13.6. In all the population groups the negative correlation between blood pressure and vital capacity appears to be accounted for by the age variable, and the partial correlation between vital capacity and blood pressure with age constant is a very small positive value in all of the samples. The corresponding analysis of the FEV ¾ figures, also summarized in table 13.6, agrees with the findings for vital capacity, and the values of the partial correlation coefficient are even closer to zero than in the case of the vital capacity.

It has been reported that heavy cigarette smoking is associated with a reduced vital capacity (Blackburn, Brozek, and Taylor, 1959; Hensler and Giron, 1963; Wilhelmsen and Tibblin, 1966; Seltzer et al. 1974). This tendency is confirmed in the seven countries data if the emphasis is on heavy smoking, that is, twenty or more cigarettes a day, and reduced vital capacity is understood to mean only a tendency to some reduction. Table 13.7 shows

Table 13.6. Partial correlation between respiratory function (volume per meter height) and systolic blood pressure (age held constant) in men free of cardiovascular disease.

Group	Vital capacity	FEV ¾
U.S. railroad	0.03	0.04
Finland	0.08	0.06
Rural Italy	0.12	0.04
Greece	0.10	0.05
Serbia	0.09	0.03

Table 13.7. Vital capacity (deciliters per meter height) at entry of men classified by cigarette smoking and then free of cardiovascular disease (mean vital capacity adjusted to age 50 by the regression of vital capacity on age in table 13.2; stopped means no smoking for at least a year).

Cohort	Never	Stopped	1–9	10–19	20–29	≥30
U.S. railroad						
N	230	176	52	307	222	22
Mean	24.5	25.5	24.7	24.0	23.4	21.4
SE	0.2	0.3	0.5	0.2	0.3	0.8
East Finland						
N	98	108	69	187	202	22
Mean	27.4	27.7	27.1	26.8	27.0	25.2
SE	0.5	0.4	0.4	0.3	0.3	0.7
West Finland						
N	184	129	105	222	115	3
Mean	26.9	27.9	27.7	27.7	27.2	24.0
SE	0.3	0.3	0.4	0.3	0.4	0.8
Crevalcore						
N	226	82	169	246	138	25
Mean	23.2	22.9	23.5	23.0	23.9	23.9
SE	0.2	0.5	0.3	0.2	0.3	0.6
Montegiorgio						
N	175	90	186	148	51	13
Mean	22.8	23.4	23.3	23.3	22.6	21.8
SE	0.2	0.4	0.3	0.2	0.5	0.9
Crete						
N	149	79	65	107	125	57
Mean	22.6	23.1	22.9	23.1	23.0	22.7
SE	0.3	0.3	0.4	0.3	0.3	0.4
Corfu						
N	125	45	68	148	95	16
Mean	22.0	22.8	23.1	22.2	22.2	23.2
SE	0.3	0.5	0.4	0.3	0.4	1.0
Velika Krsna						
N	185	31	42	116	60	4
Mean	24.1	23.4	24.4	23.9	23.2	23.5
SE	0.3	0.8	0.7	0.4	0.4	2.2
Zrenjanin						
N	89	74	33	168	67	30
Mean	23.7	23.6	23.2	23.0	22.5	22.8
SE	0.3	0.4	0.5	0.3	0.4	0.5
Belgrade						
N	213	64	24	77	58	61
Mean	24.5	24.5	25.5	24.3	24.8	23.6
SE	0.2	0.4	0.7	0.4	0.4	0.4

the mean values for the entry vital capacity in deciliters per meter of height, adjusted to age 50 by the regressions of vital capacity on age given in table 13.2, for men without evidence of cardiovascular disease at the time.

There is no regular relationship between vital capacity and smoking habits except for a tendency for the vital capacity to be somewhat low in the relatively few men smoking thirty or more cigarettes daily, and even that rule does not hold for the men of Crevalcore, Crete, and Corfu. In general, the mean vital capacity of men who had never smoked regularly did not differ from that of men who had not smoked for a year or more or from men who smoked fewer than ten or from ten to nineteen cigarettes daily. Even the men who habitually smoked twenty to twenty-nine cigarettes a day did not have significantly smaller vital capacities, on the average, than the nonsmokers in the same cohorts in Finland, rural Italy, and Greece.

We have not dealt with the question of the respiratory function of pipe and cigar smokers because only in Zutphen were those smoking habits common, and even at Zutphen the majority of men who smoked pipes or cigars also smoked cigarettes. A small minority of the American railroad men smoked pipes or cigars, but many of those men also smoked cigarettes. In the other cohorts few or no men smoked pipes or cigars.

Summary

The vital capacity (maximal expiratory volume) was recorded at entry in ten cohorts and the ¾ second forced expiratory volume (FEV ¾) was recorded in eight of them. The coefficient of correlation between the two measures of respiratory function ranged from $r = 0.75$ to $r = 0.77$ in all cohorts except in rural Italy where a gasometer with high airflow resistance was used and a low value of $r = 0.62$ was found.

Both measures of respiratory function were highly correlated with height and, negatively, with age. At age 50 an increase of one year of age was associated with an average decrease of 1.03 percent in vital capacity and of 1.36 percent in FEV ¾. At age 50 an increase in height from 170 to 172 cm was associated with an average increase of 2.5 percent in the vital capacity. In every cohort over one-fourth of the total variance in vital capacity was accounted for by age and height.

In all areas the measures of vital capacity were negatively related to blood pressure. Partial correlation analysis showed that the reduction of vital capacity with increasing blood pressure was almost entirely accounted for by the correlation of both variables with age.

In all areas the measures of respiratory function had a low negative correlation with serum cholesterol concentration and the resting pulse rate; the average coefficients with vital capacity were $r = -0.11$ and $r = -0.03$, respectively. Except in Serbia, the men most active physically tended to have slightly higher vital capacities, but the average coefficient of correlation between vital capacity and activity class was only $r = 0.07$.

The few men smoking thirty or more cigarettes daily tended to have somewhat reduced vital capacity at entry in seven cohorts but not in Crevalcore, Crete, or Corfu. Compared with nonsmokers, the men smoking twenty to twenty-nine cigarettes daily had slightly smaller average vital capacities in four cohorts, but there was no difference between heavy smokers and the nonsmokers in the six cohorts in Finland, rural Italy, and Greece. In general, the relation of vital capacity to smoking habits was smaller than is popularly supposed.

For men with no evidence of cardiovascular disease at entry, in each area the average vital capacity and FEV ¾ per meter height for each category of the ten-year death and disease experience was adjusted to age 50 using the calculated regression of the respiratory function on age specific to each cohort. That adjustment was necessary because the men who died or developed coronary heart disease tended to be older than the other men in the same cohorts. This age-standardized vital capacity proved to be a negative risk factor for all-causes ten-year deaths in all areas. The mean vital capacity of the men who died was significantly low (t values of 3.7 to 4.4) in all areas except in Greece, where the observed difference in the mean vital capacity could occur by chance in 1 out of 4 trials.

Among men with no cardiovascular disease at entry those who died from coronary heart disease in the United States and in rural Italy had significantly smaller average entry vital capacities than the men in their cohorts who stayed well. The seven cohorts in Finland, Greece, and Serbia showed no significant relationship in this respect. The total ten-year incidence of coronary heart disease among men judged to be healthy at entry was not significantly related to the entry vital capacity in any of the areas.

The entry averages for FEV ¾, similarly adjusted to standard average age 50, of the men classified according to their ten-year status, showed that this measure of respiratory function tended to be smaller in the men who died (all-causes) than in those who survived. The difference was highly significant ($t = 4.3$ to 6.7) in all areas except Greece. The men who died from coronary heart disease had low average values for FEV ¾ in the United States, Finland, and rural Italy but not in Greece or Serbia. The men who were given any diagnosis of the incidence of coronary heart disease in the follow-up period had a significantly low average for FEV ¾ at entry in Finland but not in the other areas. It is suggested that FEV ¾ may be more useful for prognosis than the vital capacity.

14 | Diet

The nutrients in the average diets of each of the cohorts, except for the railroad men, were estimated from surveys on statistical subsamples. The diets of the railroad men in the United States and Italy were estimated at the time of the entry examinations from a short questionnaire. For the railroad men and the Japanese, the estimation of nutrients was made from tables of food composition. For the other twelve cohorts the nutrient contents of the diets were estimated both by calculation with tables of food composition and by chemical analysis of duplicates of the meals as eaten by the individual men in seven-day periods, the surveys being repeated in different seasons on the same men. The methods have been published in detail (Hartog et al. 1968; Keys et al. 1970).

Systematic comparisons of the various methods of making dietary surveys were made as a part of the Seven Countries Study in Yugoslavia (Buzina et al. 1964; Buzina et al. 1966), in Finland (Roine, Pekkarinen and Karvonen 1964; Pekkarinen, Kivioja and Jortikka 1967; Pekkarinen 1967), in Italy (Fidanza et al. 1964; Fidanza and Fidanza-Alberti 1967), the Netherlands (Hartog et al. 1965), and Greece (Keys, Aravanis and Sdrin 1966). These studies showed that surveys that record the weights of the foods eaten over a seven-day period and convert this to nutrients with food composition tables specific for the region concerned agree with surveys that use the much more difficult and costly method of collecting replicates of all meals eaten and analyzing the seven-day composite chemically. The methods and problems of dietary surveys have been reviewed by Keys (1979).

As expected, there were striking differences in the habitual diets among cohorts but the diets were relatively homogeneous within cohorts. An important feature of the dietary findings was that the intraindividual variation, revealed in repeated surveys on the same individuals, was of the same order of magnitude as the interindividual variation within the cohort (Keys, Aravanis, and Sdrin 1966; Buzina et al. 1964; Fidanza and Fidanza-Alberti 1967; Keys 1965). The implications of that variability will be examined later in this chapter.

The cohort mean concentration of cholesterol in the blood serum at entry was correlated ($r = 0.67$) with the mean percentage of dietary calories from total fats and more highly correlated ($r = 0.87$) with the percentage of calories from saturated fatty acids. In general, this conforms to the experimentally demonstrated fact of the overriding influence on the blood serum cholesterol of the saturated fatty acids in the diet, but the question arises as to the quantitative agreement with expectation from controlled dietary experiments.

From many such experiments, each involving subsistence of groups of sixteen to twenty-four men in locked metabolic wards for ten to twelve weeks on chemically analyzed diets, the average finding from multiple regression analysis was cholesterol (in milligrams per deciliter serum) = $164 + 1.35 (2S - P) + 1.5Z$, where P and S are percentages of diet calories from saturated and polyunsaturated fatty acids, respectively, and Z is the square root of the cholesterol in the diet expressed as mg per 1,000 kilocalories (Keys, Anderson, and Grande, 1965, p. 770).

The results of dietary experiments on prisoners reported by Hegsted et al. (1965), who similarly applied multiple regression analysis to their data, were satisfactorily predicted by this formula (Keys and Parlin 1966). Jeremiah Stamler (personal communication, August 1978) stated that the findings from dietary and serum cholesterol studies on middle-aged Japanese men in California, Hawaii, and Japan are in good agreement with this formula. The mean serum cholesterol concentration of the men in Hawaii was observed to be 9.9 mg/dl lower than the California mean; the difference predicted by our formula was 8.8 mg/dl. The difference observed between the mean in California and that in Japan was 47.1 mg/dl; the difference predicted was 54 mg/dl.

The seven countries diet survey data provide mean values for S and P for each of the cohorts, but the diet cholesterol values are only estimates from tables of food composition with no control by chemical analysis. Accordingly, for each of the cohorts we have calculated only the value of $164 + 1.35 (2S - P)$ for comparison with the observed mean serum cholesterol values (figure 14.1). For the sixteen cohorts, the mean observed serum cholesterol was 202.2 mg/dl (SD = 33.4); the mean of the sixteen values of $164 + 1.35 (2S - P)$ is 189.5 mg/dl (SD 15.4). The difference between the two means, 12.7 mg/dl, may be ascribed to dietary cholesterol and anything else besides the fatty acids in the diet that may influence the serum cholesterol concentration, including what we have called the "intrinsic personal characteristic." (Keys, Anderson, and Grande 1965, p. 766). If only dietary cholesterol were responsible for the difference, its mean value may be calculated as $1.5 (12.7)^2 = 72$ mg of cholesterol per 1,000 kilocalories of diet, or around 200 mg a day for the average of the sixteen cohorts. More important is the fact that the correlation between the mean observed serum cholesterol and the value of $164 + 1.35 (2S - P)$ is $r = 0.90$ and the calculated mean, not allowing for dietary cholesterol, is only 6 percent lower than the observed value.

Other relevant characteristics of the cohorts at entry were not significantly correlated with the nutrient composition of their diets. The mean percentage of calories from proteins in the diet ranged only from 11 percent (Corfu, Crete, Montegiorgio) to 14 percent (Belgrade, Slavonia, Zrenjanin), so this material is not suitable for judging the possible influence of differences in protein percentage on other characteristics of the men. Mean systolic blood pressure and body mass index were correlated, but not significantly, with the mean percentage of calories from saturated fatty acids in the diet. With systolic blood pressure, the correlation was $r = 0.25$, but with only sixteen

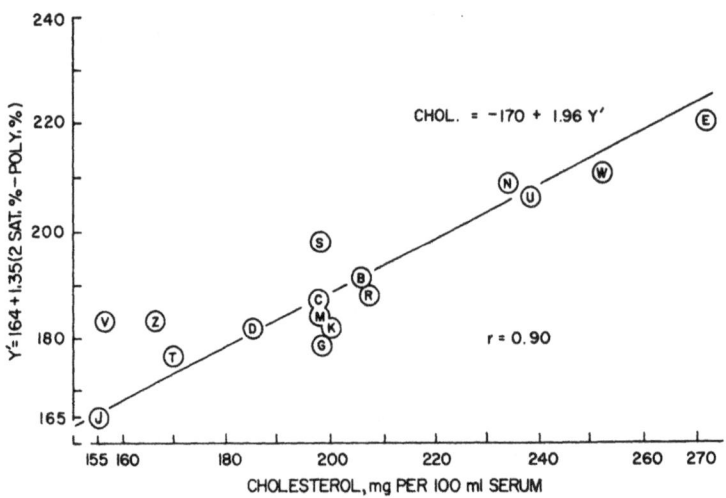

Figure 14.1. Relation of mean serum cholesterol concentration of the cohorts at entry to fat composition of the diet expressed in the multiple regression equation derived from controlled dietary experiments in Minnesota. B = Belgrade; C = Crevalcore; D = Dalmatia; E = east Finland; G = Corfu; J = Ushibuka; K = Crete; M = Montegiorgio; N = Zutphen; R = Rome railroad; S = Slavonia; T = Tanushimaru; U = American railroad; V = Velika Krsna; W = west Finland; Z = Zrenjanin.

pairs of variables the 95 percent confidence limits are −0.28 and +0.66. With body mass index, $r = 0.37$ and the 95 percent limits are −0.23 and +0.70.

Incidence Rate

In men with no evidence of cardiovascular disease at entry, the ten-year age-adjusted coronary death rate was correlated with the total fats in the diet, $r = 0.50$ (98 percent limits, +0.01 and +0.80), but the correlation with saturated fatty acids was much more significant, $r = 0.84$ (95 percent limits, +0.59 and +0.94). The ten-year incidence rate of coronary heart disease, accepting any diagnostic criterion, was less highly correlated with the dietary percentage of calories from fats; the coefficient with total fats is $r = 0.39$, with saturated fatty acids, $r = 0.73$. The first correlation is nonsignificant and the latter has 95 percent confidence limits of 0.37 and 0.90. Figures 14.2 and 14.3 display the relationships of coronary death rate to diet fat. The relationships of the incidence rate of any CHD to mean percentage of calories from diet fat are shown in figures 14.4 and 14.5.

The ten-year experience confirms and extends the five-year experience previously reported (Keys 1970). The percentage of calories supplied by saturated fatty acids in the diet is confirmed to be an important risk factor for the incidence of coronary heart disease, especially for the most serious and secure diagnosis, namely, death from that disease. The incidence rate of soft coronary heart disease (diagnosis based on criteria other than coronary death or nonfatal myocardial infarction) was also correlated with the average per-

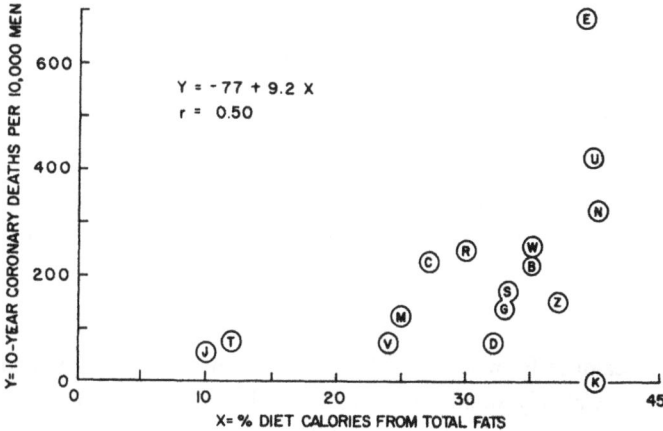

Figure 14.2. Ten-year coronary death rates of the cohorts plotted against the percentage of dietary calories supplied by total fats. Cohorts as in figure 14.1.

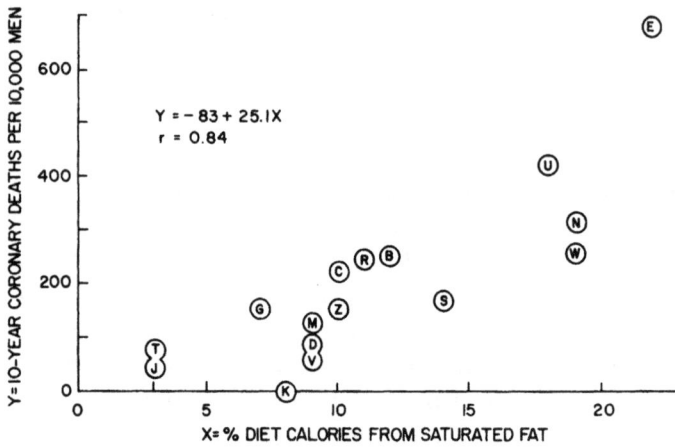

Figure 14.3. Ten-year coronary death rates of the cohorts plotted against the percentage of dietary calories supplied by saturated fatty acids. Cohorts as in figure 14.1.

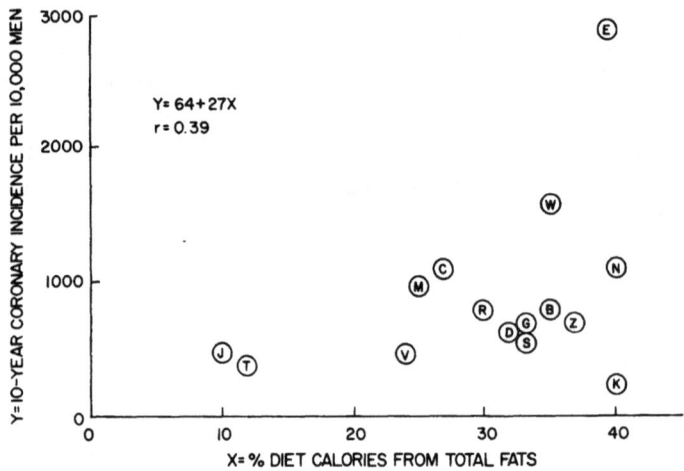

Figure 14.4. Ten-year incidence rate of coronary heart disease, by any diagnostic criterion, plotted against the percentage of dietary calories supplied by total fats. Cohorts as in figure 14.1.

centage of calories from saturated fatty acids in the diet, but the coefficient, $r = 0.64$, is relatively small compared with the coefficient for hard CHD, $r = 0.79$, and for coronary death, $r = 0.84$.

The ten-year incidence rate of coronary heart disease was significantly correlated with the percentage of calories supplied by sucrose in the average

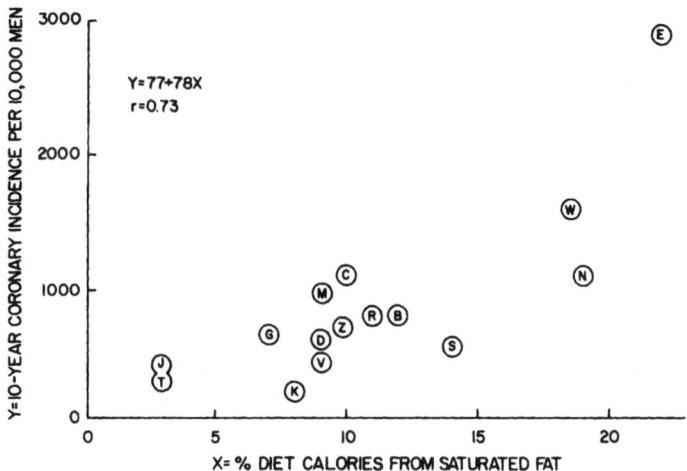

Figure 14.5. Ten-year incidence rate of coronary heart disease, by any diagnostic criterion, plotted against the percentage of dietary calories supplied by saturated fatty acids. Cohorts as in figure 14.1.

diets of the cohorts. However, as found in the analysis of the five-year follow-up data (Keys 1971), the correlation is accounted for by the intercorrelation of sucrose with saturated fatty acids in the diet. Partial correlation analysis showed that, with dietary saturated fat held constant, the correlation between dietary sucrose and the incidence of coronary heart disease is not significant ($r = 0.13$). On the other hand, with sucrose held constant in the partial correlation analysis, the correlation of the coronary incidence rate with the mean percentage of calories from saturated fat is $r = 0.62$.

The coronary incidence rate of the cohorts was not significantly correlated with the percentage of calories in the diet provided by proteins or by polyunsaturated fatty acids. In regard to the latter, the averages for the cohorts ranged from 3 percent to seven percent of calories from linoleic acid, with only trivial contributions from other polyenes. These findings conform to the general picture that in no natural diet of man so far studied do polyunsaturated fatty acids contribute more than a very small fraction of the total calories. Accordingly it must be expected that in such natural diets variations in the amount of polyunsaturated fatty acids will have at most only a trivial effect on the concentration of cholesterol in the blood serum or risk associated with it. As indicated above, the very narrow range of the average protein contribution to the diet calories in these cohorts precludes judgment of the possible effect of important differences in dietary protein.

Besides differing in the kind and amount of fats, the diets of the cohorts tended to differ in other respects that conceivably could affect the blood lipids and atherogenesis, but is is not now possible to pinpoint in quantitative detail the items of the greatest relevance. Fruits and vegetables other than roots and tubers are much more prominent in the average diets in Italy and Greece than in those of Finland, the Netherlands, and the United States. But because of the variety of fruits and vegetables involved, there is no obvious way of deciding what characteristics may be relevant. The original dietary records of some of the cohorts are currently being examined with a view to the estimation of fiber content.

Correlation with Serum Cholesterol in Individuals

In spite of elaborate efforts to obtain reliable figures for the nutrient composition of the diet consumed by the men in the special dietary subsamples in the Seven Countries Study, there was no significant correlation in those subsamples between the nutrient composition estimated for the individual men and the serum cholesterol values recorded for those individuals (Hartog et al. 1968). We have explained these negative findings as an expected result in the situation, as in these surveys, where the intraindividual variation in the dietary variables is of the same order of magnitude as the interindividual variation (Keys 1965, 1979). When this is the case it is not possible to classify the individuals reliably in respect to their position in the array of dietary variables. This was proved in repetitions of the surveys on the same men. On the other hand, the group mean values of the dietary variables were in satisfactory agreement in repeated surveys. Thus it appears that such surveys can reliably characterize the central tendency of the group, though they fail to place the individuals in reliable order within the group. This is the common situation when surveys are made of individuals in a given ethnic group in which dietary habits are relatively homogeneous. This principle was notably documented in repeated week-long surveys made in 1953 and 1954 on men in the long-time prospective study on Twin City executives (Adelson and Keys 1962). The differences between serum cholesterol values of the individual men were not "explained" by the reported differences in their diets (Adelson and Keys 1962). Results in dietary surveys on persons in the Framingham Study were similar (Mann et al. 1962; Dawber et al. 1962).

The inadequacies of the methods commonly used in dietary surveys certainly contribute to the failure of the surveys to reliably place the individuals in the array of the distribution of the diets, and therefore to relate to the individual cholesterol levels; however, they do not necessarily invalidate the averages for groups. We have reported on the good correspondence between group average changes in the diet and the average changes in serum cholesterol, not only in metabolic wards and fully controlled experimental studies but also in free living population samples (Keys 1967).

Examination of the report on a survey of 10,000 civil servants in Israel (Kahn et al. 1969) provides a good example of conformity of group averages to theoretical expectation in spite of lack of success in the attempt to relate individual diets to individual serum cholesterol levels. No data on intra-individual variation were obtained for either dietary variables or serum cholesterol, but the mean values were tabulated for each of the six geographical areas of origin of the Jews in the survey—Israel itself, eastern, central, and Southern Europe, Asia, and Africa. With these averages for the six areas of origin, the correlation between serum cholesterol and the estimated dietary saturated fat as percentage of total calories is $r = 0.94$. The dietary estimates for those samples of men of Israel are unusual in that they indicate a total fat intake of less than 30 percent of calories from that source, with polyunsaturated fatty acids accounting for 24 percent of those fat calories. It is interesting, then, to relate the serum cholesterol averages of the areas of origin to the expression $2S - P$, where S = percentage of total calories from saturated fatty acids and P that from polyunsaturated fatty acids (Keys, Anderson, and Grande, 1957, 1965). The correlation between average serum cholesterol and the average for $2S - P$ in the Israel data proves to be $r = 0.93$, essentially identical with that for saturated fatty acids.

In spite of the difficulties in relating the serum cholesterol values of individuals to their estimated diets (Antonis et al. 1965), correlations have been found in a number of studies. In a detailed study of 100 men with coronary heart disease in Ireland it was found that "the serum cholesterol of the patients was correlated with their fat, carbohydrate, calorie, and cholesterol intakes" (Finegan et al. 1968). However, the correlations observed are not statistically very important.

In a study of twenty-four young men on a year-long expedition to Antarctica, 200 measurements of the diet were made by the direct twenty-four-hour weighing method (Easty 1970). The accuracy of the estimations of the nutrient content of the diets was favored by the fact that, except for fresh meat eaten weekly, the diet was almost entirely composed of "tinned" and dehydrates. According to Easty, "apart from this characteristic [the diet] did not vary from the normal diet that would have been expected in the United Kingdom." The average nutrient composition of the diets for the year were: 3,597 kcal per day, 12.1 percent protein calories, 39.8 percent fat calories. The coefficient of correlation between total serum cholesterol and fat calories was $r = 0.53$ and that between beta lipoprotein cholesterol and fat calories was $r = 0.58$. The probability of chance explanation for both cases is less than 0.01. The correlation between the ratio of cholesterol to phospholipid in the serum to the percentage intake of fat in the diet was $r = 0.78$ ($p = 0.001$). It is interesting that in this material the intraindividual variance in the dietary nutrients was similar to the interindividual variance; obviously the many repetitions of the estimates for each individual allowed reasonably reliable placement of the individuals in the distribution of the diets. There was a slight average increase in body weight and skinfold thickness in the first two months of the stay in Antarctica with no change thereafter.

In New Zealand 517 Seventh-Day Adventists among about 2,000 attending a camp convention participated in a survey of the diet and blood pressure and serum cholesterol measured in blood from the fasting state (Fraser and Swanell 1979). The data, analyzed by the method of stepwise multiple regression, showed serum cholesterol to be significantly related to age, spread fat (butter and margarine), and ice cream. For each diet an estimate was made of $2S - P$, where S and P are the percentages of dietary calories provided by saturated and polyunsaturated fatty acid calories, respectively. In the multiple regression analysis with serum cholesterol versus age and $2S - P$, the coefficients for both age and $2S - P$ proved to be highly significant for men, but for women the relationship of serum cholesterol to $2S - P$ was less clear. It should be noted that those Seventh Day Adventists included strict vegetarians, partial vegetarians, and meat eaters, so there was a good deal more dietary heterogeneity than is commonly found in samples of people in most dietary surveys. It seems likely that such large interindividual variation was important for the positive finding obtained. A study on Seventh-Day Adventists in the area of Washington, D.C., compared vegetarians with nonvegetarians matched for place of residence, sex, age, marital status, height, weight, and occupation; serum cholesterol was significantly higher in the nonvegetarians, and the difference was seen at all ages from 25 to 72 (West and Hayes 1968).

In 1955 we surveyed Italian policemen and firemen in two cities of Italy reputed to differ in the local dietary habits, Bologna and Cagliari. In each area we also added to the survey a few men in more sedentary jobs in the medical schools and a few men doing rather heavy manual labor, making a total of 327 apparently healthy men aged 20 through 59 years of age. The dietary information was obtained by interview about the number of servings per week of meat and of fish, the number of eggs weekly, estimated amounts of butter, milk, olive oil, cheese, and wine. Each man received a standard medical examination including measurement of serum cholesterol, skinfold thickness, height, and weight. From multiple regression analysis, serum cholesterol, as the dependent variable, proved to be related to age and sum of the skinfolds, and among the dietary variables butterfat was the most significant of the dietary variables. When all the men were taken as the sample, the individual serum cholesterol value proved to be significantly correlated with the individual diet, but when Cagliari and Bologna data were analyzed separately the diet serum cholesterol correlations were not significant, illustrating the rule that within a population with high homogeneity in dietary habits it is extremely difficult to demonstrate a significant correlation between the dietary pattern of the individuals and the serum cholesterol values of those individuals.

The most recently reported study on the relationship between the blood plasma lipids and the diets of free-living individuals concerns the Tarahumara Indians of the mountains of Mexico, an unacculturated people who have attracted attention because of their remarkable endurance in kickball races, often lasting for several days, and a diet with very little food from animal sources (Connor et al. 1978). The nutrient intakes of a sample of 103 adult Indians, excluding pregnant and lactating women, were estimated from standard dietary interviews, supplemented by observations of the actual foods eaten. The plasma cholesterol concentrations of those Indians proved to be positively correlated, with probability of chance explanation less than $p = 0.01$, with dietary cholesterol ($r = 0.90$), animal fat ($r = 0.50$), total fat ($r = 0.55$), eggs ($r = 0.55$), animal protein ($r = 0.46$), and sugar ($r = 0.32$). The plasma cholesterol concentration was negatively correlated, with less than $p = 0.01$ of chance explanation, with vegetable protein ($r = 0.72$), vegetable fat ($r = 0.40$), and fiber ($r = 0.38$).

With partial correlation analysis, it seems certain that at least some of these lower correlations would lose statistical significance because of intercorrelations among the dietary variables. Plasma cholesterol was not correlated with body weight. The average diet of the adult Tarahumara provided 3 percent of calories from saturated fats, 4 percent from mono-enes, and 5 percent from polyunsaturates. The average cholesterol for adult men was 134 mg/dl plasma. A letter from W. E. Connor (August 29, 1978) advises, "We have since done a metabolic study with Tarahumara Indians and have found similar effects from dietary cholesterol as in other Americans."

The fact that most attempts to find a significant relationship between serum cholesterol values of individuals and estimates of the composition of their diets have been unsuccessful has cast doubt on the validity of the whole theory of the role of diet as a risk factor for disease. The difficulty lies in the intraindividual variability in both serum cholesterol and the diet, the latter variability being of the same magnitude as the interindividual variability in culturally homogeneous societies (Keys 1965; Buzina et al. 1964). Where significant relations have been found for free-living individuals, success may be ascribed to the reduction of intraindividual variability. This is done by making many observations on each individual, as in the young men of Antarctica, or by studying a sample with large interindividual differences, as in the case of the Seventh-Day Adventists in New Zealand (Fraser and Swanell 1979). The basic statistical theory has now been examined in mathematical detail.

The role of intraindividual variation in causing low-order or no correlation between lipids in the diet and serum cholesterol levels has been examined at length by Liu et al. (1978) who also provide detailed advice about the need to disclose true relationships often obscured by intraindividual variation. Besides insisting on the greatest precision for each cholesterol analysis and dietary estimate, more measurements on each individual are needed. "Increased numbers of measurements do not reduce intraindividual variation, but they can make possible reliable estimation of the individual's mean and thus allow accurate characterization of the individual, if validity of the data be assumed" (Liu et al. 1978). For an analysis based on food records for 448 men in Chicago to have a probability of less than 0.05 of misclassifying men of quintile five versus quintile one in regard to dietary cholesterol, at least seven days of food records would be needed. To avoid an error of over 10 percent in the accuracy of the estimation of the correlation coefficient between saturated fat and serum cholesterol due to intraindividual variation, the Chicago data indicate the need for nine food records on each man. In other samples the numbers of records needed may, of course, vary.

Jacobs, Anderson, and Blackburn (1979) also addressed themselves to the theoretical explanation of the apparent paradox between the relationship abundantly proved in controlled experiments and the frequent failure to find those relationships in surveys. They proposed a mathematical model and showed that the facts of intraindividual variation mean that "a cross-sectional study has near zero power for detecting such a relationship. It is expected that correlations near zero would arise between diet and serum cholesterol whether they are related or not. Thus cross-sectional observation of this relationship seems to be inappropriate." It may be remarked, however, that cross-sectional analyses are often appropriate for comparing groups and need not be misleading when the true interindividual variation is large, as in the case of the New Zealand Seventh-Day Adventists or the combined samples of men of Cagliari and Bologna.

The importance of these insights into the relationship of the serum cholesterol level to the diet of free-living individuals has been stressed by Stamler (1978) because they remove one of the more stubborn obstacles to the acceptance of arguments in favor of dietary management in efforts at primary prevention of coronary heart disease.

Vital Statistics

Comparisons of death rates from coronary heart disease in different countries with official data on the average diets of those countries were first made in 1952 when apparently comparable data were available from only six countries (Keys 1952, 1953a). That comparison indicated that the coronary death rate is directly related to the percentage of calories supplied by fats in the average diet. The objection that animal protein in the diet could be just as consequential as the fat content (Yerushalmy and Hilleboe 1957), concerned a similar comparison of twelve countries, but some of the data cited did not, in fact, conform to the official figures from the respective governments. The mortality data were for all heart diseases, not only for coronary heart disease, and they referred to years before the dietary data, a period in which the diet was rapidly changing in many of the twelve countries. Those same discredited data on twelve countries for the early 1950s were published again (Hilleboe 1967) ten years after their gross errors had been exposed (Keys 1957).

After it became clear that saturated rather than simply total fats should be the focus, Jolliffe and Archer (1959) made a detailed analysis of the dietary and mortality data then available from twenty countries. They concluded that, "of all the factors considered, the intake of saturated fat was most important in accounting for the differences in coronary heart disease death rates between countries." More recent analyses concerning more countries and increasingly comparable data are in agreement (Masironi 1970; Stamler, Stamler, and Shekelle 1970; Stamler 1973). Such epidemiological findings cannot prove cause and effect, but they are impressively consistent with the theory that saturated fats in the diet promote atherogenesis in man.

Although official statistics in the developed countries of the western world are increasingly reliable, questions still arise about the comparability in different countries of diagnoses and ascription of the cause of death. However, within countries with common nationwide standards of medical education and of legal certification of the cause of death, considerable credence can be given to regional differences in mortality in the vital statistics. In Italy, where a single system of medical services (socialized medicine) and death certification prevails throughout the country, the reported coronary death rate varies substantially among the sixteen regions (Menotti 1973; Mancini and Di Marino 1973). Considering persons over 40 years of age and taking the all-Italy rate for each sex as 100, the highest coronary death rate prevails in Lombardy, with 132 for men and 126 for women; the lowest rate, in Sardinia, with rates of 67 for men and 75 for women. The regions of Italy also differ in diet, notably in respect to the use of meats and dairy products, so it is interesting to examine the relationship between the coronary death rate and the dietary variables in the regions.

Table 14.1 summarizes the regression analysis of the relation of the coronary death rates of the regions of Italy to the per capita consumption of meat, milk, and cheese in those regions. The correlation between coronary death rate and meat consumption is $r = 0.59$ for men, $r = 0.40$ for women. The correlation between the coronary death rate and the consumption of milk and cheese is $r = 0.79$ for men, $r = 0.66$ for women. When both dietary items are considered in multiple regression, coronary death rate $= a + bX + cY$, where X is meat consumption and Y is consumption of milk and cheese. The least-squares result is death rate of men $= -11 + 0.41X + 5.37Y$, where the coefficient of multiple correlation is $R = 0.80$. The very small increase in the correlation when both dietary variables are considered together reflects the fact that in the regions of Italy the consumption of meat and that of dairy products are rather highly correlated ($r = 0.57$). The partial correlation between meat consumption and the coronary death rate of men, holding the dairy product consumption constant, is only $r = 0.28$, which is not statistically significant with only 15 degrees of freedom. The partial correlation of death rate with diary products consumption, holding meat constant, is highly significant ($r = 0.67$). Again, no claim is made that these correlations prove cause and effect, but the facts are consistent with the theory.

The differences in the consumption of meat and dairy products in the regions of Italy reflect climatic and economic differences. Sardinia and the southern regions are least suited to dairy farming and animal husbandry because there is little pasture land and a chronic shortage of water in the long rainless summer. Although with modern transport meats and dairy products can be shipped to the south and the islands, those items are expensive and the people in those regions are poorer than their countrymen in the north of Italy. In all parts of Italy the family expenditure for meats and dairy

Table 14.1. CHD death rate, y, from coronary heart disease of men and women over 40 years of age in fourteen regions of Italy (percentage of national average for age and sex as related to average consumption of meat, x_1, and of milk and cheese, x_2; $y = a + bx$).

Food	Men			Women		
	a	b	r	a	b	r
Meat (x_1)	35	1.1	0.59	62	0.6	0.40
Milk, cheese (x_2)	−5	6.3	0.79	26	4.4	0.66

products is closely related to the family income. According to the official statistics for 1974 (ISTAT, *Annuario di statistiche del lavoro*, vol. 15, Rome), the richest families spend an average of two and a half times more for meats than the poorest families, and the discrepancy in expenditure for milk and cheese is almost as great.

Summary

The nutrients in the average diets of the American and Italian railroad men and the Japanese were estimated from questionnaires answered by each man, using tables of food composition. For the other twelve cohorts the nutrients consumed in seven-day periods were estimated for statistical subsamples of the men in the cohorts both from tables of food composition and from chemical analysis, made in Minnesota, of lyophilized duplicates, collected in the homes, of all foods consumed. Those surveys were repeated in several seasons, but although food items changed, the averages of the several nutrients as percentage of dietary calories were relatively constant.

The average dietary composition differed greatly among cohorts, but within cohorts it was relatively homogeneous. Within the cohort the intraindividual variation was commonly of the same order as the interindividual variation within that cohort. Statistical theory shows that in this situation a significant correlation cannot be expected between individual serum cholesterol values and estimated nutrient composition of their diets unless the surveys of those individuals are repeated many times so as to reduce the effects of intraindividual variation.

Mean values of percentage of dietary calories provided by saturated and polyunsaturated fatty acids in the sixteen cohorts were used to calculate expected mean serum cholesterol concentrations from the regression equation derived from many controlled dietary experiments in closed metabolic units. The correlation between observed and expected mean values of the cohorts is $r = 0.90$. Making no allowance for dietary cholesterol, not measured in the surveys, the mean predicted serum cholesterol concentration for all sixteen cohorts was 189.5 mg/dl; the observed mean was 202.2 mg/dl. The mean difference of 12.7 mg/dl could be explained if dietary cholesterol provided an average of 72 mg of cholesterol per 1,000 kcal, or around 200 mg per man per day, a reasonable figure.

Other characteristics of the cohorts were not significantly correlated with the mean nutrient composition of their diets. Because the mean dietary calories from proteins in the cohorts varied only from 11 percent to 14 percent of calories, this material is not suitable for judging possible influence of dietary proteins. The coefficient of correlation of the average percentage of calories from saturated fats in the diets of the cohorts with systolic blood pressure was $r = 0.25$ and with body mass index $r = 0.37$. But with only sixteen pairs of values, these correlations are only suggestive.

The ten-year rate of death from coronary heart disease was correlated with the mean percentage of dietary calories from total fat ($r = 0.50$). The correlation of coronary death rate with mean percentage of calories from saturated fatty acids was $r = 0.84$, statistically much more significant. The correlation of the ten-year incidence rate of any diagnosis of coronary heart disease with total fat as a percentage of calories was only $r = 0.39$. With percentage of dietary calories from saturated fat $r = 0.73$.

The fact that the incidence rate of coronary heart disease was significantly correlated with the average percentage of calories from sucrose in the diets is explained by the intercorrelation of sucrose with saturated fat. Partial correlation analysis shows that with saturated fat constant there was no significant correlation between dietary sucrose and the incidence of coronary heart

Comparisons of coronary death rates with estimates of national diets in international statistics indicate a strong direct relationship with saturated fat in the diet, but the comparability of death certificates from different countries may be questioned. Comparisons of regions within a country with national standards and a single system of certification should be more acceptable. In the fourteen regions of Italy, the correlation of coronary death rate of men with per capita consumption of meat is $r = 0.59$; with per capita consumption of milk and cheese, $r = 0.79$.

15 | Multivariate Analyses

The simplest approach to the evaluation of the relationship of a characteristic to the prospect of future disease is to classify persons in regard to the characteristic and compare classes in their incidence rates of disease in the follow-up. But most characteristics of interest are continuous variables; to force them into discontinuous classes means a loss of information and the implication that risk, too, is discontinuous. A more serious problem arises when, as is commonly the case, several characteristics are simultaneously involved to influence the development of the disease. Cross tabulation in respect to each of the characteristics of interest may be used, but as pointed out by Truett et al. (1967), this loses much information by forcing continuous distributions into a few arbitrary classes and becomes wholly impractical with more than a few broadly classed variables.

The alternative to classification is to examine the possible relationship between a characteristic and eventual disease with a mathematical model. Linear regression is the simplest model, giving a value of zero to the absence of disease and one to its presence. The univariate form is $y = a + bx$, where x is the measurement of the characteristic. This does not dispose of the problem of simultaneous influence of other variables that may be interrelated, but the model may be expanded to the multiple regression, $y = a + b_1 x_1 \ldots b_k x_k$, in which the coefficient of each x variable is an estimate of its independent contribution. The computation can also yield values for the standard errors of the coefficients. The ratio of the coefficient to its standard error is the t value from which the statistical significance of the coefficient, and therefore of the variable, is gauged.

In the analysis of risk factors for coronary heart disease a substantial advance was the replacement of the multiple regression equation with the logistic; this yields a solution in terms of probability: $p = 1/1 + e$ to the power $-(\alpha + \beta_i x_i \ldots \beta_k x_k)$, α being the intercept and β the coefficients for the corresponding independent x variables. Truett, Cornfield, and Kannel (1967) devised a method for solving the multiple logistic equation for observed values and applied it with notable success to data from Framingham. Walker and Duncan (1967) provided a theoretically superior iterative method for solving the equation without the assumptions about the character of the distributions of the variables required in the method of Truett, Cornfield, and Kannel.

The special virtue of the logistic equation is that from the solution it is simple to estimate the risk probability of individuals or groups knowing their characteristics in regard to the independent x variables. A value of $p = 0.05$ simply means that the risk is 1 in 20. In many parallel applications of the methods of Truett et al. and of Walker and Duncan, we have never found any appreciable difference between the results. However, we prefer the latter method for its theoretical elegance in spite of its much greater demand for computer time. Moreover, in many comparisons with the ordinary multiple regression equation, we have never found the logistic to have any greater discriminating power but prefer it for the immediate ease of interpretation of the results.

Both the multiple regression and logistic models assume linear relationships between x and y or x and p, but curvilinear relationships can be examined by suitable transformations of x. An example is detailed in the next section concerning relative weight or body mass index in which the use of the square of the body mass index as an additional x variable portrays a curvilinear, U-shaped relationship that seems to fit the data more closely than the simple rectilinear relationship otherwise assumed.

Computer solutions of both the multiple regression and the logistic equations yield estimates of the standard errors of the coefficients. The ratio of the coefficient to its standard error is a t value indicating the likelihood that the difference of the coefficient from zero could result by chance. The common convention is to insist on a value of $p = 0.05$ or less before concluding significance. However, we object to rigid use of a convention that would reject a value of $p = 0.06$ as nonsignificant and therefore meaningless and would emphasize a value of $p = 0.05$, as though it were a different order of magnitude of probability.

Various methods are available for the estimation of the discriminating power of the solution of a model such as the multiple logistic. There is no difficulty in deciding whether the solution has significant discriminating power; it is more difficult to decide whether one solution or one model is better than another when both, in fact, clearly have high discriminating power. The likelihood ratio of Neyman and Pearson, the ratio of a conditional maximum of the likelihood function to its unconditional maximum, has wide applicability; it increases with the numbers involved and with the agreement between observation and expectation or prediction. Another measure, proposed by Menotti et al. (1977), measures the distribution of observed cases in the decile classes of the calculated probability. The first moment, M1, is defined as the sum of the decile class numbers multiplied by the number of cases in the corresponding decile classes, divided by the total number of cases in all ten decile classes. M1 has limits of ten, when all cases are found in the tenth decile, and one, when all cases are in the first decile. Higher orders of moments can be calculated. The second moment, M2, is calculated by taking the square of the decile class number as the multiplier. The likelihood ratio statistic (LRS) and the moments of Menotti et al. are alike in that with equal numbers the higher the value, the better the discrimination.

In chapter 7 the correlation of the cohort ten-year coronary death rate with median entry systolic blood pressure was shown to be $r = 0.64$. Chapter 8 showed a similar correlation of the coronary death rate with the cohort median serum cholesterol concentration, $r = 0.65$. Both of those correlations are highly significant, and when both of the entry variables are considered simultaneously it would be expected that together they would account for a larger proportion of the variance of the cohort coronary death rates. Figure 15.1 summarizes the result of the solution of the multiple regression equation. Because the coefficient of multiple correlation is $r = 0.81$, two-thirds of the variance of the cohort coronary death rates is accounted for by these two entry variables. The variable of age was taken care of by the use of age-standardized death rates, but age is a minor variable in the comparison of cohorts because the cohorts are so closely similar in age. Consideration of other entry variables does not significantly improve the discrimination of ten-year coronary death rates of the cohorts.

Relative Body Weight

The report on the five-year experience of the men in the Seven Countries Study presented graphs indicating that the incidence of coronary heart disease and of death was not linearly related to relative body weight or skinfold thickness, but a curvilinear relationship might hold, at least for the men of Croatia, Finland, rural Italy, and Zutphen (Keys 1970, pp. 46, 61, 73, 86). Accordingly, in the analysis of the ten-year data both the body mass index itself and the quadratic were examined with multiple regression and multiple logistic solutions, the independent variables, in addition to body mass index, being age, systolic blood pressure, serum cholesterol concentration, cigarette

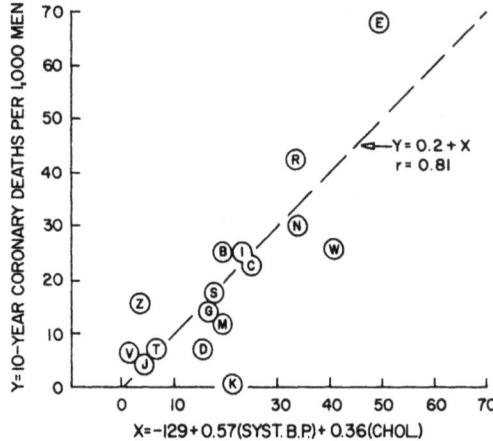

Figure 15.1. Cohort systolic blood pressure and serum cholesterol concentration medians at entry versus ten-year age-standardized death rate from coronary heart disease of men without cardiovascular disease at entry. The multiple regression solution indicates agreement with the observed coronary death rate of $r = 0.81$, and the slope, $b = 1.00$, has SE=0.19. B = Belgrade; C = Crevalcore; D = Dalmatia; E = east Finland; G = Corfu; I = Italian railroad; K = Crete; M = Montegiorgio; N = Zutphen; R = American railroad; S = Slavonia; T = Tanushimaru; V = Velika Krsna; W = west Finland, Z = Zrenjanin.

use, and resting pulse rate. In the quadratic both BMI and the square of BMI were included as variables.

Table 15.1 gives the t values of the coefficients for the BMI in the linear and for BMI and its square in the quadratic expression, together with two measures of the discrimination achieved. For the American railroad men the linear version indicates a significant negative relation between the body mass index and the probability of death from any cause in ten years. In the quadratic version the probability that the coefficient for body mass index truly differs from zero is about 11 to 1, and the corresponding figure for the square of BMI is 7 to 1. Those probabilities, of course, are smaller than the 20 to 1 odds commonly demanded to insist on statistical significance. Still, both the first moment and the likelihood ratio are smaller in the linear than in the quadratic version, suggesting better discrimination with the latter.

The corresponding analysis of the data from northern Europe does not identify any BMI coefficient as being significantly different from zero for any of the three end points. However, for all end points the values are slightly greater for the first moment and for LRS in the quadratic than in the simple linear expression of BMI. For southern Europe the coefficient for simple

Table 15.1. Values of t (β coefficient/SE) of the coefficients for body mass index (BMI) and its square in solutions to the multiple logistic equation for ten-year events in three major population groups (men free of cardiovascular disease at entry; M_1 = first moment; LRS = likelihood ratio statistic).

Ten-year event by group	N cases	Linear BMI			Quadratic BMI			
		t, BMI	M_1	LRS	t, BMI	t, BMI^2	M_1	LRS
U.S. railroad								
All-causes deaths	199	−2.31	7.29	118.0	−1.63	1.38	7.30	119.7
CHD deaths	93	.11	7.65	70.9	1.08	1.07	7.66	72.2
Northern Europe[a]								
All-causes deaths	242	−.20	7.00	100.2	−1.74	1.71	7.00	104.1
CHD deaths	91	1.18	7.76	55.9	.40	−.21	7.78	56.0
Hard CHD	217	.59	7.33	100.5	.57	−.49	7.34	100.8
Southern Europe[b]								
All-causes deaths	439	−2.16	7.40	275.2	−3.73	3.49	7.43	286.0
CHD deaths	72	.68	7.95	52.9	−.28	.38	7.98	53.0
Hard CHD	162	1.80	7.17	51.6	−.17	.43	7.20	51.7

a. Finland and Zutphen.
b. Italy, Greece, and Yugoslavia.

BMI indicates a significant negative correlation between BMI and the probability of death from all causes. In the quadratic form the coefficients for BMI and the square of BMI are both indicated to have high statistical significance, but none of the coefficients for coronary death or hard CHD is significant. Again the first moment and LRS favor the quadratic version.

The upshot of all this is to indicate that the risk of death in ten years decreases with relative body weight according to the linear model of BMI, but that the quadratic model is more appropriate. Neither the linear nor the quadratic model points to relative body weight as being of interest in regard to the risk of dying from coronary heart disease or suffering myocardial infarction.

The character of the relationship of ten-year death rate to body mass index, indicated in the linear and quadratic models, is graphically shown in figures 15.2–15.4. In those graphs the ten-year risk probability of death is plotted against body mass index for men free of cardiovascular disease, starting at age 45 and again at age 55, with the same characteristics, corresponding to the mean values for all men in the group at entry, for systolic blood pressure, serum cholesterol, cigarette smoking, and resting pulse rate.

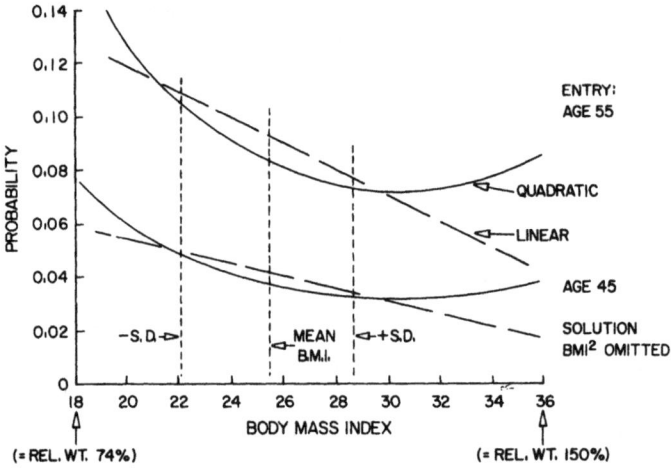

Figure 15.2. Probability of death in ten years of United States railroad men, free of cardiovascular disease at entry, calculated from multiple logistic solutions with the independent variables age, systolic blood pressure, serum cholesterol, smoking, pulse rate, and body mass index, and the same variables plus the square of BMI. Probability of death plotted against body mass index for starting ages 45 and 55, with mean values at entry of other variables for both linear and quadratic expressions of BMI.

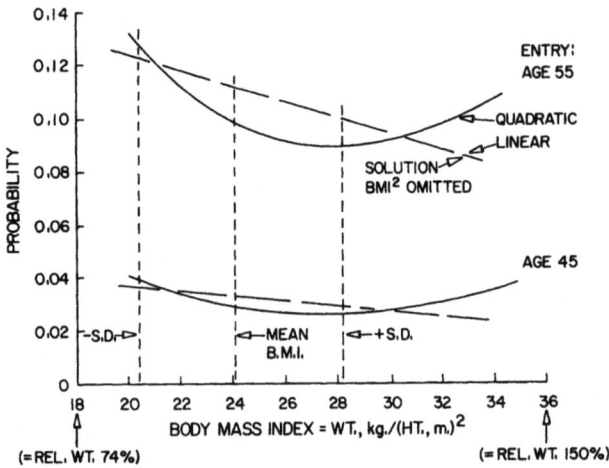

Figure 15.3. Probability of death in ten years of men in southern Europe (Italy, Greece, and Yugoslavia), free of cardiovascular disease at entry, calculated from multiple logistic solutions as in figure 15.1.

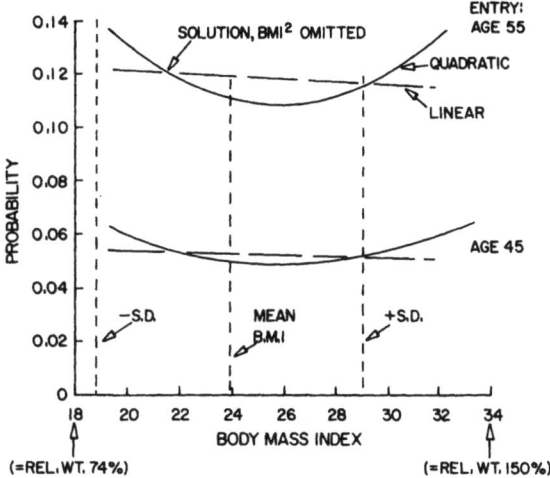

Figure 15.4. Probability of death in ten years of men in northern Europe (Finland and Zutphen), free of cardiovascular disease at entry, calculated from multiple logistic solutions as in figure 15.1.

In all cases except for coronary death among United States railroad men, the simple linear model indicates decreasing risk of death with increasing body mass index. For the United State railroad men there is no indication that the risk of coronary death is significantly related to the body mass index.

With the data from the Japanese men of Tanushimaru and Ushibuka for all-causes death in ten years, the multiple logistic equation was solved with age, systolic blood pressure, serum cholesterol, cigarette smoking, and body mass index as the independent variables and again with the same variables plus the square of the body mass index. In the first case, BMI proved to be a negative risk factor, but with $t = -1.14$, the coefficient is not significant. In the solution with BMI in the quadratic form, neither BMI nor BMI-squared coefficients were statistically significant ($t = 0.87$ and -0.95, respectively), but the net effect is also to indicate that over most of the range of BMI it is a negative risk factor. Figure 15.5 shows both quadratic and linear indications for men age 45 and 55 with systolic pressure, cholesterol, and smoking at the average values for all the Japanese men. The quadratic result is an inverted U.

On the face of it, the suggestion is that to avoid early death it is best for these Japanese men to be either thin or fat; the worst prospect applies to the middle of the distribution of relative body weight. But no such conclusion is justified. Though the graph is based on the best mathematical solution, the coefficients are far from being significantly different from zero. In the linear

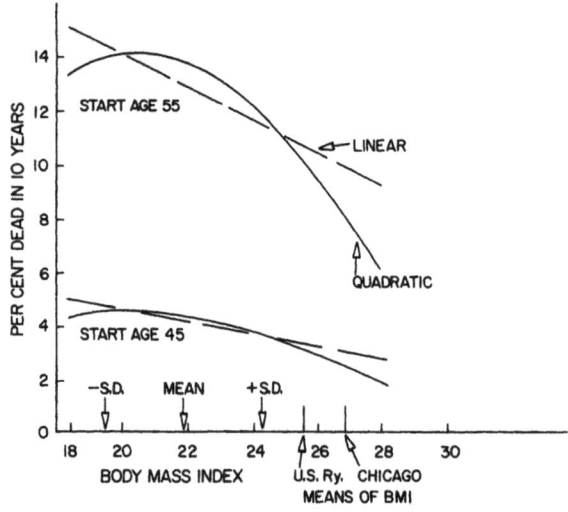

Figure 15.5. Probability of death in ten years for the Japanese men of Tanushimaru and Ushibuka, starting free of cardiovascular disease, calculated from multiple logistic solutions as in figure 15.1. None of the coefficients for BMI and BMI squared is statistically significant.

use of the body mass index, the result is a negative coefficient for body mass index. This means that the probability of death tends to decrease with increasing body mass index. But because the standard error of that coefficient is just as large as the coefficient, the t value is -1.0. Thus the data from the Japanese men fail to show any significant relationship of death rate to relative body weight. With body mass index used as the quadratic, the t values for the index and for its square are 0.8 and -0.9, respectively; again the conclusion is that no significant relationship was found.

Figure 15.6 gives the corresponding figure for ten-year deaths of American railroad men ascribed to coronary heart disease. Here again, like the all-causes deaths of the Japanese men, the quadratic indicates an inverted U, suggesting that the middle of the distribution of the body mass index is associated with the greatest likelihood of dying from coronary heart disease. The limitation is the same as with the all-causes deaths of the Japanese; neither in the linear nor in the quadratic use of the body mass index are the resulting coefficients significantly different from zero. Thus there is no indication of any relationship of coronary death to relative body weight.

The solution to the logistic equation that produced the coefficient used in making figure 15.6 gave coefficients for age, systolic blood pressure, and serum cholesterol of very high significance, with t values of 3.4, 3.4, and

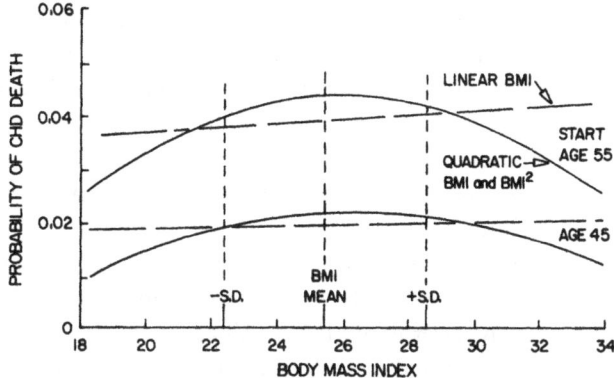

Figure 15.6. Probability of death in ten years from coronary heart disease of American railroad men, free of cardiovascular disease at entry, calculated from multiple logistic solutions as in figure 15.1.

4.5, respectively. The coefficient for cigarette smoking had a t value of 1.5, about a 6 percent chance that it is really not different from zero. The coefficient for the resting pulse rate in that same solution had a t value of 1.3, or odds of about 10 to 1 that the probability of coronary death increases with resting pulse rate at the entry examination. The conventional conclusion is that a probability 0.1, as indicated here, is too large for significance.

Other studies. In the Framingham study the relative body weight as a risk factor was examined with the multiple logistic and the data from sixteen years of experience (Shurtleff 1974). The Framingham relative body weight is the percentage of the desirable weight of the Metropolitan Life Insurance Company table in which age is ignored. This means that, to some extent, the relative weight and age are confounded, but this is probably not too important here because over the age range of most interest—40 to 60 years—the Framingham data indicate only a small correlation between age and relative weight. However, ignoring this complication, the multivariate analysis of the Framingham data indicates that relative weight is a significant risk factor for men, but not for women, for incidence of coronary heart disease if soft as well as hard diagnoses of the disease is accepted. For the more serious and secure diagnoses of myocardial infarction or death from coronary heart disease, relative weight was not a significant risk factor for either men or women, even when other risk factors were ignored.

The data on relative weight and the incidence of coronary heart disease concerned Framingham subjects starting free of evidence of coronary heart disease. Apparently men with other cardiovascular disease were not excluded. Shurtleff also examined relative weight as a risk factor for all-causes death and found highly significant negative relationships with univariate, bivariate (age and relative weight as the independent variables), and multivariate versions of the logistic. However, these indications of a marked decrease in the risk of death with increasing relative weight were obtained from the follow-up of persons only specified as being alive at the last examination preceding death.

The fourteen-year experience of men employed by the Chicago Peoples Gas Company free of definite CHD was analyzed in detail using the multiple logistic function (Dyer et al. 1975). All-causes deaths were negatively related to relative weight and to body mass index, and the negative coefficient was significant when age, serum cholesterol, smoking, and systolic blood pressure were considered. However, it was concluded that the data fitted better when the quadratic of BMI was used in the logistic equation. Figure 15.7 displays the results from both linear and quadratic use of BMI in the logistic for men aged 45 and aged 55 at entry with systolic blood pressure 130 mm.

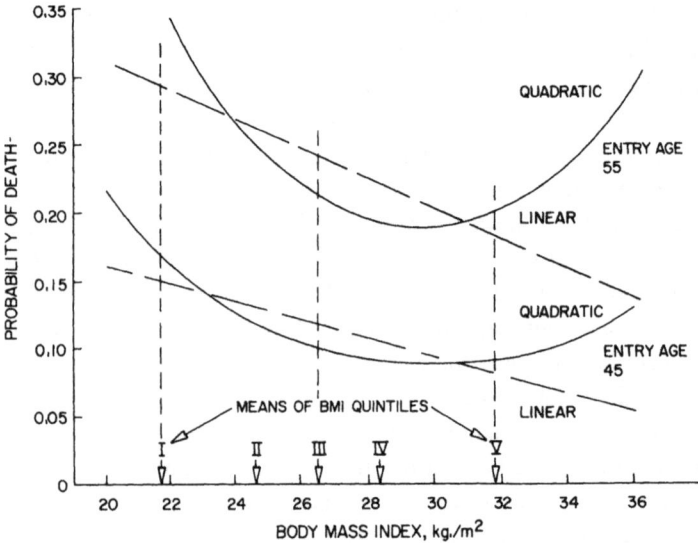

Figure 15.7. Probability of death in fourteen years of Chicago Gas Company men, initially free of definite coronary heart disease, calculated from multiple logistic solutions with the independent variables age, systolic blood pressure, and body mass index and with the same variables plus the square of BMI, for starting ages 45 and 55. With systolic pressure = 130 in all cases. Data from Dyer et al. (1975) and personal communication from A. R. Dyer.

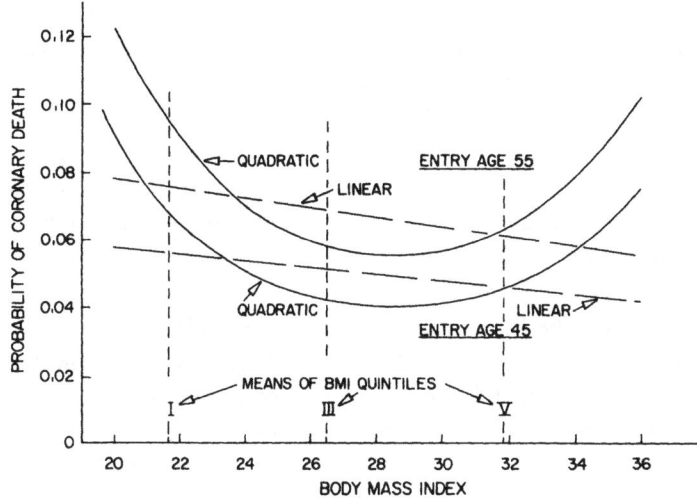

Figure 15.8. Probability of coronary death in fourteen years of Chicago Gas Company men, initially free of definite coronary heart disease, calculated from multiple logistic solutions with the independent variables age, systolic blood pressure and body mass index and with the same variables plus the square of BMI, for starting ages 45 and 55, taking systolic pressure as 130 in all cases. Data from Dyer et al. (1975) and personal communication from A. R. Dyer.

For coronary heart disease deaths, linear BMI was not significantly related. In the quadratic form there was a significant relation with body mass index as the measure but not with relative weight from the Metropolitan Life tables. Figure 15.8 gives the probability of coronary death. It was concluded that "the men with the lowest mortality in the Gas Company are those who are moderately overweight or obese. Thus for this cohort moderate overweight does not appear to be a risk factor for mortality."

The Pooling Project. In the Pooling Project the entry data and the ten-year follow-up experience of major prospective studies in the United States were pooled to provide larger numbers for the analysis of the relationship of entry characteristics to the incidence of major coronary events (death from coronary heart disease or nonfatal myocardial infarction, what we term hard CHD) (Pooling Project Research Group 1978). Pool 5 is emphasized in the Pooling Project report because it comprises the five studies most nearly identical in protocol, methods, and diagnostic criteria. Unfortunately, relative body weight was defined as percentage of desirable weight from tables of the Metropolitan Life Insurance Company, which makes no allowance for age. Since at given height the average body weight of American men, like that of most other men in the developed countries, increases with age until the middle or late fifties, this means that age and true relative weight are confounded to some extent whenever age is disregarded or ages over a span of years are grouped. The Pool 5 data (Table 28, Pooling Project Research Group 1978) show a steady increase with age of average weight as percentage of desirable weight, both for men who later stayed well and those who had "major events." Taking Y to be the weight as percentage of desirable weight, the regression for the Pool 5 men is $Y = 107.3 + 0.194$ Age for ages 40–59, all men at entry in Pool 5.

The analysis of the Pool 5 data for the relationship between incidence rate and percentage of desirable weight found that when age was considered only by five-year age group, relative weight seemed to be a risk factor for men aged 40–44 and 45–49 but not for men 50–54 or 55–59. In the multivariate analysis using the logistic function with age, serum cholesterol, diastolic blood pressure, smoking, and relative weight (as defined in terms of desirable weight) as independent variables, relative weight was not a significant risk factor for the Pool 5 men aged 40–59, but all other independent variables were significant with $p = 0.01$ or less.

The view that the risk of premature death is directly related to relative body weight, so long and widely accepted by the health professions and the general public, is the result of persuasion by a segment of the life insurance industry. In chapter 10 it was pointed out that the basic life insurance material involves biased samples, unreliable measurements, and inadequate statistical analysis. Most of the more acceptable prospective studies have been so focused on coronary heart disease as to neglect the more vital question of death, but where mortality data are reported they do not confirm the insurance company thesis.

The concordance of the follow-up findings in the Framingham, Chicago Gas Company, Pooling Project, and Seven Countries studies, with no dissenting evidence from other scientifically acceptable investigations, justifies some important conclusions, at least for middle-aged men: (1) The popular insurance company claim about mortality is grossly wrong; relative body weight is associated with risk only at the two ends of the distribution of relative weight. (2) More risk is associated with underweight than with overweight. (3) Men in the middle of the relative weight distribution but somewhat heavier than the average have the best prospect of avoiding premature death. Finally, unless it is extreme, overweight is not a risk factor for serious coronary heart disease.

Obesity

In chapter 10 it was emphasized that overweight is by no means the same as obesity or body fatness. The best simple estimate of body fatness seems to be the sum of the skinfold thickness. The coefficient of correlation between that measure and the body mass index averaged $r = 0.77$ for the sixteen cohorts; this means that some 40 percent of the total variance of skinfold thickness is not accounted for by the body mass index or relative weight. So it is desirable to examine the sum of the skinfolds separately as a possible risk factor.

Table 15.2 summarizes results from solutions to the bivariate logistic equation with sum of the skinfolds and, separately, the body mass index, with age as the other independent variable, in terms of t values. In only one of the twelve sets of data is this measure of fatness significant, namely, for the incidence of any CHD at Zutphen. Note that the body mass index is also indicated to be significant for any CHD at Zutphen. It is interesting, also, that in five of the twelve comparisons the sign of the coefficient is different for the two variables, but this is not remarkable because they are all in the zone of no significance. The finding in Zutphen of apparent statistical significance must be evaluated with consideration of the fact that this is a

Table 15.2. Sum of skinfold thickness at entry as a risk factor in men free of cardiovascular disease (t values of the coefficient for skinfold thickness and body mass index in separate bivariate logistic solutions, with age as the other variable).

Ten-year event by group	BMI	Skinfold
U.S. railroad		
All-causes deaths	−1.88	0.45
CHD deaths	0.39	1.38
Finland		
All-causes deaths	−0.35	−1.40
CHD deaths	0.77	−0.62
Hard CHD	0.65	−0.34
Any CHD	−0.38	−0.74
Rural Italy		
All-causes deaths	−0.98	0.38
CHD deaths	−0.19	1.20
Hard CHD	0.34	1.24
Any CHD	1.08	1.32
Zutphen		
All-causes deaths	1.60	1.55
Any CHD	2.27	2.46

single result among what might be viewed as twelve trials. With 89 cases of any CHD the t value of $2.46 = 0.008$ (one-sided because the positive coefficient corresponds to the direction of the prior theory) *if* it were only a single trial.

Physical Activity

Chapter 11 reported marked differences among cohorts in the relationship of habitual physical activity to the ten-year age-standardized incidence of death or coronary heart disease when other variables are ignored. Table 15.3 summarizes the result of analyses with the multiple logistic model taking account of age, systolic blood pressure, serum cholesterol, smoking habit, and resting pulse rate, as well as physical activity. The table is directed to the question of whether the physical activity recorded at entry is significantly related to the incidence of death or of major coronary heart disease in the following ten years after allowing for the other five variables. The answer is indicated by the t value, the ratio of the coefficient found for activity to its standard error. Estimation of the probability that the coefficient is not zero is made from that t value.

For the American railroad men, no support is given to the theory that risk is increased by inactivity. For all-causes death the coefficient for activity is positive. Although this suggests that increased activity increases the risk of

Table 15.3. Physical activity versus ten-year incidence of death or major coronary heart disease, men free of cardiovascular disease at entry (significance of activity indicated by the activity coefficient/SE where the coefficient is from the solution of the multiple logistic equation with variables age, systolic blood pressure, serum cholesterol, smoking, resting pulse rate, and habitual physical activity at entry).

Ten-year event by group	N cases	t	p
U.S. railroad			
All-causes deaths	210	1.3	0.10
CHD deaths	93	−0.1	0.46
Northern Europe			
All-causes deaths	287	−2.5	0.01
CHD deaths	89	−1.0	0.16
Hard CHD	156	−1.4	0.08
Southern Europe			
All-causes deaths	533	−2.1	0.02
CHD deaths	64	−2.5	0.01
Hard CHD	114	−0.6	0.27

premature death, the value found could be a result of chance in about 1 out of 5 trials (two-tailed). Moreover, an elevated death rate for the more active men was accounted for by an excessive mortality from violence. For death from coronary heart disease the data from the American railroad men give a t value for the activity coefficient that is very close to zero.

In contrast, in northern Europe (Finland and Zutphen) the all-causes death rate was inversely related to physical activity to a degree that would be expected by chance in only 1 in 100 trials. A negative relationship is also indicated in the data for coronary death and hard CHD, with a probability of chance explanation of 1 in 6 and 1 in 12 trials, respectively. In southern Europe, too, physical activity was inversely related to subsequent mortality, and the relationship is significant both for all-causes and for coronary death. For hard CHD, there was no significant relationship to activity in southern Europe.

Resting Pulse Rate

Chapter 12 showed a highly significant regression of the ten-year age-standardized death rate, both from all-causes and coronary heart disease, for American railroad men, Croatians, Finns, Italians, and Greeks, but not for Serbians or the Dutch of Zutphen. The incidence of hard CHD was less convincingly related to the pulse rate, and the incidence of coronary heart disease other than coronary death or myocardial infarction was unrelated to the pulse rate except in the group of 167 Italians and Greeks who developed other CHD. Univariate regression indicated for the Italians and Greeks a direct relationship with only $p = 0.02$ of chance explanation. But chapter 12 also showed that resting pulse rate was consistently correlated with blood pressure, physical activity (negative), and, to a lesser degree, the serum cholesterol concentration. Clearly, then, multivariate analysis is required to assess the independent relationship of resting pulse rate and incidence.

Table 15.4 summarizes the multiple logistic analyses in which the independent variables are age, systolic blood pressure, serum cholesterol, smoking habit, and physical activity as well as resting pulse rate. For the American railroad men the resting pulse rate is found to be a significant risk factor for all-causes deaths even when the other variables are controlled. The t value is only 2.5 as compared with $t = 4.8$ when the other variables are disregarded; for coronary deaths t is not significant, but ignoring other variables $t = 2.4$ (see table 12.3).

For northern Europe the resting pulse rate was not statistically significant for any of the kinds of ten-year incidence but, as table 15.4 shows, resting pulse was significant for all the kinds of incidence in southern Europe. No explanation is suggested for these regional differences.

Table 15.4. Resting pulse rate versus ten-year incidence of death or major coronary heart disease, men free of cardiovascular disease at entry (significance of resting pulse rate indicated by the pulse rate coefficient/SE where the coefficient is from the solution of the multiple logistic equation with variables age, systolic blood pressure, serum cholesterol, smoking, physical activity, and resting pulse rate at entry).

Ten-year event by group	N cases	t	p
U.S. railroad			
All-causes deaths	210	2.5	0.01
CHD deaths	93	0.9	0.19
Northern Europe			
All-causes deaths	287	1.3	0.10
CHD deaths	89	1.4	0.08
Any CHD	181	0.3	0.38
Southern Europe			
All-causes deaths	533	5.9	0.001
CHD deaths	64	2.7	0.01
Any CHD	163	2.0	0.02

Blood Pressure

In chapter 7 it was noted that in the discrimination of men who later developed coronary heart disease from those who stayed well at Framingham there was no important difference between systolic and diastolic blood pressures, though, except for the youngest men, there was a tendency in favor of the systolic pressure (Kannel, Gordon, and Schwartz 1971). Data from the five-year experience in the Seven Countries Study were substantially in agreement, but reexamination with the much larger number of events after ten years is warranted because many clinicians persist in emphasizing the diastolic pressure in evaluating risk, for example, the protocol of the ongoing MRFIT (Multiple Risk Factor Intervention Trial) study.

One method of examining the question is to use the multiple logistic equation as the model, solve it using systolic blood pressure together with the other relevant characteristics, and with the same data, repeat the solution with the addition of the diastolic blood pressure. The comparison, then, is the distribution of the observed incidence cases in the decile classes of risk probability estimated from the two solutions. We have applied this method to the ten-year seven countries data with two sets of independent variables: (1) the entry characteristics of age, serum cholesterol, smoking habit, physical activity, and systolic pressure and (2) these variables plus diastolic pressure.

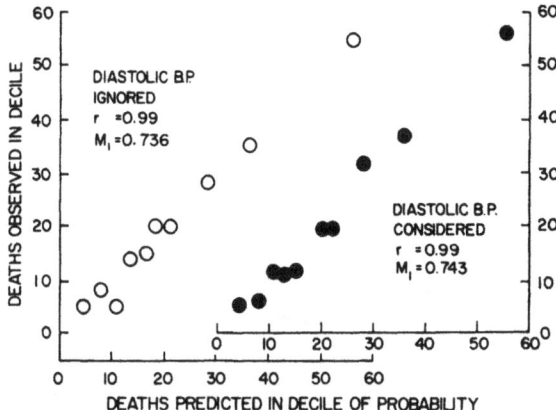

Figure 15.9. For American railroad men free of cardiovascular disease at entry, discrimination by the multiple logistic equation solution of all-causes deaths in ten years from the surviving men with independent variables of age, cholesterol, smoking habit, resting pulse rate, physical activity, and systolic blood pressure, and again with those variables plus the diastolic pressure, comparing the numbers of deaths predicted in the deciles of estimated probability and the numbers observed.

Figure 15.9 summarizes the comparison for all-causes deaths in ten years among the American railroad men who were free of cardiovascular disease at the entry examination. The addition of diastolic pressure to the systolic pressure and the other characteristics recorded at the entry examination does not significantly improve the highly satisfactory discrimination achieved without it. The first moment is slightly higher where both blood pressures are included in the logistic solution.

Figures 15.10 and 15.11 show the results of the corresponding analyses of the ten-year mortality among men in northern and southern Europe. The results are almost identical with those from the American railroad men.

Instead of all-causes death as the end point, coronary heart disease death was examined with the same method of analysis. The results for the ten-year experience of the American railroad men are graphically summarized in figure 15.12. Again the indication is that consideration of diastolic as well as systolic blood pressure does not improve the discrimination obtained when only systolic pressure is considered. Figure 15.13, the corresponding summary of discrimination of coronary heart disease death in northern Europe, is in agreement with the American experience. The result of the same analysis with the data from the men in southern Europe is similar but less important because of the smaller number of coronary deaths in southern Europe.

280 | Seven Countries

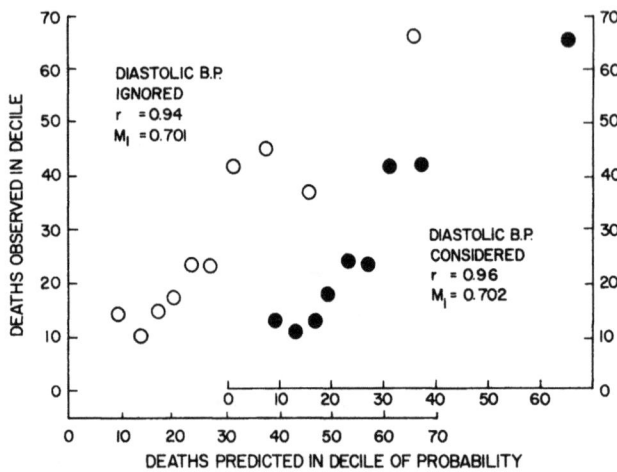

Figure 15.10. For men in northern Europe (Finland and Zutphen) free of cardiovascular disease at entry, comparison of the discrimination, as in figure 15.8, with and without consideration of the diastolic blood pressure.

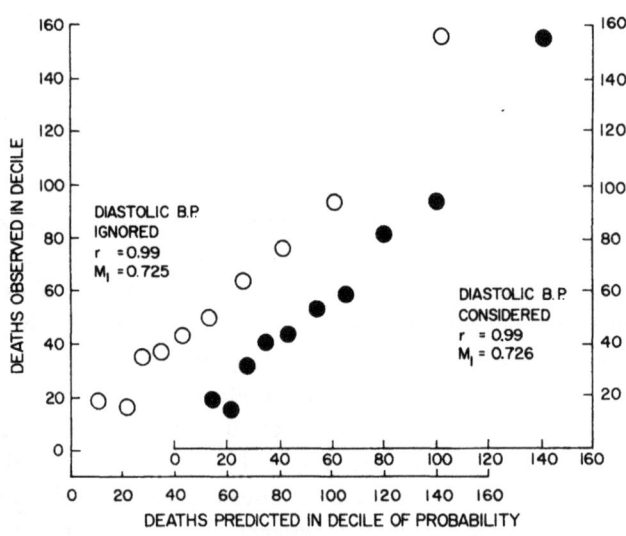

Figure 15.11. For men in southern Europe (Yugoslavia, Italy and Greece) free of cardiovascular disease at entry, comparison of the discrimination, as in figures 15.9 and 15.10, with and without consideration of the diastolic blood pressure.

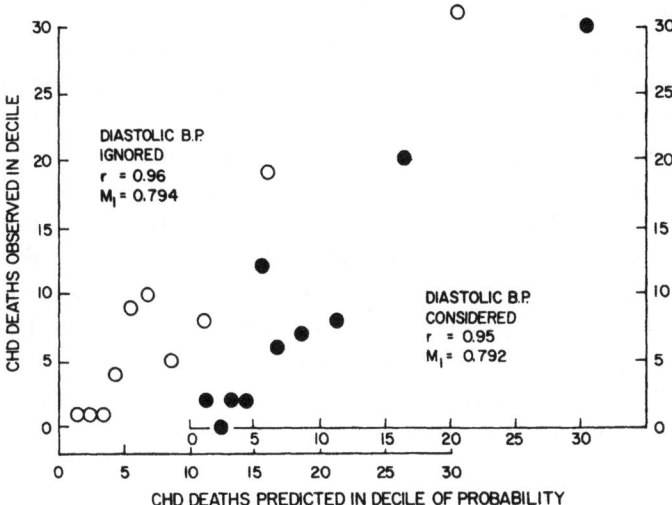

Figure 15.12. For American railroad men free of cardiovascular disease at entry, discrimination by the multiple logistic equation solution of deaths from coronary heart disease in ten years. The number of coronary deaths predicted in the deciles of estimated probability is compared with and without diastolic pressure included among the independent variables.

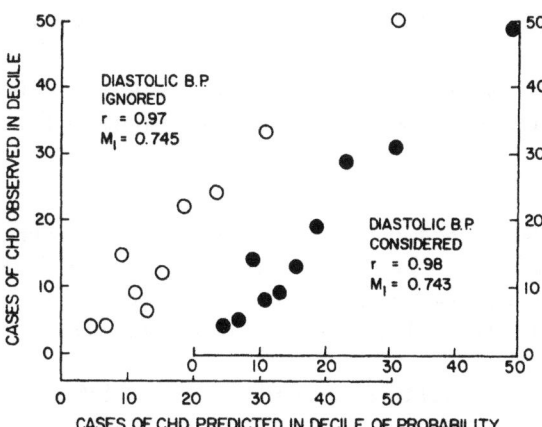

Figure 15.13. For men in northern Europe (Finland and Zutphen) free of cardiovascular disease at entry, ten-year incidence of coronary heart disease. The discrimination achieved with and without entry diastolic blood pressure is compared as in figure 15.11.

Another method of examining this question takes advantage of the fact that all men were classified at entry separately for both blood pressures specific for the cohort and each five-year class. With this information we have calculated the mean incidence rate for each decile class and the regression of the rate on the decile class. Since we are interested in the relative blood pressure of the men as a risk factor, use of the decile class number as the independent x variable allows combination of the cohorts in the analysis. For Europe, with thirteen cohorts, there are 130 pairs of values of x, the decile class, and y, the incidence rate. The result of this form of analysis is given in table 15.5. The regression of both hard and any CHD on blood pressure is highly significant as shown by the ratio of the slope, b, to its standard errors, SE_b. For hard CHD systolic pressure gives $t = 4.67$ and diastolic $t = 4.75$; for any CHD the corresponding values are 3.42 and 2.67. Besides noting that the t values are larger for hard than for any CHD, table 15.5 shows no indication of any difference between systolic and diastolic blood pressure as a discriminator between men who later developed coronary heart disease and those who did not.

For hard CHD the slope of the regression on systolic pressure is almost identical with the slope for diastolic pressure. For any CHD the slope is greater for systolic pressure, but the standard error of that difference is very large and the t value of the difference in slopes is only 0.59.

The concordance of the findings in the Seven Countries Study with those at Framingham shows that for the prediction of coronary heart disease or premature death of apparently healthy men the diastolic pressure is certainly no better, and may be less discriminating, than the systolic pressure. Moreover, from such analyses as illustrated in figures 15.9–15.13, there is no indication that considering both pressures improves the discrimination. However, the statistical methods lack sensitivity for estimating the probability of

Table 15.5. Systolic or diastolic blood pressure versus coronary heart disease incidence (regression $y = a + bx$, where y = ten-year incidence per 1,000 in the decile class, x = age- and cohort-specific decile class of blood pressure; data from 8,743 men in thirteen cohorts in Europe all free of cardiovascular disease at entry).

Blood pressure	429 Cases hard CHD				866 Cases any CHD			
	a	b	SE_b	r	a	b	SE_b	r
Systolic	36.6	5.98	1.28	0.38	89.6	7.97	2.33	0.29
Diastolic	37.5	5.79	1.22	0.39	99.8	6.04	2.26	0.23
Difference	—	0.19	1.77	—	—	1.93	3.25	—

an indicated small improvement when both discriminators are considered together.

For the latter question it is interesting to examine the values of various indicators of discrimination applied to follow-up data first with only systolic and then with both pressures in a multiple logistic analysis including other major risk factors as independent variables. Table 15.6 summarizes such comparisons in the estimation of the risk of death, of coronary death, and the incidence of coronary heart disease. Three indicators of the discrimination achieved are the first and second moments, which compare predicted and observed numbers of cases in the deciles of probability, and the likelihood ratio statistic. In all but 2 of the 24 comparisons slightly better discrimination was achieved when both blood pressures were considered with age, serum cholesterol, smoking habit, and physical activity. With the addition of the resting pulse rate, the result was essentially the same; among 24 comparisons 22 indicated slightly better discrimination when the diastolic pressure was included. Although a trend for improvement with both pressures is indicated, the difference is trivial.

Table 15.6. Discrimination between ten-year incidence cases and noncases with the multiple logistic equation using data on age, cholesterol, smoking, physical activity, and systolic pressure at entry, and with the solution using those data plus the diastolic pressure (men free of cardiovascular disease at entry; increasing discrimination is indicated with increasing values of the first and second moments and the maximum likelihood statistic).

Ten-year event by group	N	5 variables			5 variables + D BP		
		M1	M2	LRS	M1	M2	LRS
U.S. railroad (2,290 men)							
All-causes deaths	213	7.36	6.04	106.66	7.43	6.14	111.15
CHD deaths	90	7.84	6.70	74.51	7.87	6.73	75.86
Northern Europe (2,303 men)							
All-causes deaths	291	7.01	5.62	103.61	7.02	5.63	104.19
CHD deaths	89	7.78	6.61	62.12	7.84	6.70	63.84
Any CHD	181	7.45	6.20	97.09	7.43	6.17	97.23
Southern Europe (5,706 men)							
All-causes deaths	589	7.25	5.94	267.97	7.27	5.95	271.18
CHD deaths	72	7.54	6.44	53.90	7.57	6.47	53.93
Any CHD	179	6.82	5.35	44.73	6.89	5.44	46.11

Predictive Value

The first test of the utility of a model such as the multiple logistic is to compare the estimated probability of an event in classes of the array of probabilities with the actual numbers of events observed within those classes. This test shows the ability of the model to discriminate within the group of persons whose entry and follow-up data were used in the solution of the model equation, but it is not a test of predictive power for another population. From the multiple logistic analysis of the five-year experience of the men in the Seven Countries Study, we reported that the multiple logistic solution from United States railroad data very well estimated the relative risk of the Europeans. Although there was a very high correlation between the numbers predicted in the probability deciles and the observed numbers, the total number of cases in Europe was grossly overpredicted (Keys et al. 1972). Conversely, the logistic from the European data grossly underpredicted the total number of coronary cases that developed in the American railroad cohort, but there was a very high correlation between the numbers predicted and those observed in the ten decile classes of probability.

Comparisons of populations with racial as well as ethnic contrasts show unexplained large differences in the frequency of the disease (Klinebaum, Kupper, and Cassel 1971; Gordon et al. 1974; Robertson et al. 1977). The ten-year follow-up in the Seven Countries Study confirms differences in incidence not accounted for by classical risk factors. A possible explanation might be found by comparing racially different populations. But a comparison of Framingham men with men of Japanese ancestry in Hawaii showed that the risk-factor contrasts were much less in the younger than in the older men, and it was suggested that "incidence may be less than predicted when high risk characteristics are not acquired until middle age" (Robertson et al. 1977). The trend of Japanese men in Hawaii to adopt American habits, including diet, occurred in the 1940s and proceeded most rapidly in the young. In 1956, when we surveyed Japanese men in Honolulu, the average diet of young men was more Americanized than that of middle-aged men, and the serum cholesterol values reflected that difference (Keys et al. 1958). We can agree with Robertson et al. (1977) that the experience of early life is important in atherogenesis, and that later measurements of serum cholesterol may be misleading when the diet has changed greatly.

Although changes in life-style may complicate comparisons of populations in the Seven Countries Study, the differences among the populations in such changes are much smaller than in the comparison of the Japanese in Hawaii and the Americans in Framingham. The Seven Countries Study showed a major difference in the incidence rate of coronary heart disease between northern and southern Europe and relatively little difference between the American men and the northern Europeans. Although great changes in life-style occurred in the sixteen cohorts over the years before the beginning of the Seven Countries Study, there is little reason to believe that there were important differential changes. Americans were spared privations suffered by the Europeans during World War II, but changes have otherwise occurred in the same direction and with something like the same pace in all populations—less physical work, richer diets, more cigarette smoking, better medical care, and so on. It would be difficult to defend the thesis of major differences in these trends in northern versus southern Europe, especially in the rural populations that were the focus of the present study.

The ten-year experience of the men in the Seven Countries Study has been examined with the multiple logistic equation to compare the incidence of death and of coronary heart disease as observed in northern and in southern Europe and as predicted from applying to one population sample the logistic coefficients obtained from the other. The mortality observed in northern and in southern Europe has been similarly compared with that predicted from the logistic coefficients obtained from the data of the American railroad men.

Figure 15.14 shows, for the northern Europeans, the distribution of observed all-causes deaths in the decile classes of probability calculated from the American railroad men's experience. A total of 272 men in northern

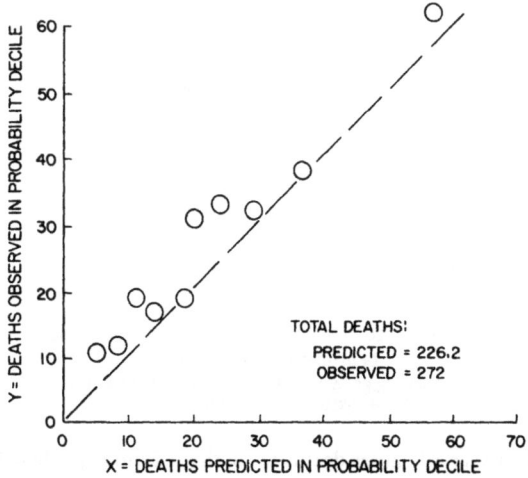

Figure 15.14. Ten-year all-causes deaths in northern Europe predicted in the deciles of probability estimated from the logistic coefficients from the data on the American railroad men and the numbers actually found in those deciles.

Europe died; only 226.2 were predicted from the railroad experience for men with the recorded entry characteristics of age, systolic blood pressure, serum cholesterol, cigarette smoking, resting pulse rate, and body mass index. In spite of the fact that the deaths in northern Europe were underpredicted by 20 percent, the correlation between the number of deaths observed in the probability deciles and the number predicted is high, $r = 0.96$. The regression of number of deaths observed on the number predicted is $y = 9.35 + 1.01x$.

The corresponding observed all-causes deaths in southern Europe and those predicted from the logistic coefficients from the American railroad experience are shown in figure 15.15. Here the total number of deaths observed and that predicted is almost identical and again the correlation between the numbers observed and those predicted in the probability deciles is very high, $r = 0.97$.

The comparison of all-causes deaths in northern Europe with those predicted for men of their entry characteristics from the experience of the men in southern Europe is summarized in figure 15.16. The total number of deaths in northern Europe was 35 percent greater than predicted from the southern European experience, but the correlation between the numbers found and those predicted in the decile classes of probability is again high,

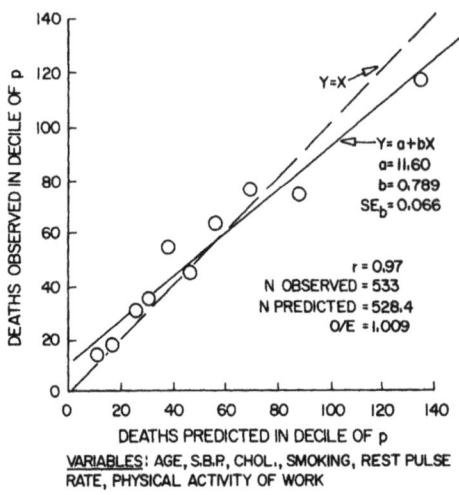

Figure 15.15. Ten-year all-causes deaths in southern Europe predicted in the deciles of probability estimated from the logistic coefficients from the data on the American railroad men and the numbers actually found in those deciles. The independent variables considered are age, systolic blood pressure, serum cholesterol, cigarette smoking, resting blood pressure, and physical activity.

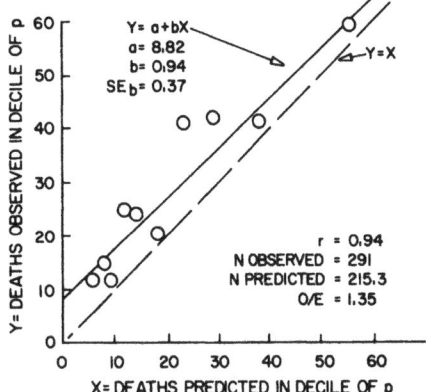

Figure 15.16. Ten-year all-causes deaths in northern Europe predicted in the deciles of probability estimated from the logistic coefficients from the data on the men in southern Europe and the number of deaths actually found in those deciles. Variables as in figure 15.15.

$r = 0.96$. The regression of observed deaths on those predicted is $y = 10.8 + 0.91x$.

In regard to death from coronary heart disease as well as from all causes, the ten-year experience of the men in northern Europe resembles that of American railroad men. Figure 15.17 summarizes the comparison from the

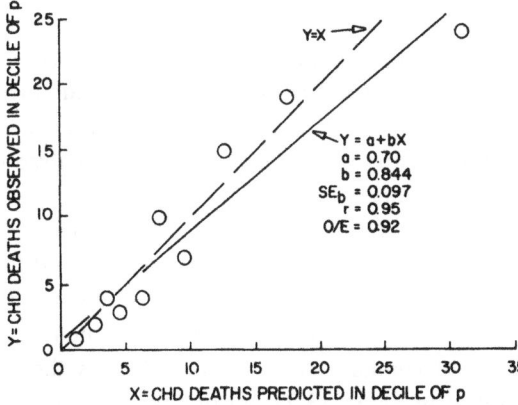

Figure 15.17. Ten-year deaths from coronary heart disease in northern Europe predicted in the deciles of probability estimated from the logistic coefficients from the data on American railroad men and the numbers of coronary deaths actually found in those deciles. Variables as in figure 15.15.

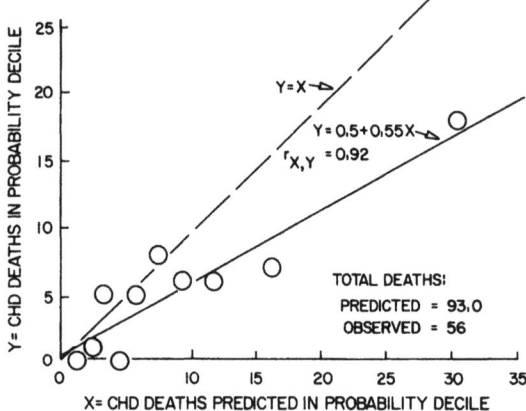

Figure 15.18. Ten-year deaths from coronary heart disease in southern Europe predicted in the deciles of probability estimated from the logistic coefficients from the data on American railroad men and the numbers of coronary deaths actually found in those deciles. Variables as in figure 15.15.

American railroad men's experience. Only a trifle fewer deaths than predicted occurred, and the correlation between the numbers observed and those predicted in the decile classes of estimated probability is $r = 0.95$.

In contrast to the comparison of observed coronary deaths in northern Europe with those predicted from the American railroad, the comparison for southern Europe, summarized in figure 15.18, shows great overprediction— 66 percent. The correlation between the numbers observed and those predicted to be in the decile classes is a little lower than in the preceding comparisons, but $r = 0.92$ is still very high. In view of the foregoing comparisons the picture in figure 15.19 is not unexpected. Among the men in northern Europe the coronary deaths in ten years were 2.5 times the number predicted for men of their entry characteristics from the analysis of the experience of the southern European men.

Figure 15.20 concerns the observed cases of hard CHD (coronary death or nonfatal myocardial infarction) in northern Europe and those predicted from the experience of southern Europe. Finally, the comparison of observation in northern Europe with prediction from southern Europe is made with any diagnosis of coronary heart disease taken as the end point; the result is summarized in figure 15.21. Again, the southern Europe experience grossly underpredicted the incidence in northern Europe, but the relative prediction is very good: $r = 0.98$. What this means is that the logistic coefficients derived from the southern European experience classify the men in northern Europe very well in regard to their relative risk among the

Multivariate Analyses | 289

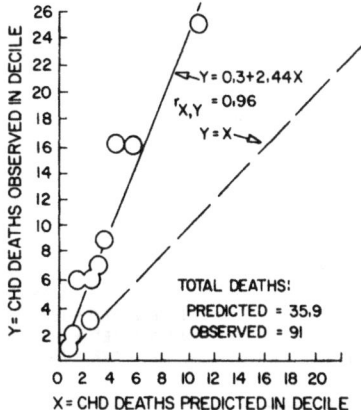

Figure 15.19. Ten-year deaths from coronary heart disease in northern Europe predicted in the deciles of probability estimated from the logistic coefficients from the data on the men in southern Europe and the numbers of coronary deaths actually found in those deciles. Variables as in figure 15.15.

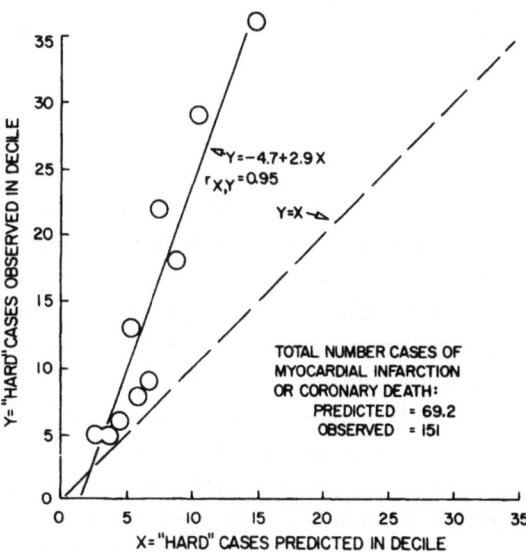

Figure 15.20. Ten-year incidence of coronary death or myocardial infarction (hard CHD) in northern Europe in the deciles of probability estimated from the logistic coefficients from the data on the men in southern Europe and the number of such incidence cases actually observed in those deciles. Variables as in figure 15.15.

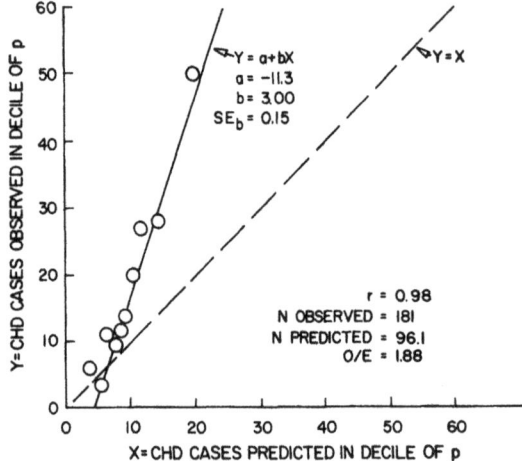

Figure 15.21. Ten-year incidence of coronary heart disease by any diagnostic criterion in northern Europe in the deciles of probability estimated from the logistic coefficients from the men in southern Europe and the number of such incidence cases actually observed in those deciles. Variables as in figure 15.15.

northern Europeans. The men who are estimated to have the highest probability of developing coronary heart disease among the northern Europeans turn out to be, indeed, the men with the worst experience among the northern Europeans.

Coefficients

Table 15.7 gives the coefficients for age, systolic blood pressure, serum cholesterol, cigarette smoking, resting pulse rate, and physical activity, and the intercept, for the ten-year incidence of death or coronary heart disease, among men free of coronary heart disease at entry, in the American railroad cohort, in northern Europe (Finland and Zutphen), and in southern Europe (Italy, Yugoslavia, and Greece). The standard errors of the coefficients, and the corresponding t values, are also tabulated.

Relative body weight (body mass index) is not included in this set of independent variables because it makes little if any contribution to the discrimination between cases and noncases with the multiple logistic model. Measures of respiratory function were also excluded from the logistic solutions in table 15.7 because entry data are lacking for Dalmatia, Slavonia, Zutphen, the Rome railroad men, and a large portion of the American cohort.

The coefficients in table 15.7 may be useful in estimating at least relative risk of death or the development of coronary heart disease in other samples.

Table 15.7. Multiple logistic coefficients, their standard errors, and t values for ten-year all-causes death, CHD death, and any CHD for men free of cardiovascular disease at entry (values are 100 times the coefficients and their SEs).

Group (N)	Risk	α	Age	S BP	Chol.	Smoking	Pulse	Activity
U.S. railroad (2,269)	All-causes death	−1200.92	9.05	1.21	0.24	27.99	1.51	19.98
	SE	108.10	1.43	0.37	0.16	4.64	0.61	15.25
	t	−11.11	6.33	3.28	1.45	6.04	2.46	1.31
(2,269)	CHD death	−1413.03	7.65	1.76	0.85	34.88	0.83	2.48
	SE	161.83	2.13	0.53	0.22	7.24	0.91	22.66
	t	−8.73	3.59	3.36	3.91	4.82	0.91	0.11
Northern Europe (2,287)	All-causes death	−928.04	8.12	1.50	0.08	17.58	0.68	−22.05
	SE	96.29	1.26	0.32	0.12	4.20	0.51	8.88
	t	−9.64	6.43	4.75	0.66	4.19	1.33	−2.48
(2,089)	CHD death	−1361.79	7.27	1.89	0.90	27.65	1.16	−24.33
	SE	169.53	2.17	0.52	0.20	7.36	0.84	15.02
	t	−8.03	3.35	3.60	4.58	3.75	1.38	−1.62
(2,103)	Any CHD	−1227.15	9.79	2.02	0.54	13.22	0.17	−7.59
	SE	123.85	1.61	0.39	0.15	5.08	0.64	11.26
	t	−9.91	6.09	5.23	3.52	2.60	0.27	−0.67
Southern Europe (5,210)	All-causes death	−1076.09	12.73	0.94	−0.37	8.56	1.89	−13.66
	SE	69.40	1.01	0.23	0.12	2.84	0.32	6.48
	t	−15.51	12.60	4.17	−3.13	3.02	5.90	−2.11
(4,741)	CHD death	−1391.49	9.00	1.68	0.59	13.93	2.26	−40.21
	SE	181.71	2.63	0.56	0.28	7.61	0.83	15.96
	t	−7.66	3.42	3.00	2.08	1.83	2.74	−2.52
(4,759)	Any CHD	−939.25	5.85	1.13	0.41	0.63	1.09	6.83
	SE	110.93	1.61	0.38	0.19	4.82	0.55	11.08
	t	−8.47	3.63	2.97	2.23	0.13	1.98	−0.62

Relative risk should be emphasized especially in dealing with individuals. The t values afford an indication of the probability that the coefficients are not actually zero. From the standard errors, the confidence intervals can be calculated as 1.96 times the standard error for the 95 percent interval; 2.58, for the 99 percent interval. The corresponding confidence limits are simply the tabulated coefficient plus and minus the confidence interval.

These solutions refer to the model in which the independent effects of the variables are taken to be additive and the variables themselves are taken to be related linearly, if at all, to the end point. A second limitation is that the coefficients and the events refer to specific times, the time of entry, which stretched over the years 1958 to 1964, and the time period of ten years thereafter. No consideration is given to the possibility that the characteristics measured at entry may not have well represented those characteristics in the preceding years. And no allowance is made for possible changes after entry. Some changes in the follow-up period are noted in chapter 16, but the relationship of such changes to the incidence of disease and death in the ten-year period is not treated here.

The men in Japan are not included in table 15.7. The incidence of coronary heart disease at Tanushimaru and Ushibuka was too low to warrant detailed multivariate analysis. Table 15.8 gives the logistic coefficients, their standard errors, and the corresponding t values from the solution for 71 ten-year all-causes deaths among 757 men of Tanushimaru and Ushibuka. The limited number of men at risk reflects the fact that there were uncertainties about the cholesterol values of many of the men at entry.

For ten-year all-causes deaths in Japan only age is indicated to be a highly significant risk factor. For systolic blood pressure the t value indicates that there is about 1 chance in 12 that the coefficient would not be different from zero if many trials were made. By the same token, the indication is that the chances are better than 10 to 1 that the systolic pressure is a positive factor. For serum cholesterol it is not surprising that it does not emerge as a significant risk factor in a sample in which the median cholesterol value is 160 mg/dl. The absence of any indication that cigarette smoking is a signifi-

Table 15.8. Japan (Tanushimaru and Ushibuka), multiple logistic coefficients, their standard errors and t values for ten-year all-causes death of men with no cardiovascular disease at entry.

Variable	Coefficient	SE	t
Age	0.1238	0.0269	4.60
Systolic BP	0.0068	0.0049	1.40
Smoking	−0.0044	0.0487	−0.09
Cholesterol	−0.0012	0.0037	−0.31
Body mass index	−0.0630	0.0551	−1.14
Intercept (α)	−8.0810	1.9905	−4.06

cant risk factor is more unexpected and, so far, totally unexplained. Finally, as for the negative coefficient for relative body weight (body mass index), the indication is that there is about a 12 percent chance that the average of many trials would be a value of zero for the coefficient. The conventional conclusion is, then, that the body mass index is not a significant factor. On the other hand, emphasis might be put on the indication that the chances are nearly nine to one that the coefficient is, indeed, negative. So the indication is that the betting odds are about nine to one that, in general, the death rate decreases with increasing relative body weight.

Summary

The interrelations among risk factors must be considered in estimating their independent contributions to the discrimination of future cases and noncases. Moreover, it is desired to estimate the combined contributions of two or more variables to the discrimination.

Although several multivariate methods were used, most emphasis was on the multiple logistic equation. The contributions of the independent variables are added in the exponent of e, the base of natural logarithms, and the solution yields coefficients for the variables which afford estimation of the probability of being a case. The iterative method of Walker and Duncan was used to solve the equation, and the result was evaluated by comparison of the numbers of cases observed with those expected from the probability calculation.

The utility of the multiple logistic approach is illustrated in the examination of the large differences among the cohorts in the mortality from coronary heart disease. The regression of death rate of the cohorts on the entry characteristics of those cohorts was calculated for each characteristic separately. Only two entry variables were significantly related to the incidence rate, blood pressure and cholesterol concentration in the blood serum. The cohort medians of those variables accounted for 41 and 42 percent, respectively, of the variance in death rate. With both blood pressure and cholesterol as independent variables and death rate as the dependent variable, 66 percent of the variance was accounted for, and both blood pressure and cholesterol proved to be significant independent, additive contributors to risk.

In the examination of relative body weight as a risk factor, multiple logistic analyses were made simultaneously considering age, systolic blood pressure, serum cholesterol, smoking habit, resting pulse rate, and the body mass index. For all-causes death, BMI was not significant in northern Europe but was a significant negative risk factor for both the American railroad men and the southern Europeans; the probability of death in ten years decreased with increasing relative weight. Repeating the analyses with the square of the BMI as an additional variable produced a U-shaped relation of incidence to the body mass index and a slightly better fit of the observed incidence to that expected from the multiple logistic solution. The indication was that the risk of ten-year death was least for men somewhat above the average in relative body weight. This finding is in agreement with the experience of the men of the Peoples Gas Company, Chicago, and is not controverted by data from other prospective studies.

Similar analyses with the sum of the skinfolds replacing the body mass index among the independent variables gave similar results. With BMI and the sum of the skinfolds as the only independent variables and the age-standardized ten-year incidence rate as the dependent variable, the logistic was solved separately for the American railroad men, the Finns, the rural Italians, and the men of Zutphen for all-causes death, coronary death and the incidence of coronary heart disease. Both BMI and the sum of the skinfolds were significant risk factors for the incidence of coronary heart disease at Zutphen, but not for all-causes death there. Neither variable was significant for any of the incidence end points in the other three regions. Because the positive finding at Zutphen for one end point was 1 out of 12 trials, it would easily be a chance variation.

Inclusion of habitual physical activity at entry as a variable in the multiple logistic equation indicated that it was not a risk factor for the American railroad men but was significant for ten-year all-causes death in northern and in southern Europe and also for coronary death in southern Europe, the death rate decreasing with increasing activity. The incidence of nonfatal myocardial infarction or other manifestations of the disease was not significantly related to physical activity in any area.

Solution of the multiple logistic equation including the resting pulse rate as one of seven entry variables showed it to be a significant factor for all-causes deaths of the American railroad men and the men in southern Europe but not of the northern Europeans. Except in southern Europe, the incidence of coronary heart disease was not significantly related to entry resting pulse rate.

Both systolic and diastolic blood pressure were highly significant risk factors for death and for incidence of coronary heart disease in multiple logistic analyses, but neither measure was superior to the other. Inclusion of both blood pressure measures in a single multiple logistic solution suggested a slightly better discrimination than with either one alone.

The vital capacity at entry was similarly added to the independent variables in the logistic equation, and the solutions were obtained for all-causes death, coronary death, and the incidence of coronary heart disease. In all areas of the Seven Countries Study, low vital capacity carried a significant risk for all-causes death, but in only one of five populations was the vital capacity related to the risk of coronary death. The incidence of coronary heart disease was not related to the vital capacity in any area.

In all areas simultaneous consideration of several entry variables in the multiple logistic equation showed great discriminatory power for coronary death in ten years, but all-causes death was less well discriminated.

The multiple logistic solution from the experience in one area gave good prediction of the relative coronary risk in other areas but produced gross errors in the prediction of absolute risk. The logistic solution for ten-year coronary death of the Americans applied to the southern Europeans classified the men very well in regard to relative risk but greatly overpredicted the numbers of coronary deaths in that area. The multiple logistic solution from the data on the southern Europeans classified the northern European men satisfactorily in relative risk, but the absolute numbers of coronary deaths and of nonfatal incidence were greatly underestimated.

It appears that some unidentified variable or variables, unrelated to those considered here, contributed to increase the risk of the Americans and the northern Europeans or to protect the southern Europeans and the Japanese. Alternatively, it could be that the measurements at entry were not equally representative of the long-time characteristics of the men in the different areas.

16 | Change at the Ten-Year Follow-up

Analyses of the relationships of the ten-year disease experience of the subjects to their personal characteristics refer to the characteristics as recorded at the entry examinations. But those entry characteristics were not static; some of them changed substantially over the years. An analysis of relationships of the incidence of disease and death to changing characteristics is beyond the scope of this book, but it is of interest to note average differences, in the same individuals, between the ten-year and the entry values of some measured variables.

Cross-sectional comparisons must be distinguished from longitudinal comparisons of the same individuals. For example, a comparison of 50-year-old men with 40-year-old men at one point in time is not necessarily the equivalent of a comparison of the characteristics of men at age 50 with their characteristics at age 40. As will be seen, some of our longitudinal findings do not correspond with the expectation from cross-sectional data at entry. During the years of follow-up important changes in life-style occurred in the population. Difference between values recorded at entry and again ten years later must reflect the effects of aging per se plus effects of changes in the mode of life. When the comparisons of entry and later measurements refer to the same individuals, possible effects of differential mortality are not involved.

In planning the Seven Countries Study, it was decided to focus on samples of rural populations because they are generally more stable than urban populations in place of residence and in working and living habits. Not long ago life in our out-of-the-way villages would have changed little, if any, in ten years. But these are times of change. From the late 1950s to the early 1970s, television, home electricity, indoor plumbing, many more telephones and motor vehicles, paved roads, and more readily available medical

Body Weight

In all cohorts men after ten years tended to be heavier. Table 16.1 shows the average percentage changes in body weight of 6,276 men in Europe classified according to age at entry. For all areas and ages combined the mean ten-year change was a gain of 3.4 kg. In all areas the weight gain tended to be inversely related to the age at entry. Combining all areas, the least-squares regression is $y = 10.3 - 0.14x$, where y is the percentage weight gained in ten years and x is the age at entry. The standard error of the slope is $r = -0.51$. The younger the age, the greater the weight gain, but at all entry ages the tendency was to gain weight during the follow-up period.

As shown in table 6.1 there was no correlation between body mass index

Table 16.1. Mean weight change (ten years minus entry) as percentage of entry weight of 6,276 men in Europe, reweighed at ten years.

Entry age	Croatia	Finland	Italy[a]	Zutphen	Greece	Serbia
40–44						
N	173	315	235	129	223	427
Mean	6.3	3.6	3.4	5.0	5.6	3.8
SE	0.6	0.4	0.5	0.5	0.4	0.4
45–49						
N	260	367	443	178	254	211
Mean	5.5	3.1	1.9	4.1	4.8	1.3
SE	0.4	0.4	0.4	0.5	0.5	0.5
50–54						
N	292	329	381	155	251	340
Mean	4.4	2.8	2.3	2.6	3.3	1.3
SE	0.5	0.4	0.4	0.5	0.5	0.4
55–59						
N	242	267	212	142	200	250
Mean	4.3	2.0	1.9	3.8	3.0	−0.6
SE	0.5	0.4	0.6	0.5	0.5	0.4
40–59						
N	967	1,278	1,271	604	928	1,228
Mean	3.7	2.9	2.1	3.8	4.2	1.8
SE	0.3	0.2	0.2	0.3	0.2	0.2

a. Crevalcore and Montegiorgio.

and age at entry, but that table included 1,789 men not covered in table 16.1, 1,013 men who had died in the ten-year period and 776 men alive but whose weights were not recorded at the ten-year anniversary. So it is necessary to compare the follow-up relationship of weight to age with the relationship at entry in the same men. In all areas, the mean body weight at entry of the men covered in table 16.1 tended to be inversely related to age. For all areas combined, the mean body weight at entry of the men reweighed ten years later was 71.7 kg for 1,502 men then aged 40–44, 71.0 kg for 1,713 men aged 45–49, 69.7 kg for 1,748 men aged 50–54, and 68.4 kg for 1,313 men than aged 55–59 years. For these 6,276 men the least-squares regression of entry weight, y, on entry age, x, is $y = 81.5 - 0.225x$.

Since at entry the body weight was significantly correlated, inversely, with age, the expectation would be, other things being equal, that the average body weight would decrease during the ten years of follow-up. Actually, the opposite was found. The discrepancy between cross-sectional and longitudinal age trends indicates an average change in metabolic balance in the postentry period, a change in the diet or in energy expenditure or both.

It is not possible to document properly either dietary or energy expenditure changes, but a strong impression was gained from repeated visits to the local areas that, in general, over those years the average diets became increasingly rich and energy expenditure decreased. In southern Europe the village shops began to offer butter and ice cream, more meat in great variety was on display, and poultry was no longer a rare treat. In talking with the man about their eating habits, the impression was that many of them were eating meat and dairy products twice as often as at the time of the entry examinations. Bakers were obviously selling less dark bread and more white bread and pastries. Signs of poverty were much less noticeable than in our first visits to the villages.

In regard to energy expenditure, the increased use of labor-saving machinery and a shorter work period were notable in all areas. In most of the areas the trend has been to change from a nine- or ten-hour day, six days a week, to an eight-hour day, five or five and a half days a week. In some areas, including all of Italy, even the private shopkeepers and small tradesmen are now forbidden to operate long hours or every day. Finally, almost no one walks to work as they did in the 1950s and early 1960s. But we infer from the data in table 16.1 that the older men were least affected by these trends in life-style.

For the American railroad men, only five-year follow-up examination data are available. For all ages combined there was no significant weight change in five years, but the younger men showed a slight gain, averaging 1 percent of the entry weight for 1,030 men under 50 years at entry, and the older men showed a slight loss. The average weight of 561 men aged 50–54 at entry decreased 0.2 kg, and the average of 599 men aged 55–59 at entry decreased 0.4 kg. There was no evidence of any significant change in lifestyle of the American railroad men.

Blood Pressure

In chapter 7 we mentioned the difficulty of assuring identical conditions for the measurement of blood pressure in the several cohorts. In the five- and ten-year reexaminations our questions about the exact comparability of blood pressure recordings in the different areas persisted, but in general the places for the examinations and most of the members of the examining teams were the same at entry and later examinations. Thus, within areas any trends of blood pressure changes over time should be valid. Still, there were wide divergences among areas in the trends over time.

Table 16.2 shows, by area of Europe, the mean systolic blood pressure of the men classified by age at entry who were reexamined ten years later, together with the mean of the ten-year blood pressure minus the entry value. In all areas there was a tendency for the entry blood pressure to increase with age at entry. When all areas and ages are combined, the least squares solution of the regression equation, $y = a + bx$ is $a = 104.4$, $b = 0.86$, where y is systolic blood pressure and x is age. Based on the 24 pairs of age and blood pressure values in table 16.2, the coefficient of correlation is $r = 0.79$ and the standard error of the slope, $b = 0.15$. This is the cross-sectional picture at entry of the men who were followed for ten years and then reexamined.

In the follow-up in all areas systolic blood pressure tended to increase, the average ten-year increase ranging from 3.7 mm Hg in Greece to 15.1 mm Hg in Croatia. For all ages and areas combined, the ten-year change in systolic pressure averaged 8.3 mm Hg. The mean age at entry of all these men was 49.8 years. From the regression equation in the preceding paragraph, relating systolic pressure at entry to age at that time, it would be predicted that ten years later, when the average age would be 59.8 years, the average systolic pressure would have increased 8.6 mm Hg. This excellent agreement between the average change observed in the follow-up and the projection from the cross-sectional data should be looked at more closely.

When all ages and areas are combined, the least-squares regression of the ten-year change in systolic pressure, y, is $y = 1.68 + 0.133x$, where x is age at entry. This indicates a blood pressure increase in ten years of 7.0 mm for men starting at age 40 and of 9.5 mm for men starting at age 59 years. The coefficient of correlation between age at entry and ten-year change in blood pressure is $r = 0.18$, calculated from the 24 pairs of values in table 16.2. It

Table 16.2. Mean systolic blood pressure and mean change (ten years minus entry, the same men).

Entry age	Croatia	Finland	Italy[a]	Zutphen	Greece	Serbia
40–44						
N	175	333	245	128	231	431
Mean at entry	145.9	141.4	142.9	142.3	133.8	138.6
SE	1.6	1.1	1.2	1.7	1.3	1.0
Mean change	13.8	6.7	5.3	5.2	0.7	8.9
SE	1.2	0.9	0.9	1.3	1.0	0.8
45–49						
N	262	390	476	178	263	212
Mean at entry	145.8	145.1	152.4	147.0	139.3	143.4
SE	1.2	1.1	1.0	1.6	1.4	1.5
Mean change	14.3	10.0	7.2	8.5	3.4	9.0
SE	1.1	0.9	0.8	1.2	1.1	1.3
50–54						
N	301	347	411	158	266	337
Mean at entry	151.5	150.1	155.6	148.0	145.3	152.2
SE	1.2	1.3	1.1	1.7	1.3	1.4
Mean change	15.1	9.1	4.0	4.5	5.4	11.8
SE	1.0	1.1	0.9	1.4	1.0	1.1
55–59						
N	246	282	248	144	207	249
Mean at entry	155.4	156.1	160.4	149.6	148.7	151.2
SE	1.4	1.6	1.5	1.9	1.8	1.4
Mean change	17.0	11.8	3.3	3.1	5.4	10.9
SE	1.1	1.2	1.2	1.3	1.4	1.2
40–59						
N	984	1,352	1,380	608	967	1,229
Mean at entry	150.0	147.7	153.1	146.9	141.6	145.7
SE	0.7	0.6	0.6	0.9	0.7	0.7
Mean change	15.1	9.3	5.2	5.5	3.7	7.3
SE	0.5	0.5	0.5	0.7	0.6	0.5

a. Crevalcore and Montegiorgio.

may be questioned whether this indicated relationship between entry age and ten-year increase of blood pressure is statistically significant because there are only 23 degrees of freedom though each pair of values represents, on the average, 271 men.

The agreement between cross-sectional and longitudinal data on the relationship of systolic blood pressure with age suggests that, whatever may have

Table 16.3. Mean diastolic blood pressure at entry and mean change (ten years minus entry).

Entry age	Croatia	Finland	Italy[a]	Zutphen	Greece	Serbia
40–44						
N	175	333	245	127	231	431
Mean at entry	88.7	82.5	87.7	88.5	81.3	85.7
SE	0.8	0.6	0.7	1.0	0.8	0.6
Mean change	6.5	−0.6	6.0	0.9	0.4	2.5
SE	1.0	0.6	0.7	1.1	0.8	0.5
45–49						
N	262	390	476	177	263	212
Mean at entry	86.8	83.1	90.2	91.3	80.8	86.1
SE	0.7	0.6	0.6	0.9	0.8	0.9
Mean change	4.5	−1.1	5.9	3.6	−0.7	2.8
SE	0.8	0.6	0.6	1.0	0.8	0.8
50–54						
N	300	347	411	158	265	337
Mean at entry	86.4	84.4	90.2	89.4	82.4	87.7
SE	0.6	0.7	0.6	1.0	0.7	0.7
Mean change	4.2	−1.8	4.5	−0.9	−0.6	3.0
SE	0.7	0.6	0.6	1.1	0.8	0.6
55–59						
N	246	282	248	144	207	248
Mean at entry	86.8	83.5	90.3	87.4	80.0	85.8
SE	0.7	0.8	0.8	1.1	1.0	0.8
Mean change	3.3	−1.7	3.3	−0.2	−2.0	0.0
SE	0.7	0.9	0.7	1.0	0.9	0.8
40–59						
N	983	1,352	1,380	606	966	1,228
Mean at entry	87.0	83.4	89.7	89.3	81.2	86.3
SE	0.3	0.3	0.3	0.5	0.4	0.4
Mean change	4.5	−1.3	5.0	1.0	−0.7	2.5
SE	0.4	0.3	0.3	0.5	0.4	0.3

a. Crevalcore and Montegiorgio.

been the changes in life-style during the ten years, they had little effect on the systolic blood pressure.

The relationship of diastolic blood pressure to age and to the years of follow-up are quite different from the systolic blood pressure. The data are summarized in table 16.3. In none of the areas was there any significant relationship between the diastolic pressure and age at entry. In the follow-up it appeared that the average diastolic pressure rose significantly in Croatia, Italy, and Serbia, but the increases were small. The change is statistically significant because the number of subjects is large, but it would not seem to be medically significant. In Finland and Greece the mean ten-year was a decrease in the diastolic pressure, and the decrease in Finland was statistically significant but trivial. These inconsistencies suggest that the average recorded changes may represent only changes in the conditions of measurement.

At entry the American railroad men showed a marked increase with age in the average systolic blood pressure of the men who were also reexamined five years later—133.1 mm Hg for 618 men aged 40–44, 135.3 mm Hg for 518 men aged 45–49, 141.8 mm Hg for 565 men aged 50–54, 144.2 mm Hg for 605 men aged 55–59. These values have standard errors of 0.7 to 0.9, so the age trend is consistent and highly significant. The least-squares regression of systolic pressure, y, on age, x, is $y = 99 + 0.80x$.

After five years the systolic blood pressure of the American railroad men tended to be slightly lower than at entry, with an average decrease of 1.3 mm Hg. The five-year change tended to be inversely related to age at entry. The mean changes, with standard errors in parentheses for increasing five-year age groups were: -3.2 (0.6), -1.8 (0.7), -0.4 (0.8), and $+0.2$ (0.7). The regression on entry age of five-year change in systolic pressure is $y = 12.9 + 0.23x$, where y is five-year change and x is entry age.

Diastolic blood pressure of the American railroad men at entry showed a distinct tendency to rise slightly with age. For the successive five-year age groups at entry, the mean diastolic pressures with standard errors in parentheses were: 83.9 (0.44), 84.9 (0.47), 86.4 (0.46), and 86.6 (0.47). The regression on age, x, of the entry diastolic blood pressure, y, is $y = 76 + 0.19x$. After five years with diastolic blood pressures of these men tended to be slightly lower at all ages, with an average fall of 2.6 mm. The average fall ranged from 2.4 mm for men aged 55–59 at entry to a fall of 2.8 mm for men aged 45–49 at entry.

Serum Cholesterol

Table 16.4 summarizes, for the same individuals in the areas of Europe, differences between serum cholesterol concentration at the ten-year and at the entry examinations. In all the European areas there was a significant average increase in serum cholesterol, but that change was much less in northern than in southern Europe. The average increase in ten years for 1,939 men in northern Europe was 6.92 mg/dl (SE = 0.95); for 3,928 in southern Europe the average was an increase of 28.44 mg/dl (SE = 0.63). This difference is in accord with the observation that the changes in the way

Table 16.4. Mean change of serum cholesterol (ten years minus entry, mg/dl).

Entry age	Croatia	Finland	Italy[a]	Zutphen	Greece	Serbia
40–44						
N	193	335	219	125	193	409
Mean change	33.2	13.4	24.2	10.6	33.2	47.9
SE	2.5	2.3	2.2	3.0	2.5	1.9
45–49						
N	218	392	415	165	218	191
Mean change	26.8	11.7	22.5	2.8	26.8	43.5
SE	2.4	2.3	1.9	2.8	2.4	3.2
50–54						
N	210	346	361	155	210	312
Mean change	18.6	1.6	22.6	4.8	18.6	42.0
SE	2.4	2.4	2.2	3.0	2.4	2.3
55–59						
N	171	282	205	139	171	232
Mean change	12.5	2.8	14.4	3.3	12.5	35.7
SE	3.2	2.5	2.8	3.2	3.2	2.4
40–59						
N	792	1,355	1,200	584	792	1,144
Mean change	23.1	7.7	21.5	5.1	23.1	43.1
SE	1.3	1.2	1.1	1.5	1.3	1.2

a. Crevalcore and Montegiorgio.

of life in southern Europe were much more marked than those in northern Europe.

Table 16.4 also indicates a tendency for the serum cholesterol changes to be inversely related to the age at entry. For the northern European men the regression of serum cholesterol change, y, on entry age, x, is $y = 43.0 - 0.73x$. The corresponding regression for southern European men is $y = 81.1 - 1.06x$. This inverse relationship suggests that the older men were more stable in their way of life, and this, too, was in agreement with the impression from related visits to the areas. It might be asked to what extent it would be possible to ascribe the ten-year cholesterol changes to aging per se. In chapter 8 it was shown that over the ages 40 through 59 in none of the areas was there a significant relationship between serum cholesterol and age. The chapter 8 material included the men who died during ten years and those alive for whom ten-year cholesterol data are not available. But the entry cholesterol data for 5,867 men covered in table 16.4 also failed to show any correlation between entry cholesterol and age.

Because the cross-sectional material at entry is limited to men aged 40–59, it may be asked whether a metabolic difference after those ages might not be involved in the trend for the ten-year cholesterol averages to be substantially greater than the entry values. That would require a general tendency for serum cholesterol to rise after age 60. But long ago cross-sectional surveys including older men showed a general tendency for serum cholesterol concentration to decrease in old age (Keys et al. 1950). In the present material the increase in serum cholesterol observed after ten years was less in the older than in the younger men. So increasing age itself cannot account for the increased serum cholesterol values observed after ten years.

Serum cholesterol was also measured at the five-year reexaminations of the same men covered in table 16.4. In general, the five-year averages were intermediate between the entry and the ten-year values. Figure 16.1 shows the picture for Croatia, distinguishing the Dalmatia and Slavonia cohorts. In Finland, most of the average serum cholesterol rise in the follow-up was accounted for by east Finland (figure 16.2). In rural Italy, the average serum cholesterol changes at the five- and ten-year reexaminations were similar in Crevalcore and in Montegiorgio (figure 16.3). For Greece, the Crete and Corfu cohorts both showed a substantially linear rise in serum cholesterol concentration from entry to the ten-year reexamination (figure 16.4). In Serbia all three cohorts showed a rather similar picture for serum cholesterol increase over the years (figure 16.5). The differences between the mean and five-year and the five-year and ten-year averages are statistically significant in all but the Belgrade five-year and ten-year comparison.

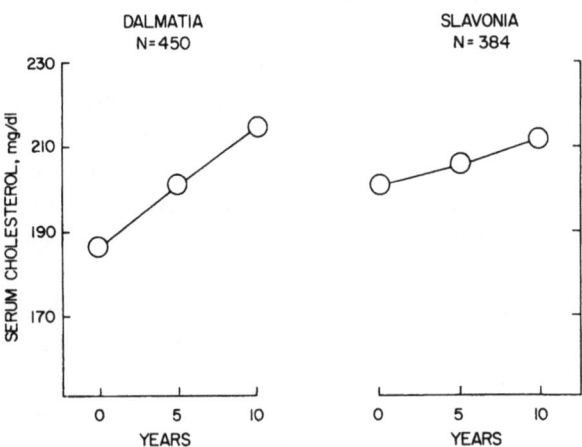

Figure 16.1. Mean serum cholesterol values of 450 men in Dalmatia and 384 in Slavonia at entry and at the five- and ten-year examinations.

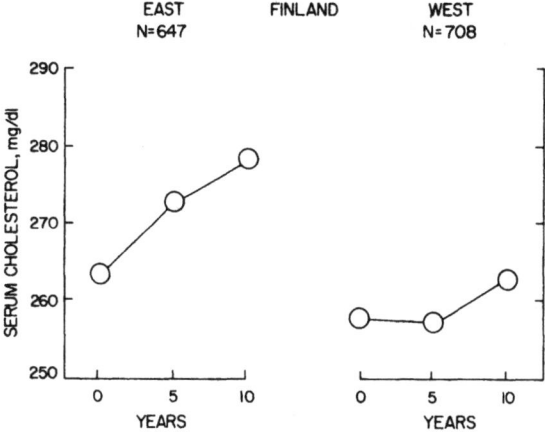

Figure 16.2. Mean serum cholesterol values of 647 men in east Finland and 708 in west Finland at entry and at the five- and ten-year examinations.

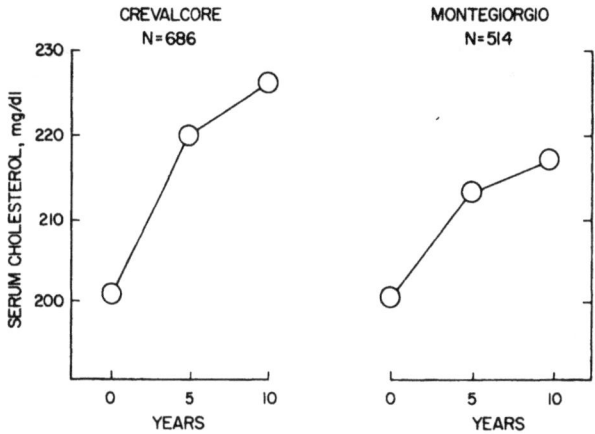

Figure 16.3. Mean serum cholesterol values of 686 men in Crevalcore and 514 in Montegiorgio at entry and at the five- and ten-year examinations.

At Zutphen there are some questions about five-year serum cholesterol data. There were no five-year blood samples for many of the subjects, and only subsamples of the material were sent to Minneapolis for analysis. The data available indicate at least rough correspondence with the change indicated in table 16.4 for ten years. Mean values for the same 584 men in 1960 and again in 1970 are shown in figure 16.6.

Only five-year follow-up values for serum cholesterol were obtained for the American railroad men. For 2,287 men aged 40–59 at entry, the

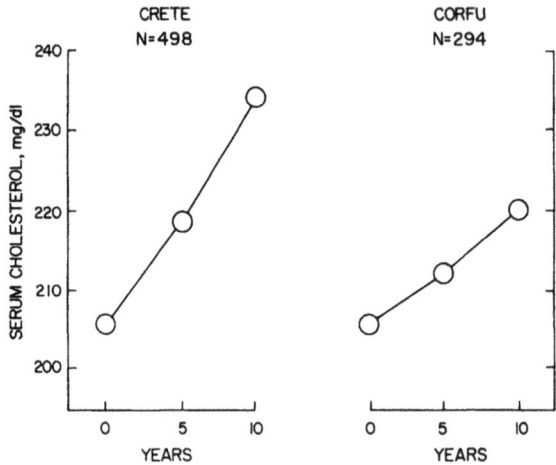

Figure 16.4. Mean serum cholesterol values of 498 men in Crete and 294 in Corfu at entry and at the five- and ten-year examinations.

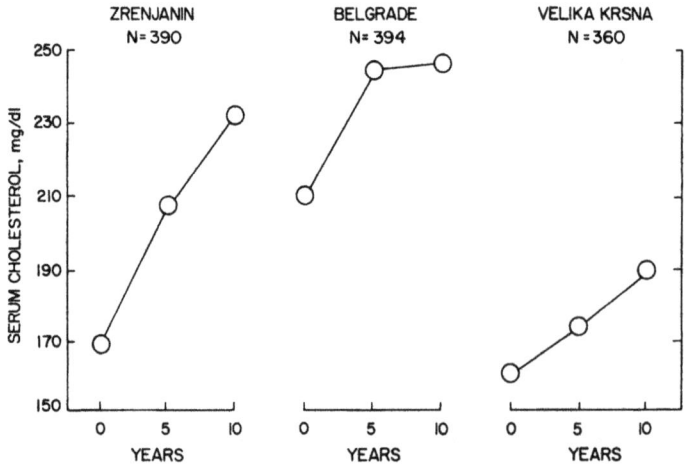

Figure 16.5. Mean serum cholesterol values at entry and at the five- and 10-year examinations. Same 390 men in Zrenjanin, 394 in Belgrade, and 360 in Velika Krsna.

average change after five years was a decrease of 2.16 mg/dl with standard error of 0.81. The change, y, is directly related to entry age, x, and the regression is $y = 11.3 - 0.27x$. The average follow-up change was very small, but it was in the opposite direction to the findings in Europe.

It should be recalled that, unlike the European men, the Americans

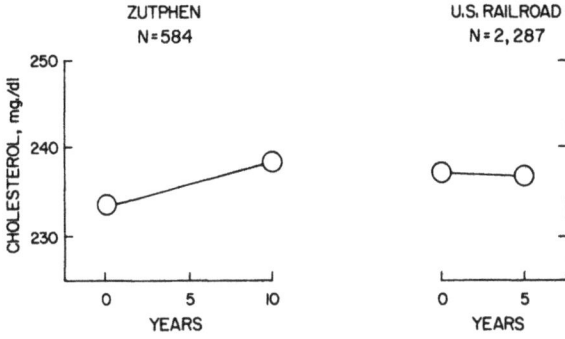

Figure 16.6. Mean serum cholesterol values of 584 men in Zutphen at entry and again ten years later and of 2,287 American railroad men at entry and again five years later.

showed no significant gain in weight during the follow-up period, although there was a trivial tendency for the younger men to gain a little and for the older men to lose a little weight. The five-year change in serum cholesterol concentration, y, tended to be positively related to the five-year change in body weight, x. The regression is $y = -2.64 + 1.80x$, where x is in kg, y in mg cholesterol per dl. Figure 16.6 shows serum concentration at entry and again five years later for the same 2,287 men.

Diet

Earlier in this chapter it was remarked that repeated visits to the rural areas of the Seven Countries Study strongly suggested important changes in the average diets of the men in rural southern Europe during the ten-year period of the follow-up. The impression that the consumption of animal products in general was increasing was gained from observing the foods offered in the local shops, talking with the men about their meals, occasionally observing the food preparation in the homes, and now and then joining the men at table. This impression was shared by all members of the teams who made such periodic visits, but such unstructured observations suffer from lack of proper documentation. However, for rural Italy, at least, the impression is born out by the data of repeated dietary surveys (Fidanza and Fidanza-Alberti 1975).

Table 16.5 summarizes the average values from seven-day dietary surveys on forty men in Crevalcore and Montegiorgio in 1960, repeated in 1965 and in 1970. The men, 40 through 59 years of age in 1960, were statistically selected to represent random samples of the cohorts. In 1970 the average percentage of the total dietary calories provided by fats was 20 percent greater than in 1960. During that same period the average percentage of the total calories in the diet provided by meats and other animal products rose by 27 percent. Our impression was that there were similar changes in the average diets of the cohorts in Croatia, in Greece, and in rural Serbia in the ten-year follow-up period.

The changes recorded in the diets of the men of Crevalcore and Montegiorgio are not peculiar to those areas of Italy. Table 16.6 summarizes estimates by A. Mariani of the Instituto Nazionale di Nutrizione (Rome) of

Table 16.5. Seven-day dietary surveys on men in rural Italy (Fidanza and Fidanza-Alberti 1975).

Year	Diet calories (%)		
	Animals[a]	All fats	Sat. fatty acids
1960	13.8	25.7	9.1
1965	14.1	26.1	11.4
1970	18.9	32.0	10.8

a. Meat, milk, cheese, eggs, fish.

Table 16.6. Per capita food consumption in Italy by year (kilograms per year and as percentage of 1901–5; figures for kg are rounded, percentages calculated from unrounded figures).

Food	1901–5	1926–30	1951–55	1965–69	1971–73
Cereal grains					
kg	161	174	145	138	144
%	100	108	91	86	90
Meats					
kg	15	22	19	46	58
%	100	147	124	300	384
Milk					
kg	34	37	52	66	72
%	100	107	153	193	211
Butter, cheese					
kg	4	6	8	11	13
%	100	143	210	283	325
Sugar					
kg	3	8	15	26	30
%	100	280	500	850	987

the per capita consumption of certain foods in Italy over the years 1928 to 1972, with the values expressed as percentages of the averages for the years 1901 to 1905. Since the 1950s the national consumption of meats, butter, and cheese has increased spectacularly and the per capita consumption of milk increased almost 50 percent from 1952 to 1972. Fidanza (1979) estimates that for Italy as a whole the percentage of total calories provided by animal proteins averaged 4.4 percent in 1954–1956, 4.7 in 1964–1966, and 5.6 in 1974–1976. That 27 percent increase in twenty years is surpassed by the estimated change in the consumption of fats in the diet. The percentage of total calories from animal fats was estimated to have been 10.4 in 1954–1956, 11.7 in 1964–1966, and 13.7 in 1974–1976. The twenty-year change in fats is a rise of 35 percent. The increase in the consumption of total fats has been even greater, averaging 23.5 percent of total calories in 1954–1956 and 33.0 percent twenty years later, an increase of 40 percent.

In Japan, the available food supply for human consumption is estimated each year, as in other countries with effective ministries of agriculture, but actual household food use is also estimated, independently, in a large national nutrition survey that covers statistical samples of all parts of the country. That annual survey, initiated by the military occupation after the surrender of Japan in 1945, provides information about the diets of all segments of society in the country in remarkable detail. Table 16.7 summarizes data from those two sources for 1955 through 1975.

The estimated calories in the available food supply somewhat exceed the figures from the household surveys, presumably reflecting waste, but the two sets of estimates are in rather good agreement for proteins and fats. The outstanding features in these data are the enormous increase over the years in the consumption of fats from animal sources, followed by a large, but less spectacular increase in animal protein in the diet. The per capita intake of animal fat in 1970 was 138 percent of that in 1955. These changes in the nutrients in the national average diet reflect an increase in the per capita intake of meats from 9 grams per day in 1955 to 43 grams in 1970 and of milk and milk products from 14 grams per day in 1955 to 79 grams in 1970. The calories of these increases were offset by decreases in cereals and potatoes, which averaged 374 and 38 grams per day, respectively, in 1970 compared with 480 grams and 81 grams per day in 1955. The dietary changes in Japan in the last twenty years include a large increase in the consumption of fruits with relatively little change in the consumption of vegetables, pulses, fish, and sea foods.

Everyone agrees that the Japanese diet has improved greatly since the time of the privation of World War II and the time before the war when vitamin deficiencies were common. It remains to be seen, however, what the result

Table 16.7. Average nutrients per capita in the diet in Japan estimated from food availability by the Japanese Ministry of Agriculture and Forestry (AF) and from household dietary surveys by the Ministry of Health and Welfare (HW) (data summarized by Tadataka Fukui for the International Symposium on Diet and Health at Osaka, December 4–5, 1978).

Nutrient	Unit	1955	1960	1965	1970	1975
Calories						
AF	kcal	2,217	2,290	2,408	2,472	2,467
HW	kcal	2,104	2,096	2,184	2,210	2,188
Total protein						
AF	g	66	70	74	76	79
HW	g	70	70	71	78	80
Animal protein						
AF	g	17	21	27	32	35
HW	g	22	25	29	34	39
Total fat						
AF	g	22	29	40	52	59
HW	g	20	25	36	47	52
Animal fat						
AF	g	8	11	18	22	25
HW	g	7	9	14	21	27

will be on the incidence and mortality of cardiovascular diseases. The change in saturated fatty acids and cholesterol in the diet has been very large, and there are many reports of increased levels of cholesterol in the blood, which, however, do not yet reach the values characteristic of the United States and northern Europe. In parallel, there certainly has been a striking increase in the frequency of diagnoses of coronary heart disease. It is unwarranted to insist that these parallelisms are simply cause and effect. Some Japanese physicians suggest that a part of the explanation is a new awareness of the disease and its symptomatology.

The data on the diet in the United States over the last twenty years are in contrast to the trends in Italy and southern Europe and in Japan. Stamler (1978) has pointed to the changes in per capita consumption of some foods in the United States that indicate an important reduction in the intake of saturated fatty acids and cholesterol in the diet. Stamler points to the indications from various surveys that the average level of cholesterol in the blood serum is falling. Enthusiasts for the dietary control of blood lipids in an effort to reduce the incidence of coronary heart disease are much heartened by the recent vital statistics for the United States that show, for the first time, a progressive decline in the death rate from coronary heart disease. It is too much, of course, to credit the indicated dietary changes with the declining coronary death rate. But the fact is that these changes are in accord with the hypothesis.

This is not the place to attempt a review of national trends in the diets and mortality from coronary heart disease in the vital statistics of our seven countries. The foregoing notes about Italy, Japan, and the United States are interjected only to illustrate the point that these are, indeed, times of change and that the characteristics of the men at the time of their entry into the Seven Countries Study imperfectly represent those men over the years of follow-up and the years before, the silent years of atherogenesis. In this and other prospective studies, the interpretation of relationships between entering characteristics and the later incidence of disease proves to be more difficult than thought at the start.

Smoking Habits

Table 16.8 summarizes the distribution of the same men by smoking habits at entry, five years later, and ten years later for all men free of evidence of cardiovascular disease at the entry examination. The men are classified according to age at entry because, as will be seen, smoking habits tended to have some relation to age.

In most of the areas, the percentage of men who were nonsmokers increased during the period of follow-up; the differences in table 16.8 between the percentages for nonsmokers at entry and at ten years indicates the men who had stopped smoking after the start of the study. The Greeks and the United State railroad men were exceptional in that the answers to the questionnaire about smoking indicate that fifteen of the older Greek men (50–59 at entry) who had been nonsmokers at entry said they were smoking at the time of the ten-year reexamination, whereas among the Americans aged 45–59 at entry, sixty-one who said they were nonsmokers at entry reported they were smoking cigarettes at the five-year reexamination.

A somewhat surprising finding in the data on cigarette smoking over the ten years was a tendency in some of the areas for the smokers to increase their smoking. If heavy smokers are defined as men who reported they habitually smoked at least twenty cigarettes a day, as the years went on there was an increasing percentage of heavy smokers in Yugoslavia and in the younger men in Greece. In the five-year follow-up of the United State railroad men there was an increase in heavy smoking in all but the oldest age group.

Without attempting to explain why men changed their smoking habits, the fact remains that a good many of them did change. It is thus not really correct to use only the entry smoking data in the estimation of the relation

Table 16.8. Cigarette smoking habits at entry and at the five-year and ten-year examinations of men free of cardiovascular disease at entry (heavy smokers use 20 or more cigarettes every day).

			Nonsmokers (%)			Heavy smokers (%)		
Area	Entry age	N	Entry	Five-year	Ten-year	Entry	Five-year	Ten-year
U.S. railroad	40–44	504	33	38	—	30	35	—
	45–49	414	37	43	—	26	30	—
	50–54	406	43	48	—	20	22	—
	55–59	397	48	52	—	20	17	—
Croatia	40–44	165	44	48	43	17	15	36
	45–49	239	42	45	48	20	18	26
	50–54	274	38	43	47	22	21	32
	55–59	218	45	51	52	24	19	27
Finland	40–44	281	40	49	50	22	31	31
	45–49	308	38	48	49	22	19	21
	50–54	248	41	51	53	18	23	20
	55–59	186	40	55	56	15	18	13
Japan	40–44	162	19	—	23	46	—	43
	45–49	186	15	—	19	52	—	49
	50–54	191	17	—	25	44	—	35
	55–59	174	20	—	26	45	—	21
Italy	40–44	346	38	38	43	24	26	20
	45–49	525	38	39	44	16	17	10
	50–54	485	40	44	49	16	16	6
	55–59	256	41	46	52	13	11	5
Zutphen	40–44	120	18	33	38	11	9	8
	45–49	164	17	31	38	12	8	7
	50–54	130	35	50	54	7	4	5
	55–59	119	35	47	55	9	4	4
Greece	40–44	219	37	37	34	28	29	33
	45–49	244	45	43	40	26	26	29
	50–54	245	35	38	39	27	25	29
	55–59	181	43	45	46	25	18	17
Serbia	40–44	399	47	50	55	22	31	30
	45–49	184	47	49	52	22	19	29
	50–54	294	45	52	60	17	24	23
	55–59	219	56	59	62	10	10	6

of smoking to the subsequent incidence of disease and death. With this, as with other variables, relationships between personal characteristics and the events during the follow-up period are somewhat blurred by the fact that the entry data cannot accurately describe the long-term characteristics of the men.

The Vital Statistics of the United States report a substantial decrease, from 1968 to 1975, in the death rate. The age-adjusted rate for the population as a whole fell 19 percent; a striking decline in deaths from coronary heart disease made a major contribution to the improvement in the all-causes death rate. The data have now been analyzed critically by Cooper et al (1979) who conclude that the change is real. They comment that trends in medical and social practices could be "contributing significantly to the observed decline in mortality: improved care for medical patients with symptomatic CHD; sizeable decreases in cigarette smoking among adult men and women; decline in consumption of saturated fat and cholesterol with concomitant fall in mean serum cholesterol level of the population; enhanced detection, treatment and control of hypertension in the population" (Cooper et al. 1979, p. 719).

Summary

This book concerns relationships of the ten-year incidence of disease and death to the characteristics of the men at the entry examinations. But some characteristics changed over the years, reflecting aging, interim events, and changes in the mode of life. For men without evidence of significant disease at entry, effects of age may be inferred by cross-sectional comparison of the average characteristics of men of different ages. For men who stayed well, longitudinal changes over the years of follow-up may reflect changes in lifestyle as well. We report average differences between ten-year and entry characteristics of the same men who showed no evidence of cardiovascular disease at entry or ten years later.

At entry the relative body weight was not related to age in any of the cohorts. In the absence of intervening disease or changes in life-style, diet, or energy expenditure, no change in average body weight would be expected in ten years, at least in men under 60 at the ten-year examination. Actually in all the areas of Europe the average weight of the men always healthy increased in ten years. The mean increase for 6,276 men was 2.9 kg and ranged from 1.8 kg in 1,228 Serbians to 4.4 kg in 928 Greeks. The gain was greatest in the youngest men, averaging 5.1 kg in men 40–44 at entry, and decreased steadily with entry age to an average of 2.3 kg in men 55–59 at entry. In the first five years the average increase in those Europeans was 2.2 kg, so most of the ten-year change was in the first five years.

The American railroad men were reweighed only after five years at which time the average for 2,290 men was a trivial 0.1 kg increase. However, like the Europeans, the tendency was for an inverse relationship with age. For 1,130 men under 50 years at entry there was an average gain of 0.9 kg while the 1,160 men aged 50 to 59 at entry showed an average loss of 0.3 kg. A change in life-style in Europe but not in the United States is suggested.

In all areas of Europe the systolic blood pressure rose during the ten years of follow-up. This change corresponded closely with the expectation indicated by the regression of systolic pressure on age at the entry examinations. At entry the diastolic pressure was not significantly related to age in any of the areas. After ten years the mean diastolic pressure was slightly higher than at entry in Croatia, Italy, and Serbia, slightly lower in Finland and Greece. It would seem that the changes in life-style in Europe had no significant effect on blood pressure.

In the American railroad men the average systolic pressure slightly decreased in five years in spite of a marked regression on age at entry. The five-year average diastolic pressure was higher than at entry. The fact that the measurements were made by different persons on the two occasions may be relevant.

In all areas of Europe there was a significant rise in serum cholesterol concentration in ten years, though at entry cholesterol concentration was independent of age and in other studies cholesterol tended to decrease after 60 years of age. The trend of cholesterol to rise was much more marked in southern than in northern Europe. The cholesterol change tended to be inversely related to age. The American railroad men showed a slight average decrease in serum cholesterol in five years. As with body weight, the indication is that the diet tended to change in Europe but not in the United States.

Quantitative information on dietary changes of the men in this study is scanty; however, all indications are that in southern Europe and in Japan there was a substantial increase in dietary fat from animal sources during the years of follow-up. In the United States the general trend, if any, was for some substitution of vegetable for animal fat and a reduction of cholesterol in the diet. It may be relevant that the current tendency is for the death rate from coronary heart disease to decrease in the United States but to increase in the other countries represented in this study.

17 | Some Conclusions

1957: The protocol and methods for the proposed international collaborative study on the epidemiology of coronary heart disease were tested in full-scale field trials in villages in southern Italy and the Greek island of Crete in 1957. Medical scientists from England, Finland, France, Japan, the Netherlands, the United States, and Yugoslavia, as well as from Italy and Greece, took part. Besides revising the methods and standardizing criteria from the practical experience, those trials showed that in such villages suitable local preparation could enlist the cooperation of almost all the men invited in the designated area. Moreover, physicians from different countries, working together in the field, could agree on standardized examination procedures and diagnostic criteria and the establishment of a central headquarters where all data would be collected and analyzed.

Those 1957 trials were in preparation for parallel prospective studies of middle-aged men to compare the incidence of coronary heart disease in diverse populations, to find and evaluate relationships between the incidence of the disease and the characteristics of the men before clinical disease was evident, and to examine the universality, or variability, of those relationships in contrasting populations. Prospective studies to observe the incidence of coronary heart disease had started a decade before in Minnesota, shortly to be followed by similar programs at Framingham, Massachusetts, Los Angeles, Albany, and elsewhere in the United States.

By 1957 those pioneer American prospective studies had accumulated over 24,000 man-years of experience which incriminated arterial blood pressure, the concentration of cholesterol in the blood serum, and cigarette smoking as what would later be called *risk factors* for clinical coronary heart disease. The subjects of those studies were a very limited sample of mankind; they were middle-class, urban, white Americans. Already there was talk of preventive programs to stop smoking and to find and somehow control hypertension and hypercholesterolemia.

In the meantime, explorations in Italy, Spain, South Africa, Japan, and Finland in 1952–1956 had produced much evidence for major differences among populations in the incidence of coronary heart disease, differences related to contrasts in the average level of cholesterol in the blood serum that, in turn, seemed to be associated with the fats in the average diets of those populations. In metabolic wards an important influence of the diet on the cholesterol level was established by rigidly controlled experiments on men. By 1957, opposing effects on serum cholesterol of saturated versus polyunsaturated fatty acids in the diet had been measured, and similar relationships between dietary fat and serum cholesterol were indicated in Bantu in South Africa, Japanese in Japan, Hawaii, and California, as well as in white Americans and Europeans. Claims that the rules were disproved by Eskimos and Navajo Indians were shown to have no basis in fact.

1958 to 1964: 12,763 Men Enrolled in the Seven Countries Study

This, in brief, was the background of the start, in 1958, of systematic prospective studies of men aged 40–59 living in two areas of Croatia (Yugoslavia), employed by railroad companies in the United States, and living in a farming area of Kyushu, Japan. The subjects were men named on rosters of all men aged 40–59 in the designated area or, in the case of the railroad men, the designated occupation. Following the same rules, new cohorts were added to make a total, by 1964, of sixteen cohorts in seven countries. The entry examinations covered 12,763 men, over 90 percent of the men on the rosters of those eligible. In each case the examinations were conducted close to the place of residence of the subjects, the examining teams including representatives from other areas of the study and the central staff in addition to the basic team of the country or region.

In order to assure comparability among cohorts, all diagnoses were based on the findings of the physicians in this study with review by central staff; secondhand medical reports were not used unless confirmed by members of the study teams. Significant diagnoses made at the time of examinations represented the agreement of two or more internists. In the incidence of coronary heart disease, the analyses commonly distinguished between hard CHD, coronary death or myocardial infarction, and soft CHD, all other diagnoses of the disease, including uncomplicated angina pectoris. For the diagnosis of cause of death, besides death certificates, local medical records were examined, and relatives and intimates of the deceased as well as local physicians were interviewed. Those diagnoses were then reviewed by central staff.

The examinations were repeated after five years and, except for the American railroad men and some railroad men in Italy, on the tenth anniversary of the entry examination. Mortality, checked each year in each cohort, was given particular attention because, though the initial focus was on coronary heart disease, it was realized that the ultimate concern for the health of a population is the age-specific death rate.

Entry Examinations

At the entry examinations 667 men were judged to be suffering from cardiovascular disease; of these 183 had old myocardial infarction and 63 uncomplicated angina pectoris. The cohorts differed greatly in prevalence; the rates for the Americans and the Finns were much higher than for the other cohorts. The 667 men with positive diagnoses at entry were excluded from most analyses of the subsequent ten-year experience, but they were followed in regard to prognosis.

During ten years, compared with all men in the same cohorts, the men with coronary heart disease at entry had an age-standardized death rate 2.7 times greater from all-causes and 4.9 times greater from coronary heart disease. On the other hand, a substantial number of men with entry diagnoses of coronary heart disease were alive with no evidence of the disease ten years later. The picture was similar for the men given a diagnosis of noncoronary heart disease at entry. Among 152 such men in Europe, 62 were dead in ten years, a death rate 4 times that of the other men, but at the ten-year reexamination no diagnosis of heart disease was recorded for 66 men.

At entry, 603 men with no evidence of clinical disease showed nonspecific abnormalities in the electrocardiogram. Those men were not excluded from the analyses of the subsequent incidence of disease. Their ten-year death rate was 167 percent of the rate for all men in the study. Although the difference is highly significant, the abnormalities included are of many types and more analysis is needed.

Ten-year Deaths

In ten years 1,507 men died, 410 from coronary heart disease. Excluding the men with cardiovascular disease at entry, there were 1,280 deaths, 290 from coronary heart disease. The age-standardized death rates varied among the cohorts, northern and southern Europeans differing most significantly. The rate was 29 percent higher in northern than in southern Europe for all-causes deaths, 265 percent higher for coronary deaths. The northern Europeans also had a much higher rate of death from lung cancer. Excluding coronary heart disease and lung cancer, there was no significant difference between northern and southern Europeans in the age-standardized death rate.

The ten-year death rates from all causes of the American and the Italian railroad men were not significantly different, but the coronary death rate of the Americans was 72 percent higher than that of their Italian counterparts. For the American railroad men the all-causes death rate of the physically active switchmen was significantly higher than that for their sedentary counterparts, but most of the difference was accounted for by deaths from violence. The coronary death rate of the switchmen also tended to be higher than that of the sedentary men, but the difference was not statistically significant.

For the sixteen cohorts in the study, the age-standardized rates of death from coronary heart disease were not correlated with the death rates from noncoronary heart disease. Analysis of mortality data reported by the World Health Organization for the countries in Europe, the United States, Canada, Australia, and New Zealand also failed to find a correlation between coronary and noncoronary death rates. The recurrent suggestion that a low coronary death rate is necessarily accompanied by a high rate from other causes has no basis in the data from the relatively developed countries.

U.S. Vital Statistics during the period of this study were used as a general basis of reference in regard to mortality. The deaths expected (E) to match the American experience for men of the same age were calculated for each cohort and compared with the numbers observed (O). For all-causes deaths the figure for the sixteen cohorts combined was $O/E = 0.82$ and for coronary deaths $O/E = 0.53$. Men with cardiovascular disease at entry were not excluded in these calculations. For the American railroad men the corresponding figures are $O/E = 0.77$ and 0.92.

The men in this study were never proposed to be statistically representative of their countries of residence, but in the outcome their death rates proved to be highly correlated with those of all men of the same age in their respective countries. Expressing the age-standardized death rates of each country as percentage of the mean rate of the seven countries, the correlation between the present experience and that reported by the World Health Organization is $r = 0.86$ for all-causes and $r = 0.98$ for coronary deaths, the slopes of the regression lines being 0.9 and 1.0, respectively. In relative death rate, then, the cohorts are not unrepresentative of men of their ages in their several countries.

Incidence of Coronary Heart Disease

Among 9,780 men with no evidence of cardiovascular disease at entry, 1,264 were given a diagnosis of coronary heart disease during the ten-year follow-up, 351 being cases of hard CHD (coronary death or myocardial infarction). The Americans are not included here because they had no ten-year reexamination. The incidence rate per 10,000 of hard CHD varied from a low of 26 on the island of Crete to a high of 1,074 for the men of east Finland. For all diagnoses of coronary heart disease in ten years, the same cohorts provided the extremes, 210 for the Cretans, 2,868 for the east Finns.

Except in the Netherlands, the distribution of the several manifestations of the disease was similar in the several regions in the study. The percentage of all coronary diagnoses accounted for by hard CHD varied only from 37 in Serbia to 42 in Finland, but at Zutphen, the Netherlands, the figure was 54 percent. This peculiarity was explained by a very low frequency of diagnoses of uncomplicated angina pectoris at Zutphen, a reflection, it seemed, of local diagnostic custom.

The experience in the several regions was consistent in regard to the relationship of nonfatal myocardial infarction to death from the disease. The coefficient of correlation between the rates of nonfatal infarction in the cohorts with their coronary death rates was $r = 0.9$. On the other hand, the coronary death rate was not correlated with the rate of incidence of the disease inferred simply from the new appearance of nonspecific changes in the electrocardiogram sometimes considered to indicate coronary heart disease.

In an attempt to find reasons for the marked differences among the cohorts in the incidence of coronary heart disease, characteristics of the men in the cohorts were examined. The cohorts were closely matched in age, and in any case the differences in incidence rates were not altered by age-standardization. Comparison of the cohorts in respect to their mean relative weights or the percentage overweight of specified degrees showed no correlation with incidence of or mortality from coronary heart disease. Similar consideration of body fatness was also unproductive. Consideration of the percentage of men sedentary or very active, or of the average degree of physical activity, in the cohorts was not helpful. Smoking habits, expressed as average cigarettes smoked per day, or as percentage of nonsmokers or of heavy smokers were equally unrelated to the subsequent incidence rates of the disease. However, three characteristics proved to be instructive.

Differences among the cohorts in arterial blood pressure and in serum cholesterol each accounted for over 40 percent of the variance of the cohorts in the ten-year coronary death rate. When the cohort median values for both systolic blood pressure and for serum cholesterol were taken as independent variables in multiple regression analysis, two-thirds of the cohort variance in coronary death rate was explained. The estimated mean percentage of calories provided by saturated fatty acids in the diets of the cohort was equally successful in explaining the variance in coronary death rate of the cohorts. Inclusion of this dietary variable in the multiple regression equation with blood pressure and serum cholesterol did not significantly reduce the unexplained variance in coronary death rate. This is understandable in view of the very high correlation ($r = 0.84$) between the average values of serum cholesterol and of saturated fats in the diets of the cohorts.

Consideration of other characteristics of the diets of the cohorts did not significantly improve the explanation of the differences among the cohorts in the incidence rate of coronary heart disease. Those incidence rates were significantly correlated with sugar and with cholesterol in the diet, but those variables make no significant independent contribution; their relationships with incidence are explained by their high correlation with saturated fats in the diets: $r = 0.84$ for sucrose, 0.89 for dietary cholesterol.

So differences among the cohorts in coronary incidence were not explained by differences among the cohorts in age, relative body weight, in body fatness, in habitual physical activity, or in smoking habits. But this does not dispose of questions about the role of those characteristics as risk factors for the individual men within the cohorts. Those questions can be answered only by comparison of the characteristics of the individuals with their subsequent experience.

Age

Age was not a factor in comparisons of the cohorts in regard to incidence rates because the cohorts were closely matched in age and any slight differences in age were compensated for by standardization of rates by single years of age. Within cohorts, however, the twenty-year range of entering ages called for careful examination of the relationship of incidence to age. Regression analysis showed that for all 12,763 men combined, the ten-year all-causes death rate per 1,000 men was $-409 + 10.52$ times entry age in years; the corresponding rate for coronary deaths was $-94 + 2.51$ times entry age. For the American railroad men free from cardiovascular disease at entry, the slopes of the regressions on age of the ten-year all-causes and coronary heart disease death rates are not significantly different. For the American railroad men free of cardiovascular disease at entry, the corresponding figures were 2.6 and 2.8 percent increase per year of age at entry for all-causes and for coronary deaths, respectively. The influence of age on the death rate of middle-aged men as reported in official vital statistics is similar. The incidence rate of major coronary heart disease also tended to be a linear function of entry age, the slope of the regression on age being somewhat less steep than the slope of the mortality rate on age.

Among the risk factor variables examined in this study, blood pressure showed a substantial correlation with age, but allowance for that relationship in solutions of the bivariate logistic equation only trivially reduced the effect of age. For men free of cardiovascular disease at entry, the ten-year incidence of hard CHD (infarction or coronary death), holding blood pressure constant, for rural Finns was 58 per 1,000 for men aged 45 at entry and 92 for men aged 55, a 59 percent increase because of age. The corresponding analysis of the experience of rural Italians, holding blood pressure constant, indicated a ten-year incidence of hard CHD of 25 per 1,000 men aged 45 at entry and 50 for men ten years older, a 100 percent increase because of age.

These facts show that reporting incidence rates of men in ten-year, or wider, age classes can be seriously misleading. Even five-year age classes are imprecise in that the implication is that the incidence rate for a man aged 50 is the same as that of a man aged 54 though in reality there is an average difference of 10 percent or more. Age is the most important of the risk factors for mortality and for incidence of major coronary heart disease, and it is a continuous variable that should be treated as such. For this reason age, by single years, is treated as an independent variable in all multivariate analyses in the present work.

Blood Pressure

In the comparison of the cohorts, their characteristic (median) systolic blood pressure at entry accounted for 41 percent of their variance in ten-year all-causes age-standardized mortality; the diastolic pressure had much the same importance, accounting for 38 percent of the variance. The median blood pressure accounted for a slightly larger percentage of variance of the cohorts in the death rate from coronary heart disease, 47 percent being explained by systolic and 42 percent by diastolic blood pressure.

Within all cohorts the two entry characteristics most significant for discriminating those who later developed coronary heart disease in ten years from those who did not proved to be age and the resting blood pressure. Since nothing can be done about age, but blood pressure can be controlled to some extent, it follows that for middle-aged men the variable of greatest interest for prevention efforts is the blood pressure.

For middle-aged men without evidence of cardiovascular disease at entry, the probability of death in ten years (all-causes) increased in the different cohorts by 15 to 22 percent with each increase of 10 mm of systolic blood pressure over the range of 125 to 165 mm Hg. For the American railroad men and for the men in Finland entering at age 50, the bivariate logistic solutions for the ten-year incidence indicates that an entry blood pressure of 150 mm is associated with a 16 percent higher death rate than a blood pressure of 140 mm. Similar analysis of the data on the Mediterraneans (Italians and Greeks) showed entering with 150 mm was associated with a 22 percent greater all-causes ten-year death rate than entering with 140 mm.

The risk of developing coronary heart disease in ten years was related to the entering resting blood pressure to much the same extent. In Finland an entry systolic pressure of 150 mm in a 50-year-old man was associated with an 18 percent greater rate of incidence of myocardial infarction or coronary death than a pressure of 140 mm at the same age. Among the Mediterranean men the risk of developing hard CHD was 16 percent greater with an entry pressure of 150 mm than with 140 mm.

The systolic blood pressure was significantly correlated with some other characteristics of interest. In this study average correlations at entry were: with relative body weight, $r = 0.21$, with serum cholesterol, $r = 0.13$, with resting pulse rate, $r = 0.20$, but with cigarette smoking $r = -.09$. When all of these intercorrelations are taken into account in the solutions of the multiple logistic equation, the importance of the blood pressure is still very large. The correlation between blood pressure and age is important, too; the average coefficient of correlation in the present material is $r = 0.23$, but, as noted above, at any given age the blood pressure has great prognostic importance.

It is commonly thought that the diastolic pressure is more significant than the systolic pressure because it is less affected by the emotional state at the moment and it changes less with age. On the latter point, in the seven countries material, the average coefficient of correlation with age in the 16 cohorts at entry was $r = 0.23$ for systolic and $r = 0.13$ for diastolic pressure. Nevertheless, in all the analyses of the present material the prognostic value of the systolic pressure was never surpassed by that of the diastolic pressure. The experience of the Framingham study was similar; the predictive power of the systolic pressure was, if anything, a little better than that of the diastolic pressure. However, in multiple logistic analyses of the ten-year seven countries experience, when both systolic and diastolic blood pressures were used as independent variables together with age, serum cholesterol, and other variables of interest, the discrimination was slightly better than when only one of the blood pressure measures was used. Though the improvement is trivial and cannot be shown to be statistically significant, the fact is that the result was similar in all regions and with various end points for ten-year events—slightly higher values for the likelihood ratio statistic and for first and second moments of the distribution of the observed cases in the deciles of estimated probability when both blood pressures were used than with either one alone. Conceivably, this could mean only that two measurements are better than one, reducing the effect of error in reading or transcription in one measurement.

The above presentation of the relationships of risk to blood pressure is based on regression analysis, which involves the assumption of a linear relation, an assumption made in substantially all previous epidemiological studies. But the examination of the data without assumptions about the character of the relationship raises a question about linearity. In the present material, taking either mortality or the incidence of coronary heart disease as end points, no significant relationship of incidence to the blood pressure at entry was found over roughly the lower two-thirds of the distribution of the blood pressure in any of the regions. The picture is much the same with either systolic or diastolic pressure. In the upper third of the blood pressure distribution the incidence rate tended to rise sharply. These findings suggest the need to reexamine epidemiological data on blood pressure and disease with no assumptions about the character of the relationship. This is not to suggest a critical level of blood pressure or a return to the old simplistic idea of the dichotomy, normal versus abnormal, or health versus disease, that dominated all medical thinking until very recently. The data suggest a curvilinear relationship, with no particular cutting point to justify classifying people as hypertensive or normotensive, but also with no justification for the common view that the lower the blood pressure the better.

Cholesterol Concentration

In the seven countries entry data the concentration of cholesterol in the blood serum was slightly correlated with relative body weight and body fatness, the coefficients of correlation in the 16 cohorts averaging $r = 0.29$ and $r = 0.19$, respectively. With blood pressure the correlation was still smaller, $r = 0.13$, and with age there was essentially no correlation, the average being $r = 0.02$. This corresponds to the common finding in that the cholesterol level of middle-aged men is independent of age.

The sixteen cohorts differed widely in the general level of cholesterol in the blood serum, from mediun values of around 160 mg/dl in three cohorts to over 250 in the Finnish cohorts. The ten-year rate of death from coronary heart disease in the cohorts, excluding the men with evidence of cardiovascular disease at entry, proved to be highly correlated with the median cholesterol values of the cohorts, with $r = 0.80$. Thus the serum cholesterol median accounted for 64 percent of the variance of the cohorts in the coronary death rate. Including nonfatal cases, the incidence rates for coronary heart disease of the cohorts were also highly correlated with their median values for serum cholesterol at entry. For myocardial infarction or coronary death (hard CHD), the coefficient of correlation is $r = 0.81$; for other (soft CHD) manifestations of the disease $r = 0.79$. All men were considered to be free of cardiovascular disease at entry. When men with cardiovascular disease at entry are included in the calculations, the correlation is not less; in fact for coronary death versus entry cholesterol $r = 0.82$.

On the other hand, the all-causes death rates of the cohorts were not significantly correlated with their cholesterol levels; $r = 0.12$. Considering only noncoronary deaths, the correlation with the median serum cholesterol values was negative, $r = -0.35$, but with only sixteen pairs of values the conclusion is simply that the noncoronary death rate was not significantly related to the entry serum cholesterol concentration.

We noted that the coronary death rates of the cohorts were related to their median blood pressures at entry, with $r = 0.64$, so it might be thought that taking account of blood pressure as well as cholesterol at entry would account for much more of the variance in coronary mortality than when only cholesterol was considered. This is not the case, however. When both entry variables are used in the multiple regression equation with mortality from coronary heart disease as the dependent variable, the result is that 66 percent of the variance in mortality is accounted for, only a trifle more than when cholesterol alone was considered. The reason is that the entry median values for blood pressure and for cholesterol in the cohorts are highly correlated ($r = 0.59$). This relationship between values for the cohorts is not to be confused with the relationship between serum cholesterol and blood pressure values of the individual men within the cohorts, which averaged only $r = 0.13$.

So we turn from comparing cohorts to comparing the experience of the individual men within the cohorts. In that comparison the incidence of coronary death was importantly related to the entry cholesterol concentration. At the upper end of the cholesterol distribution, the likelihood of becoming a coronary victim increased sharply with the cholesterol level. For the American railroad men the risk of all-causes death was also directly related to the entry cholesterol level, but this was not true in any of the other areas of the study. In Italy, Greece, and Yugoslavia the ten-year all-causes risk of death tended to decrease with increasing serum cholesterol concentration at entry. In Finland there was no clear-cut trend for all-causes deaths to be related to cholesterol but the noncoronary death rate decreased with increasing serum cholesterol, the rate for the men in the top quintile of the cholesterol distribution at entry being roughly half that of the men in the bottom quintile.

The experience of the American railroad men in the seven countries study is similar to that reported from other prospective studies in the United

States. The consideration only of the American experience, with the customary assumption of linear relationships, has led to the view that the lower the cholesterol concentration, the better for the individual and the public health, a view engendered by concentration on coronary heart disease and the current situation in the United States. That view would appear to have serious limitations for other populations.

The idea that the risk of developing coronary heart disease rises steadily with the serum cholesterol level was promoted by the early reports from studies in the United States which simply compared the experience of men classified as high and low and then graduated into broad groupings such as tertiles of the cholesterol distribution. That view seemed to be nicely verified from the results of regression analysis, especially with the multiple logistic equation. But the ordinary use of such regression analyses automatically guarantees answers in terms of linear relationships. The solutions are simply the response to the demand for the best straight lines to fit the data.

When assumptions about normal distributions and linear relations are abandoned and age-standardized death rates are simply calculated for classes of serum cholesterol concentration, the current data indicate that the all-causes death rate tends to rise with serum cholesterol only at levels of the order of 275 mg/dl and above. For coronary deaths no relationship to serum cholesterol is indicated at levels below around 230 or 240 mg/dl. It would seem that a more critical examination of cholesterol-versus-incidence data in other studies might be rewarding.

Smoking Habits

For the past thirty years or so most men have been cigarette smokers, though in middle age a substantial percentage are ex-smokers. At entry in the present study more than half of the men were cigarette smokers except in two Serbian cohorts and even in those groups over 40 percent were smoking every day. Still, the cohorts were not identical in smoking habits. In five cohorts 30 percent of the men smoked at least twenty cigarettes daily, and in four other cohorts 15 percent or fewer were in that heavy smoking class. However, differences in the all-causes mortality or coronary death rate or the coronary incidence rates of the cohorts could not be shown to be related to any measure of the smoking habits of the cohorts—the proportion of the men who were nonsmokers, the proportion who were heavy smokers, the average cigarettes per day, and so on.

Various prospective studies on middle-aged men have found that cigarette smoking is an important risk factor for coronary heart disease. Accordingly, other things being equal, it would be expected that differences in the smoking habits of the cohorts would be reflected in the death or incidence rates of coronary heart disease. But other things were not equal in the several cohorts. They differed in the general level of blood pressure and cholesterol in the blood serum, and those two variables alone accounted for two-thirds of the variance in incidence rate of the cohorts. Only a third of the variance is left for all other variables, known or unknown, including smoking habits. Incidentally, in these sixteen cohorts smoking habits were not significantly related to the median values of blood pressure and serum cholesterol.

Besides the fact that the median blood pressures and cholesterol values preempted, so to speak, the major part of the variance in the incidence rates, it must be emphasized that the differences in smoking habits among the cohorts were not great. The cohort average for cigarettes smoked per day varied from 7.1 (Montegiorgio, Italy) to 14.8 (Tanushimaru, Japan). Omitting the Japanese cohorts, the highest average was 12.7 cigarettes daily in east Finland. The comparison, then, is like comparing light with moderate smokers, a comparison that, in studies comparing individuals, is not reported to show large contrasts in the incidence of death or coronary heart disease.

Within cohorts the picture is different. The ten-year experience of the American railroad men was the same for the men who had never smoked regularly and for those who had stopped. The incidence of death, all-causes or coronary, was roughly three times greater for men who smoked twenty or more cigarettes daily than for nonsmokers. In Finland and in the Netherlands the relationship between smoking habits and ten-year incidence was similar except that the former smokers had about twice the death rate of the men who had never smoked. In Yugoslavia, the death rate of heavy smokers was twice that of men who never smoked and clearly greater than the rates of the rest of the men, but ex-smokers did not differ significantly from men smoking up to 19 cigarettes daily. In Italy and Greece cigarette smoking could not be shown to be a very important risk factor for ten-year death, though the mortality of the heavy smokers was 34 percent higher than that of the men who had never smoked. In Japan the ten-year death rate was unrelated to smoking habits.

The ten-year incidence rate of coronary heart disease of the Americans with no evidence of cardiovascular disease at entry is unknown. The five-year experience showed no difference between never- and stopped-smokers, but there was a steady rise in incidence rate with the number of cigarettes smoked daily. In contrast, in all the European regions the ten-year incidence of the disease among heavy smokers was roughly double that of the rest of the men in the same cohorts, but there were no differences among men who had never smoked, who had stopped, or who were only light smokers at entry.

Both in northern and southern Europe the rate of death from cancer and other neoplasms tended to be a linear function of cigarette smoking. The northern Europeans were more prone than the southerners to die from cancer of the respiratory system, and that fact accounted for a significantly higher death rate from neoplastic disease in general in the north.

The indication of relatively little risk of smoking in the Japanese is puzzling, but the numbers are not large enough to rule out the possibility of a modestly excessive death rate of smokers in the Japanese population from which the two samples were drawn. It cannot be maintained that the smoking habits at entry were unrepresentative of earlier years or the ten years of follow-up of the Japanese. The answers to questions about smoking habits at entry indicated that in almost all the men the smoking habits had been much the same for many years, and in the follow-up questionnaires the answers were little changed.

These analyses of the relationships of smoking habits to ten-year incidence of death or disease take no account of the possibility that differences in the type of tobacco or its cure or in the manner of smoking are important. In southern Europe until recently only a small fraction of the cigarettes smoked were of the flue-cured Virginia type, different varieties of *Nicotiana tabacum* being dominant and sun curing the rule. Also, in southern Europe cigarettes are commonly smoked to a shorter length and are often allowed to stop burning to be relit from time to time. The latter custom is made possible by the absence of additives that keep the tobacco burning once it is lit. There are, it appears, important questions about the kind of tobacco, its cure, additives used, and the way the cigarettes are smoked that need careful study in connection with the long-time effects of smoking.

In the absence of good evidence that cigarette smoking independently promotes atherogenesis, it can be suggested that its importance in regard to death from coronary heart disease may be in its effect on myocardial irritability, an effect that could be fatal if the blood supply to the myocardium is severely compromised but relatively inconsequential in the absence of severe atherosclerosis.

Relative Body Weight and Fatness

An important direct relationship between relative body weight and the risk of early death has long been a popular view in America, a view seldom questioned in medical circles and vigorously championed by some insurance companies that produced almost the only evidence for such a relationship. Repeated demonstrations of serious defects in the insurance company material have been largely ignored. It is also commonly thought that the risk of developing coronary heart disease tends to be a direct function of relative body weight though no claim to that effect was made by the insurance company actuaries.

In the Seven Countries Study the entry data showed great differences among the cohorts in relative weight and in relative fatness, two correlated but by no means identical characteristics. In comparing the ten-year experience of the cohorts, no indication of increasing death rate with increasing frequency of overweight or obesity could be found. Except at Zutphen, the Netherlands, where no relationship of mortality was indicated, the tendency in all regions was for the death rate to decrease with increasing relative weight and fatness. Among the American railroad men, those in the upper half of the relative weight distribution had a ten-year death rate only 80 percent that of the other men, a disproportion that would be expected to occur by chance in only about 11 out of a 1,000 trials. In Croatia, Finland, Italy, Greece, Serbia, and Japan the decrease of mortality with increasing relative weight was even more pronounced.

More detailed examination of the relationship of mortality to relative body weight indicated that the data might be better fitted by a curve than a straight line. Accordingly, relative body weight and its square were used as two variables, together with age, systolic blood pressure, serum cholesterol, smoking habits, and the resting pulse rate, in the solution of the multiple logistic equation to discriminate men who died from those who did not. The results indicate that using the quadratic of the relative body weight produced a somewhat better fit, with the indication that the lowest mortality is for men slightly above average relative weight, the death rate increasing progressively for the lightest and the heaviest men. These findings agree very well with the long-time follow-up of men employed by the Peoples Gas Company, Chicago. While the results support the view that extreme overweight is a major hazard, they indicate that extreme underweight is even more dangerous. They do not support the view that men somewhat above the average weight for men of their height and age should be urged to reduce; such men, at least in middle age, tend to have a better prospect of avoiding early (ten-year) death than their fellows in the same population.

In regard to death from coronary heart disease, the picture is less clear. For the Americans, Finns, and Yugoslavs the ten-year coronary death rate showed no statistically significant relationship, linear or curvilinear, to relative body weight or fatness, although the lowest coronary death rates tended to be in the middle of the relative weight and fatness distributions. For the Italians and Greeks, the coronary death rate tended to increase with increasing relative weight and especially with body fatness. Among men free of evidence of cardiovascular disease at entry, 58 died from coronary heart disease in ten years, 37 being in the upper half of the relative weight distribution,

36 in the upper half of the body fatness distribution. The difference is significant by chi-square, but this takes no account of other variables.

The ten-year incidence of coronary heart disease, including all manifestations, showed no consistent relation with either relative weight or relative fatness though in most of the areas there was a trivial tendency for the incidence to be somewhat higher in the upper than in the lower halves of the distributions of relative weight and body fatness. This tendency disappeared when other variables were simultaneously considered in solutions of the multiple logistic equation.

A critical examination of data from other prospective studies failed to find any important disagreement with the conclusions from the present study. Except for men at the extreme upper end of the distribution, overweight is not an important risk factor for coronary heart disease nor for premature death.

Physical Activity

Proponents of the theory that physical activity helps prevent coronary heart disease took their clue from the death rates of men in the "social classes" as reported in British vital statistics. It was an easy step to emphasize the importance of occupational activity. Retrospective studies reported that London bus drivers were more apt to die from the disease than the more active conductors; the coronary death rate was higher for postal clerks than for letter carriers; stevedores were relatively protected as compared with their foremen; farmers had fewer heart attacks than the less active townsmen. Prospective data with details of predisease characteristics of men differing in physical activity have been scanty. The protocol of the Seven Countries Study included provisions to examine the question of the relationship of long-time physical activity to mortality and the incidence of coronary heart disease.

Thirteen of the cohorts in the Seven Countries Study included men in all occupations in the prescribed areas. At entry each man was asked about his habitual occupation and his physical activity. From the answers they were classified as: (1) sedentary or only engaged in light activity, (2) moderately active, meaning that their work required some nonstrenuous physical effort, and (3) heavy work much of the working week. No probing questions were asked about vigorous recreational exercise for the simple reason that middle-aged men in the areas under study almost never engaged, then or now, in what they would consider curious behavior.

The Belgrade professors were all essentially sedentary. The railroad men in the United States and in Italy were deliberately selected by character of their occupation to provide contrasts in habitual physical activity in a single industry where the occupation is unusually stable, all men enjoy good medical services, and none of the men suffer real economic privation. The American railroad men fell into two classes, relatively sedentary indoor workers and more active men working outdoors. The Italian railroad men provided a third class, maintenance-of-way men whose work demanded a good deal of physical effort.

In recent years propaganda to activate men in sedentary jobs in the United States and other highly developed countries has been increasingly pervasive, with much stress on the theory that nonoccupational vigorous exercise, especially of the anaerobic kind, will protect against heart attacks. In some countries many men, otherwise sedentary, are taking up tennis and jogging, but this vogue did not affect the men in any of the cohorts in this study up to the end of the ten-year follow-up. As for the idea that anaerobic exercise to the point of getting out of breath is protective, the data from the Seven Countries Study are not relevant. It is a rare emergency that provokes anaerobic work in any ordinary occupation, including bus conductors, letter carriers, and stevedores as well as the farmers, masons, loggers, and so on, in the Seven Countries Study.

Another point to be noted before summarizing the current findings regarding the activity variable is the fact that men differing in occupational activity are rarely fully comparable in other relevant respects. Multivariate analysis is usually required before arriving at a positive conclusion about any independent effect of physical activity.

Comparison of the cohorts in mortality and incidence indicated that their ten-year all-causes death rates were negatively related to the proportion of men in the cohorts who were sedentary—the larger the proportion of sedentary men, the lower the death rate. However, the statistical significance of that comparison depends on the very low death rate of the sedentary Belgrade professors. The rates of coronary death and the incidence of coronary heart disease were not related to the activity composition of the cohorts. All that can be concluded from these comparisons of the cohorts is that consideration of their activity characteristcs does not help to explain their differences in rates of disease incidence and death.

Analysis of the experience of the sedentary versus the more active American railroad men is facilitated by the fact that at entry the two classes did not differ in blood pressure or serum cholesterol and a trivial difference in age is taken care of by age-standardization of incidence rates. The ten-year death rate of the more active railroad men, compared with that of their sedentary colleagues, was 15 percent higher from coronary heart disease, 46 percent higher from all causes. But the difference in coronary death rate is not statistically significant, and most of the unfavorable all-causes mortality of the more active men is accounted for by an excess of deaths from violence.

In contrast, in the Italian railroad men, both all-causes and coronary death rates were inversely related to physical activity. Interpretation is complicated by some other differences among the activity groups, but multivariate analysis indicated that, independent of other variables, mortality decreased with increasing habitual activity.

The findings in rural Italy are in general agreement with those of the Italian railroad men. Although the rates of mortality and the incidence of coronary heart disease of moderately and very active men were not significantly different, the sedentary men were unduly prone to death and heart attacks. In Greece, too, the sedentary men had a higher all-causes death rate, but there was no difference between the moderately and very active men. For the incidence of coronary heart disease a similar trend was indicated, but the numbers are small and no statistically significant differences were found.

The results of the ten-year follow-up in Finland, Croatia, the Netherlands, Serbia, and Japan emphasize the inconsistency of relationships between physical activity and the incidence of death and disease. In Finland, where the number of cases of incidence was relatively large, the coronary incidence and death rates were higher in the moderately active men than in either their sedentary or very active compatriots. Finally, only a small proportion of the Finns were sedentary, but they had a greatly excessive rate of death from causes other than coronary heart disease.

At Zutphen, the Netherlands, the sedentary and moderately active men did not differ in either all-causes or coronary death rate. The very few (98) very active men had a remarkably low death rate but suffered the highest incidence of coronary heart disease. In Yugoslavia, neither all-causes nor coronary heart death rates were related to physical activity, but the sedentary men had the highest incidence of coronary heart disease. In Japan there were too few sedentary men to yield a useful rate for the incidence of coronary heart disease, but the very active men did not differ from their less active compatriots in all-causes death rate.

Some, but not all, of the inconsistencies in the seven countries data on physical activity as a variable related to subsequent disease and death might be charged to small numbers in some cohorts. What seems to be the most reasonable conclusion is that the habitual physical activity, or its lack, cannot be an independent, universal causative factor in promoting or protecting from early death or the development of coronary heart disease.

Resting Pulse Rate

The resting pulse rate, determined from measurements on the electrocardiograms of men without evidence of cardiovascular disease, was not related to age over the range 40–59 years, and had only small correlations with blood pressure, serum cholesterol, a slight negative correlation with the vital capacity, and no consistent relationship with smoking habit. The men most active physically had the lowest average pulse rates in all cohorts.

In comparisons of the cohorts, considering the 12,095 men without cardiovascular disease at entry, neither the ten-year mortality rate nor the incidence rate of coronary heart disease was related to the average resting pulse rate of the men at the entry examination.

Within each of the areas, however, the ten-year death rate was linearly related with the entry pulse rate, and this was indicated both for all-causes and for coronary deaths. However, the total incidence of coronary heart disease among men free of cardiovascular disease at entry was much less closely related to the pulse rate. In none of the cohorts was there any indication of a critical pulse rate; the relation to future incidence appeared to be linear, at least over 90 percent of the distribution of pulse rates.

Respiratory Function

At the entry examinations the vital capacity was measured in ten of the cohorts, and the timed (¾ second) forced expiratory volume (FEV ¾) was also measured in eight of them. In all cohorts both measures of respiratory function were closely related to height and, inversely, to age. In all analyses the respiratory function per unit height was used. In comparisons among cohorts the regression of the respiratory function on age found for each cohort was used to adjust to mean age 50. The same adjustment was made in comparing the values for respiratory function of the men in different classes according to their ten-year experience.

Comparison of the cohorts in regard to their mean vital capacity and ten-year incidence rate was unrewarding; vital capacity did not help explain the differences in incidence rates. The apparatus and technique of measurement could have contributed to that negative finding because exact comparability among cohorts in those respects could not be guaranteed. Within each cohort, instruments and technique were constant.

In every cohort the all-causes ten-year death rate of men free of cardiovascular disease at entry increased with decreasing vital capacity. In the United States and in rural Italy, but not in the other cohorts, the mortality from coronary heart disease was also significantly related to the vital capacity. The ten-year incidence rate of coronary heart disease (all diagnoses) was not significantly related to the vital capacity in any of the nine cohorts with available data. In the American railroad men, where five-year but not ten-year data were available for all coronary heart diagnoses, the incidence of the disease tended to increase with decreasing vital capacity, but the trend was not statistically significant.

The corresponding analyses using the FEV ¾ as the measure of respiratory function gave similar results plus the indication that the timed forced expiratory volume may be a better discriminator than the simple vital capacity in indicating the risk of early death. In multiple logistic analyses, comparison of the solutions using the vital capacity versus those using the FEV ¾, all other variables in the equations being the same, the t values for the discrimination of ten-year deaths were larger with FEV ¾ than with the vital capacity.

Respiratory function tended to be reduced in the heaviest smokers (twenty or more cigarettes every day) but had little or no relation to smoking habits in the rest of the men in any of the cohorts. Smoking habits were allowed for in the analyses, summarized above, of relationships of respiratory function to the incidence of disease and death.

Respiratory function has received relatively little attention in prospective studies concerned with the coronary problem. The subject merits more, and more critical, attention.

Diet

One of the considerations in selecting the areas for inclusion in the Seven Countries Study was the desire to have cohorts differing in their habitual diets. Early in the planning of the approach to getting data on the dietary variables it was agreed that resources were lacking to attempt to characterize accurately the individual men in regard to their diets. However, in populations where dietary habits are relatively homogeneous, it should be possible to characterize their diets by the averages from random samples of men whose diets could be studied in careful detail, with checks on the chemical composition by chemical analysis. The suitability of the method adopted, based on these considerations, was demonstrated in the experience in repeated seven-day surveys on the same individuals in most of the cohorts.

The averages for the men in the dietary subsamples were reasonably stable in repetitions, but the placement of the individual men in the arrays for the several dietary variables was not. The intraindividual variance was of the same order as the interindividual variance, so it was not possible to classify the individual men reliably even into broad classes as high, medium, or low in calories from saturated fatty acids, and so on. But the stability of the subsample averages encouraged the belief that they should be reasonably representative of the averages for the habitual diets of the cohorts. Evidence of the utility of those estimated cohort averages came from two tests.

First, the estimated mean percentages of calories from saturated and polyunsaturated fatty acids in the diets of the cohorts were used to calculate mean serum cholesterol concentrations, using the multiple regression equation summarizing data from very many controlled dietary experiments on men in metabolic units. The coefficient of correlation between observed and calculated cholesterol values for the sixteen cohorts is $r = 0.9$. The difference between the average observed values and those calculated only from the saturated and polyunsaturated fat calories, 12.7 mg/dl, corresponds with a reasonable estimate of the dietary preformed cholesterol, which was not chemically measured and therefore not included in the calculations.

The second test of the estimates of the average diets of the cohorts is the comparison of the dietary figures with the ten-year experience. The correlation of the ten-year coronary death rate of the cohorts with the estimate of percentage of calories from total fat in the diets is $r = 0.50$, but the correlation with the percentage of calories from saturated fats is $r = 0.84$. With the ten-year incidence rate of coronary heart disease, accepting all manifestations of the disease, the correlation with total fat colaries is only 0.39 but with saturated fat calories the result is $r = 0.73$.

The incidence rate of coronary heart disease was also significantly related to the average percentage of calories from sucrose in the diet, but this was accounted for by the high correlation between sucrose and saturated fat in the diets. Partial correlation analysis showed that with saturated fat constant, coronary heart disease incidence was not significantly related to the amount of sucrose in the diet.

The percentage of calories provided from total proteins in the diet was not related to ten-year incidence rate, but this negative result would be expected in view of the small variation among the cohorts in the total protein percentage of diet calories. Incidence was significantly related to the percentage of dietary calories from animal proteins but that would be expected from the correlation of animal protein with saturated fatty acids and with dietary cholesterol.

Dietary fiber, currently of much interest, was not directly estimated in the dietary surveys. However, most of the original raw data on amounts and kinds of foods eaten are still preserved in the several area headquarters, in the original languages, and efforts are under way to make estimates of fiber in the diets. It may be remarked, at this time, that the common diets of the United States and northern Europe are generally much lower in fiber than the habitual diets in Italy, Greece, Yugoslavia, and Japan.

Two recent publications call for a note on the interpretation of surveys on the diets of individuals. We have repeatedly found that a dietary survey on men in an ethnically homogeneous population does not allow a valid classification of the individual men in regard to their habitual intake of specific nutrients such as the several kinds of fatty acids. Other surveys indicate that this is the rule; where high reliability for data on individuals are claimed, the repetitions involve the same dietitians who were fully aware, in the repetition, of the answers given in the first survey. At Framingham, a repetition of the survey by another dietitian gave values for fatty acids having little correlation with the first survey. Now reports from Chicago and Minneapolis have set forth the statistical theory. In ethnically homogeneous populations, such as industrial employees in Chicago, Minneapolis business men, residents of Framingham, rural folk in Italy, many repeated surveys, of the order of seven or more, on the same individuals would be required to allow satisfactory classification in their intakes of nutrients.

Critics of the diet-cholesterol-atherogenesis theory have pointed to the lack of correlation between serum cholesterol values of individual men with their answers to questions about their diets. Long ago we pointed out that this must be expected where intraindividual variability is of the same order of magnitude as the interindividual variability, a common situation in our experience.

Mathematical Models and Multivariate Analyses

Responsible students of the coronary problem long ago abandoned the idea of seeking *the* cause of the disease, agreeing that several, perhaps many, variables are involved in almost all cases. The demonstration in prospective studies that the risk of heart attack in a few years increases with the blood pressure, the concentration of cholesterol in the blood serum, and cigarette smoking raised some questions still unresolved.

For each of these so-called risk factors, what is the character of the risk variable relationship to the development of the disease? The first tendency, following the ancient tradition of medicine to put things into two classes, good or bad, was to look for cutting points, critical values, that would separate hyper- from normo-. But it was apparent that the risk factors are continuous, quantitative variables that should be related quantitatively to the risk. So it was natural to ask for a formula to relate the amount of risk to the amount of the risk factor. The obvious first suggestion is a linear regression in the form $y = a + bx$, where y is the risk of heart attack or other end point and x is the value of a variable such as the blood pressure. With suitable follow-up data the values of the constant a and the coefficient b are found which best relate y to x in *this linear model*. Other models, parabolic, exponential, quadratic, and so on, might fit better, but their exploration is only beginning to attract interest.

Since it is agreed that a number of risk factors are involved and at least some are interrelated, the question is how to put the risk factors together to pool their contribution to the total risk. The first answer is simply to extend the regression idea to the multiple regression equation: $y = a + b_1 x_1 + b_2 x_2$ . . . to cover any number of x variables, blood pressure, serum cholesterol, smoking habit, and so on. Here each of the variables is assumed to make a contribution to the risk in proportion to the size of the variable multiplied by its coefficient, and all of those contributions are simply added together. Or the more elaborate multiple logistic equation may be favored, but this too simply adds the estimated contributions of each variable, contributions which are taken to be linearly related to the size of the variable.

Here again the simple linear model may not most effectively take account of the several influences that promote the disease, but so far little exploration has been done with other models or with various transformations of the variables in the multivariate equations. In Chicago and in the Seven Countries Study, both the relative body weight (body mass index) and its square were used together with other variables in the multiple logistic equation in the attempt to discriminate men who later died from those who did not. With both sets of data the result was to indicate that the risk of death is curvilinearly related to the body mass index, the least risk of early death being that of the men in the upper middle part of the distribution of body mass index. The implications are far-reaching, of course.

Still, even in their simplest forms the multiple regression and the logistic equations greatly help to discriminate between persons who later do or do not develop the clinical disease, with no demonstrated difference between the two equations in discriminating power. As commonly tested, this discrimination is descriptive, not a test of prediction. But if the study has been made on a fair sample of a population, it is reasonable to propose that the results allow useful predictions for other unbiased samples from the same or similar populations. This proposition has been tested successfully in predicting the outcome for patients surviving myocardial infarction in one part of the United States from the multiple logistic solution of the findings in another part of the country. More specific for the present interest, the multiple logistic solution from the American railroad men in the Seven Countries Study well predicted the outcome of men similarly studied at Framingham and at Chicago. But these examples of successful cross-prediction concern samples of men from the same general population of Americans.

One of the purposes of the Seven Countries Study was to see the result of the application of these multivariate methods to different populations.

Within populations, the solution of the multiple logistic equation was similarly successful in discriminating between men who later became coronary victims and those who did not. And the same variables were important in the various populations—age, blood pressure, serum cholesterol, cigarette smoking habit. The next test, the attempt to predict the outcome in one population from the results in another, produced interesting results.

The application to the entry data of the multiple logistic coefficients obtained by solving the equation with data from the southern Europeans well classified the northern Europeans in regard to their relative risks of developing coronary heart disease. The Finns and Dutch rated most at risk from application of the southern European coefficients to their entry characteristics proved, indeed, to be the men with the highest incidence rate in their cohorts. It may be helpful to explain the procedure of calculation.

The solution of the multiple logistic equation makes it possible to estimate the probability of coronary death, or whatever end point was used in the solution, of an individual in the population represented by the sample tested, from his values for the independent variables in the equation, his age, blood pressure, serum cholesterol, and so on. If the application of the coefficients in the equation to his values yield a probability of $p = 0.03$, it is estimated that he has 3 out of 100 chances of dying in the time span covered by the test equation. For 100 men all with values of $p = 0.05$, the estimate is that 5 of them will die from the disease within the specified time.

When all the individuals in the test are arrayed in order of their estimated probabilities of coronary death, those in the bottom 10 percent, in the bottom decile, of the distribution, and so on, then the sum of the values of p for the men in each decile gives an estimate of how many of the men will die in each decile class. The accuracy of the discrimination achieved is measured by the correspondence of those estimated numbers with the actual numbers of deaths within each decile class.

Test was made of the application of the multiple logistic solution for the ten-year experience of southern Europeans to the entry data of the northern Europeans. The number of coronary deaths predicted in each of the decile classes of probability was compared with the number actually observed; the coefficient of correlation was $r = 0.95$; the prediction of *relative* risk was excellent. Absolute risk is another matter. In this test the sum of the probabilities for all of these northern Europeans was 35.9, meaning that the southern Italian experience would predict 35.9 deaths among the northern Europeans. But actually 91 deaths were observed. The reverse test, predicting coronary death among the southern Europeans from the northern European experience, greatly overestimated the deaths in southern Europe.

Cross predictions for northern Europeans from American logistic solutions, and vice versa, well classified the men in relative risk and also gave reasonably good estimates of the total coronary deaths.

What does all this mean? One possibility is that there are factors, as yet unknown, that increase the risk of Americans, Finns, and Dutch or help protect the southern Europeans. In that case the unknown factors must be substantially independent of the risk factors so far identified. Another possibility is that the long-time characteristics of the southern and northern Europeans were differently represented in the entry examinations in the two areas. In any case, it seems that the risk factors so far studied have universal importance, but not necessarily the same quantitative effect in all populations. It is also clear that it is not justifiable to estimate absolute risk in various populations from multivariate relationships observed in other populations.

Changes over Time

A major premise of prospective studies that seek to learn about relationships between predisease characteristics and the development of disease is that those characteristics recorded at the start of the follow-up are descriptive of the subjects at more than just the moment of the entrance examination. But, apart from measurement error, many items of measurement show substantial intraindividual variation, even over short periods of time, so the recorded characteristics at the start of follow-up are imperfect indications of the average or most representative features of the individuals. Measurements on the same individuals repeated over a few weeks indicate average intraindividual standard deviations up to 10 percent or more in such items as blood pressure, serum cholesterol concentration, and other physiological and biochemical variables. True relationships between predisease characteristics and the subsequent development of disease will be blurred to the degree that the recorded characteristics fail to be truly representative of the individuals. For this reason, a relationship found in the eventual analysis will usually be an underestimate of the true relationship.

More troublesome is the fact that people change over the years, even while they are still apparently healthy. Their smoking habits, diets, use of drugs or alcohol, the level of physical activity change, so over the years of follow-up their characteristics may depart importantly from those recorded at the start. The Seven Countries Study provides some examples.

Some changes observed at the five-year and ten-year reexaminations may be considered normal responses to aging. A moderate rise in systolic but not in diastolic blood pressure and a decrease in vital capacity are in that category and should not complicate analyses of the relationships between entry characteristics and the incidence of disease and death. But in the Seven

Countries Study some changes were observed that cannot be explained in that way nor ascribed to changes in the state of health.

In the European cohorts, a progressive average gain in weight was recorded averaging 2.9 kg in ten years, a change contrary to the expectation of a small decrease as the effect of aging observed in cross-sectional comparisons. That small change in weight in itself would not be expected to have any significant effect on the likelihood of disease or early death, but there are indications that there was not only a little change in energy balance but also a more important change in the character of the diet.

The most interesting fact is that there were substantial changes in the serum cholesterol concentration, particularly in the cohorts in southern Europe where the same individuals showed average increases of ten percent or more when no change or a decrease would be expected simply as a result of middle-aged men getting ten years older. And it is in those areas, Italy, Greece, and Yugoslavia, where the general population is progressively consuming more meat and dairy products than at the start of the Seven Countries Study. Vital statistics of those countries report an important increase in the age-specific rate of death from coronary heart disease. It is possible, of course, that the reported increases in coronary deaths reflect increasing awareness of the coronary problem and changing diagnostic custom of the local physicians. But the parallels in the changes in food consumption, in serum cholesterol concentration, and in death rates in the vital statistics are cause for thought.

Characteristics of the Subjects before the Study

The average values for cholesterol in the blood serum of the southern Europeans rose progressively in the ten years of follow-up, so it is pertinent to wonder about the years before the entry examinations. There is much reason to believe that the cholesterol averages in that area were substantially lower. There is no doubt that the average diets were lower in meats and dairy products. The Italian statistics, which may be typical for the whole region, indicate that the per capita consumption of meats in the early 1960s was double that of ten years earlier. Serum cholesterol data from explorations in Italy in the early and middle years of the 1950s indicate averages for middle-aged men in the working class around 170 mg/dl instead of the average of 200 mg/dl or a little more at the entry examinations in this study. It is interesting to calculate what such a difference might mean for the incidence of coronary heart disease.

Taking the average values of the rural Italians recorded at entry for age, systolic blood pressure, serum cholesterol, cigarette smoking, and physical activity, the probability of ten-year coronary death can be estimated with the coefficients obtained from the solution of the multiple logistic equation for the experience of the American railroad men. The result is $p = 0.0190$. With all other variables the same but cholesterol of 170 mg/dl the estimate is only $p = 0.0142$. Making the same calculations using the coefficients from the solution for the experience in Finland, the result is similar; with cholesterol of 170 mg/dl the probability of coronary death is about three-fourths that with cholesterol of 200 mg/dl.

Although these calculations are speculative, they do point to the likelihood that some part of the discrepancy between the incidence of coronary heart disease observed in the southern Europeans and that expected from the American and northern European experience could reflect lower serum cholesterol values in the years before the entry examinations. This is an example of the problems faced by the epidemiologist in a changing world.

Omissions

Students of the epidemiology of cardiovascular disease will point to omissions in the Seven Countries Study, the characteristics of the men not recorded at the examinations, variables suggested to be risk factors for coronary heart disease that were not examined. We are well aware of these shortcomings and regret them. For the most part, the variables we now wish we could report were fully in mind when the work was in the planning stage and protocols were being drafted; financial limitations caused their omission.

In the list of variables to be considered for inclusion in the ultimate protocol, the first to be eliminated were roentgenograms of the chest and lipoprotein fractionation of the blood serum. Both items would have been too costly to be included in the standard examinations but, in several cohorts chest roentgenograms were made on local initiative. The resulting films have not been provided to our central headquarters nor, to our knowledge, have they been locally used for other than detection of conditions for referral to local physicians.

Lipoprotein fractionation was omitted not only because of expense and difficulty in doing such work in the remote locations of the villages but also because previous trials of such measurements suggested that relevance to the coronary problem would not justify the effort. Paper electrophoresis of serum followed by cholesterol measurement of the separated alpha and beta lipoproteins (Anderson and Keys 1956) was applied in 1956 surveys on middle-aged men in Hawaii and Japan (Keys et al. 1958) and in Finland (Keys, Karvonen, and Fidanza 1958). The Finns and Japanese differed greatly in beta lipoprotein cholesterol but very little in the alpha cholesterol, a finding suggesting that the alpha fraction is not important in the epidemiology of coronary heart disease. Now, in view of the recent interest in high-density lipoprotein in the plasma, we regret that lipoprotein separation was not attempted in the Seven Countries Study.

Financial limitations also ruled against inclusion of glucose tolerance tests and serum uric acid measurement in the standard protocol. Another argument against glucose tolerance tests was the insistence of advisers in the villages that the response rate to participate in the study would be much reduced if we insisted on the subjects remaining an extra hour or two at the examination place to be subjected to another venepuncture.

Where We Stand in 1979

A list of things not done is the negative side of the picture; the positive accomplishment is measured in terms of new knowledge and insight gained. Before the start of the program we felt confident that we would find differences in the incidence of coronary heart disease among the populations sampled, but the fact remained to be proved. In the outcome, the ten-year experience did show important differences. In the meantime, other workers were confirming population differences in the incidence of the disease in Puerto Rico, Hawaii, Japan, and Massachusetts.

The differences found in the Seven Countries Study were partly explained by differences in the blood pressure, serum cholesterol, and the typical diets of the cohorts. The differences in incidence rates among the cohorts could not be shown to be related to the characteristics of the cohorts in relative body weight, smoking habits, or physical activity, a fact that may be disappointing to some workers, but it is a gain to recognize that the relationships are more complex than previously supposed.

Our ten-year findings, and concordance with other studies, make it clear that the big three risk factors for coronary heart disease now established are age, blood pressure, and serum cholesterol. The findings about cigarette smoking as a risk factor indicate that here, too, relationships are not as simple as first supposed. The same may be said about habitual physical activity; the inconsistencies among cohorts about this characteristic as a risk factor indicate simply that it is not independently and universally important.

Critics of attention to the epidemiology of coronary heart disease have long suggested that a low incidence of that disease involves a trade-off for other and less acceptable causes of death. That specter is now laid to rest by the demonstration that the incidence rate of death from coronary heart disease is unrelated to the rate of death from other causes, at least in relatively developed populations.

Relative overweight was the first characteristic proposed as what we now call risk factors. The opinion of some insurance company actuaries is still accepted almost without question by most members of the health professions as well as the general public, although the defects and deficiencies of the evidence have been repeatedly pointed out. It is now clear that the facts are quite different, at least for middle-aged men, from the common belief. Gross obesity is bad, but worse is a corresponding degree of underweight; men near or slightly above the average relative body weight have the best prospect of avoiding premature death. The question of the relation of body fatness and relative body weight to the prospect for health needs complete reexamination with better samples and measurements and more sophisticated analyses than used by the actuaries in the past.

The use of multivariate methods in the discrimination between cases and noncases in different populations, and the application of the results to cross predictions between populations show the strengths and the weaknesses of our present knowledge on risk factors for coronary heart disease. The findings in one population are satisfactory for classifying the individuals in other populations in regard to relative risk but absolute risk is another matter. The major risk factors identified so far seem to have universal importance, at least in Europe and America, but their weight may differ among populations. Compared with the experience in the United States, the southern Europeans suffer much less from coronary heart disease than would be expected from their characteristics of age, blood pressure, serum cholesterol, smoking habits, and physical activity.

The Future

The epidemiological approach to the problem of coronary heart disease, initiated barely thirty years ago, has now amply demonstrated great power in finding relationships, unearthing clues to etiology, and suggesting preventive measures. But many of the relationships are proving to be more complex than first proposed.

There is much interest in applying what is known and seems to be prudent in preventive trials, preventive practice, and guidelines to the general public. Irrespective of such public health advice, it is clear that many people are already changing their habits of diet, smoking, and exercise on their own accord.

The period of epidemiological exploration of these matters is not over, and there is still much to be learned from the study of experiments of nature. The need for more and better epidemiological studies has never been more obvious. Until now, all prospective studies, including the Seven Countries Study, have dealt with too few persons; the standard errors of the means and rates are too large. The instability of lifestyle in many populations greatly complicates the collection of representative data and their analysis, but perhaps the instability itself should be included in the analysis as a risk factor. Moreover, the almost universal assumption that risk is a linear function of the characteristics of interest must give way to less restrictive ideas and mathematical models. Finally, besides our great concern about the incidence of coronary heart disease, new epidemiological programs should be more broadly concerned with all disease and death.

Appendix

Table A.1. Distribution of men in characteristics measured at entry (shown by the decile cutting points below which were 10 to 90 percent of the men).

Age	N	\multicolumn{9}{c}{Decile}
		1	2	3	4	5	6	7	8	9

U.S. RAILROAD

Age	N	1	2	3	4	5	6	7	8	9
\multicolumn{11}{c}{Height (cm)}
40–44	525	167	170	173	174	175	177	178	180	182
45–49	501	167	170	173	174	174	176	177	180	181
50–54	502	166	169	172	173	174	174	177	179	180
55–59	569	165	168	171	172	173	174	176	178	179
\multicolumn{11}{c}{Relative body weight (%)}
40–44	525	87	93	97	102	104	108	111	114	120
45–49	501	86	94	97	101	103	107	110	116	120
50–54	502	87	93	96	100	103	107	110	115	121
55–59	569	86	91	96	101	103	106	109	114	120
\multicolumn{11}{c}{Sum of skinfolds (mm)}
40–44	525	16	21	25	29	33	35	39	43	47
45–49	501	18	23	25	28	32	36	38	43	46
50–54	501	21	23	26	29	33	36	39	42	48
55–59	570	20	23	26	30	32	35	37	44	49
\multicolumn{11}{c}{Systolic blood pressure (mm Hg)}
40–44	526	115	120	125	127	130	136	140	146	158
45–49	501	116	123	127	130	134	140	147	160	162
50–54	503	116	124	129	138	137	143	150	161	170
55–59	571	118	127	130	135	140	149	157	163	175

Table A.1. (continued)

| Age | N | \multicolumn{9}{c}{Decile} |
		1	2	3	4	5	6	7	8	9
\multicolumn{11}{c}{Diastolic blood pressure (5th phase, mm Hg)}
40–44	526	70	75	79	80	83	87	89	94	99
45–49	501	70	78	81	83	84	86	92	94	100
50–54	503	71	77	82	84	84	90	92	98	100
55–59	571	72	81	83	85	86	89	93	98	105
\multicolumn{11}{c}{Serum cholesterol (mg per 100 ml)}
40–44	517	182	197	211	213	234	245	258	276	298
45–49	496	183	196	215	218	234	250	258	280	296
50–54	498	186	209	216	219	236	250	268	278	296
55–59	565	190	207	220	222	244	259	270	281	297

DALMATIA, YUGOSLAVIA

Age	N	1	2	3	4	5	6	7	8	9
\multicolumn{11}{c}{Height (cm)}
40–44	85	166	169	171	173	175	176	178	179	182
45–49	183	166	168	170	171	173	174	176	178	182
50–54	211	165	169	170	172	173	175	177	179	182
55–59	190	165	166	169	170	172	174	175	177	180
\multicolumn{11}{c}{Relative body weight (%)}
40–44	86	82	84	86	90	94	98	102	103	108
45–49	184	80	85	88	90	93	95	98	104	111
50–54	212	78	83	85	87	90	92	96	100	107
55–59	189	77	79	82	85	88	91	97	103	111
\multicolumn{11}{c}{Sum of skinfolds (mm)}
40–44	85	10	11	12	13	15	17	21	24	34
45–49	184	10	10	12	13	15	17	20	25	31
50–54	212	9	10	11	12	14	16	18	23	28
55–59	189	9	10	10	11	13	15	17	24	32
\multicolumn{11}{c}{Systolic blood pressure (mm Hg)}
40–44	84	115	126	130	131	136	140	141	147	160
45–49	184	120	121	125	130	135	138	140	150	164
50–54	212	120	122	130	131	137	140	145	155	165
55–59	192	120	124	130	130	135	140	150	152	165
\multicolumn{11}{c}{Diastolic blood pressure (5th phase, mm Hg)}
40–44	84	70	70	76	80	85	89	90	92	95
45–49	184	70	70	75	79	80	82	88	92	96

		Decile								
Age	N	1	2	3	4	5	6	7	8	9
50–54	212	70	70	75	79	82	85	90	92	98
55–59	192	70	74	77	80	82	85	88	92	99
Serum cholesterol (mg per 100 ml)										
40–44	84	146	155	163	176	182	200	214	227	251
45–49	181	141	156	168	176	185	198	208	220	237
50–54	211	136	155	166	174	186	198	208	225	241
55–59	190	142	152	164	177	188	198	208	222	246

SLAVONIA, YUGOSLAVIA

		Decile								
Age	N	1	2	3	4	5	6	7	8	9
Height (cm)										
40–44	102	161	164	166	168	170	172	173	175	178
45–49	182	162	163	165	166	168	169	170	173	175
50–54	197	159	161	163	165	166	168	170	172	175
55–59	216	161	163	165	166	168	169	171	173	176
Relative body weight (%)										
40–44	102	81	85	88	93	95	100	103	106	112
45–49	181	80	84	88	91	94	97	103	107	120
50–54	197	77	81	83	86	88	92	98	103	114
55–59	215	77	80	84	88	91	93	98	104	111
Sum of skinfolds (mm)										
40–44	102	10	10	12	13	15	18	20	23	28
45–49	181	9	10	11	13	15	17	22	26	33
50–54	197	9	10	10	12	13	14	16	22	31
55–59	215	9	10	11	12	14	15	17	22	27
Systolic blood pressure (mm Hg)										
40–44	102	111	120	125	130	130	135	140	146	165
45–49	180	116	120	125	130	130	137	140	151	163
50–54	197	115	120	128	130	131	139	144	152	161
55–59	216	115	123	130	138	140	146	152	162	171
Diastolic blood pressure (5th phase, mm Hg)										
40–44	102	68	70	75	78	79	80	85	90	97
45–49	180	69	72	77	78	80	85	89	90	100
50–54	197	68	70	76	78	80	82	86	89	96
55–59	216	68	72	78	80	84	86	90	95	100
Serum cholesterol (mg per 100 ml)										
40–44	95	149	162	178	186	196	210	217	232	249
45–49	176	147	159	177	186	197	207	218	237	255
50–54	192	152	164	176	186	200	206	217	232	260
55–59	213	146	162	174	182	194	202	220	234	256

Table A.1. (continued)

| | | \multicolumn{9}{c|}{Decile} |
Age	N	1	2	3	4	5	6	7	8	9
TANUSHIMARU, JAPAN										
					Height (cm)					
40–44	112	155	157	159	160	162	163	164	165	167
45–49	117	154	156	158	160	161	162	164	165	168
50–54	137	153	155	157	158	159	161	163	165	167
55–59	143	152	154	156	159	160	161	162	163	165
					Relative body weight (%)					
40–44	111	80	82	85	87	89	91	94	95	98
45–49	116	77	79	82	84	86	88	90	93	100
50–54	137	75	79	80	82	84	87	90	93	100
55–59	143	75	79	81	82	84	86	89	92	99
					Sum of skinfolds (mm)					
40–44	110	11	12	12	14	15	16	18	22	23
45–49	113	10	12	13	14	15	17	18	21	24
50–54	136	10	11	12	14	14	16	17	21	26
55–59	140	11	12	12	13	15	16	18	21	26
					Systolic blood pressure (mm Hg)					
40–44	112	102	110	112	117	120	124	132	138	145
45–49	117	108	114	118	120	128	132	136	142	152
50–54	137	110	114	120	125	132	137	140	146	160
55–59	143	112	120	124	132	138	148	156	166	183
					Diastolic blood pressure (5th phase, mm Hg)					
40–44	112	51	58	62	64	68	70	74	78	83
45–49	117	58	62	68	70	70	74	78	84	90
50–54	137	60	64	68	70	72	75	80	82	90
55–59	143	60	64	70	71	78	80	88	92	100
					Serum cholesterol (mg per 100 ml)					
40–44	109	109	140	147	157	167	183	212	237	277
45–49	111	111	131	147	155	165	185	198	220	259
50–54	132	114	133	149	164	178	187	216	231	266
55–59	139	116	134	144	155	168	183	205	225	257
EAST FINLAND										
					Height (cm)					
40–44	207	161	164	165	167	168	170	172	174	177
45–49	234	161	163	165	166	168	169	171	173	177

		Decile								
Age	N	1	2	3	4	5	6	7	8	9
50–54	196	160	163	165	167	168	170	171	172	174
55–59	168	159	162	163	165	167	169	170	172	175
Relative body weight (%)										
40–44	205	83	86	90	92	94	97	101	104	110
45–49	230	82	86	89	92	94	98	102	106	110
50–54	194	79	83	86	89	93	95	99	105	111
55–59	168	78	82	85	89	90	93	96	101	110
Sum of skinfolds (mm)										
40–44	207	10	11	12	13	13	15	18	22	28
45–49	239	10	11	12	13	15	18	20	25	31
50–54	197	9	11	11	13	14	17	21	24	30
55–59	172	8	10	11	12	14	16	18	22	32
Systolic blood pressure (mm Hg)										
40–44	206	124	130	135	138	141	145	150	154	164
45–49	235	125	130	134	138	140	145	150	160	173
50–54	197	130	135	139	143	149	154	158	169	179
55–59	171	130	139	144	148	153	160	166	174	184
Diastolic blood pressure (5th phase, mm Hg)										
40–44	206	75	80	80	85	87	90	90	95	100
45–49	235	78	80	82	85	88	90	92	98	102
50–54	197	77	80	85	88	90	92	96	100	104
55–59	170	78	81	86	90	90	94	98	100	107
Serum cholesterol (mg per 100 ml)										
40–44	207	193	220	232	248	265	276	288	302	328
45–49	239	208	222	239	259	272	284	295	313	335
50–54	196	208	220	238	251	262	280	302	315	340
55–59	172	190	211	231	245	259	268	280	292	317

WEST FINLAND

		Decile								
		1	2	3	4	5	6	7	8	9
Height (cm)										
40–44	166	164	168	169	171	173	174	175	177	180
45–49	221	164	167	168	170	171	173	174	176	178
50–54	240	163	167	168	170	172	173	174	176	178
55–59	220	162	165	167	169	170	171	173	175	178
Relative body weight (%)										
40–44	164	86	90	93	95	98	101	104	107	115
45–49	216	82	86	90	94	96	100	105	109	115
50–54	238	82	85	89	92	97	101	104	109	115
55–59	217	80	85	88	92	95	98	101	105	114

350 | Appendix

Table A.1. (continued)

| Age | N | \multicolumn{9}{c}{Decile} |
		1	2	3	4	5	6	7	8	9
\multicolumn{11}{c}{Sum of skinfolds (mm)}
40–44	168	11	12	13	15	16	19	21	25	32
45–49	224	11	12	13	15	16	19	21	26	32
50–54	245	11	12	13	15	16	19	23	27	35
55–59	222	10	11	12	14	16	19	21	24	31
\multicolumn{11}{c}{Systolic blood pressure (mm Hg)}
40–44	168	112	120	125	130	133	136	141	147	159
45–49	224	119	122	126	130	135	139	142	148	156
50–54	245	118	124	130	134	139	143	146	152	165
55–59	222	121	129	132	139	143	150	155	164	177
\multicolumn{11}{c}{Diastolic blood pressure (5th phase, mm Hg)}
40–44	168	67	70	74	78	80	80	83	86	92
45–49	224	70	74	77	78	80	81	85	88	92
50–54	245	70	73	78	80	82	84	88	90	100
55–59	222	72	76	78	80	82	86	89	90	97
\multicolumn{11}{c}{Serum cholesterol (mg per 100 ml)}
40–44	168	201	216	227	238	248	260	278	293	314
45–49	223	201	216	228	242	255	267	277	300	319
50–54	244	197	214	231	245	257	277	284	306	323
55–59	222	195	216	228	238	251	258	269	282	305

USHIBUKA, JAPAN

Age	N	1	2	3	4	5	6	7	8	9
\multicolumn{11}{c}{Height (cm)}
40–44	107	153	156	157	159	160	161	162	165	167
45–49	114	153	156	157	159	160	162	163	165	167
50–54	129	151	154	156	157	158	160	161	163	165
55–59	107	150	153	156	157	159	160	162	165	168
\multicolumn{11}{c}{Relative body weight (%)}
40–44	107	77	82	85	88	91	93	96	99	102
45–49	114	78	81	84	87	89	91	93	96	101
50–54	129	77	80	82	85	87	88	90	92	97
55–59	107	72	77	80	82	84	86	88	92	96

Sum of skinfolds (data not available)

| | | \multicolumn{9}{c}{Decile} |
Age	N	1	2	3	4	5	6	7	8	9
\multicolumn{11}{c}{Systolic blood pressure (mm Hg)}
40–44	115	110	114	120	120	126	132	135	140	152
45–49	128	107	114	120	120	128	135	145	155	165
50–54	139	112	118	125	130	135	140	150	156	176
55–59	118	114	120	128	135	140	144	154	165	181
\multicolumn{11}{c}{Diastolic blood pressure (5th phase, mm Hg)}
40–44	115	60	66	70	72	75	78	80	82	90
45–49	128	64	68	70	74	76	80	80	90	97
50–54	139	65	70	72	75	80	80	84	87	96
55–59	118	67	70	74	77	80	84	86	90	96
\multicolumn{11}{c}{Serum cholesterol (mg per 100 ml)}
40–44	112	99	134	142	150	162	170	175	184	201
45–49	127	101	134	144	153	163	173	178	189	202
50–54	136	104	134	142	152	157	16–	178	188	204
55–59	118	116	136	146	154	164	172	181	191	204

CREVALCORE, ITALY

Age	N	1	2	3	4	5	6	7	8	9
\multicolumn{11}{c}{Height (cm)}
40–44	174	161	163	166	167	169	171	173	174	176
45–49	303	160	162	165	167	168	169	170	172	175
50–54	291	160	162	165	166	168	170	171	173	176
55–59	219	158	161	163	165	167	168	170	173	175
\multicolumn{11}{c}{Relative body weight (%)}
40–44	175	88	92	96	101	105	110	114	120	128
45–49	300	86	91	96	100	103	107	111	116	124
50–54	288	87	91	96	99	102	105	110	114	122
55–59	216	86	90	94	98	101	104	112	118	125
\multicolumn{11}{c}{Sum of skinfolds (mm)}
40–44	176	12	14	17	21	23	26	29	32	40
45–49	303	11	14	17	18	21	26	30	34	38
50–54	294	12	15	18	20	22	25	28	32	37
55–59	218	12	14	17	20	22	25	30	36	41
\multicolumn{11}{c}{Systolic blood pressure (mm Hg)}
40–44	175	120	125	130	132	136	140	146	154	161
45–49	299	120	130	133	138	142	147	150	157	169
50–54	290	127	132	138	141	147	151	160	166	180
55–59	218	130	139	143	150	157	161	169	174	185

Table A.1. (continued)

Age	N	\multicolumn{9}{c}{Decile}

Age	N	1	2	3	4	5	6	7	8	9
\multicolumn{11}{c}{Diastolic blood pressure (5th phase, mm Hg)}
40–44	175	73	76	79	80	84	88	90	92	98
45–49	299	75	78	80	84	87	90	91	95	100
50–54	289	77	80	81	85	88	90	92	97	104
55–59	218	78	80	82	87	90	90	94	98	104
\multicolumn{11}{c}{Serum cholesterol (mg per 100 ml)}
40–44	170	156	166	174	184	194	202	215	226	256
45–49	294	146	167	178	186	194	204	217	238	257
50–54	284	150	172	182	190	198	207	216	232	246
55–59	214	152	170	179	190	204	216	226	241	257

MONTEGIORGIO, ITALY

Age	N	1	2	3	4	5	6	7	8	9
\multicolumn{11}{c}{Height (cm)}
40–44	123	159	162	163	164	165	167	168	170	174
45–49	246	157	160	162	164	165	166	168	169	172
50–54	217	156	158	160	162	163	164	167	169	171
55–59	130	156	158	160	161	162	164	166	168	171
\multicolumn{11}{c}{Relative body weight (%)}
40–44	123	82	89	92	96	99	102	107	110	117
45–49	246	84	88	92	95	98	102	108	112	120
50–54	217	81	84	89	92	94	99	103	107	114
55–59	130	79	82	86	88	94	97	102	108	121
\multicolumn{11}{c}{Sum of skinfolds (mm)}
40–44	123	9	10	11	13	15	18	21	24	28
45–49	247	10	11	12	14	16	18	20	25	32
50–54	216	9	10	11	13	14	16	20	22	28
55–59	130	9	10	11	12	14	16	18	22	26
\multicolumn{11}{c}{Systolic blood pressure (mm Hg)}
40–44	123	112	118	120	124	128	130	135	139	145
45–49	247	119	123	129	130	134	138	140	146	158
50–54	217	119	123	129	131	137	140	146	154	161
55–59	131	120	130	135	139	142	146	151	160	173
\multicolumn{11}{c}{Diastolic blood pressure (5th phase, mm Hg)}
40–44	123	70	70	72	76	78	80	80	82	91
45–49	247	70	74	76	79	80	82	84	90	93

| | | \multicolumn{9}{c}{Decile} | | | | | | | | |
Age	N	1	2	3	4	5	6	7	8	9
50–54	217	70	75	78	80	81	83	89	90	98
55–59	131	72	76	80	81	83	85	88	90	97

Serum cholesterol (mg per 100 ml)

Age	N	1	2	3	4	5	6	7	8	9
40–44	122	157	165	175	184	192	201	210	224	249
45–49	244	155	169	183	192	200	208	219	235	257
50–54	216	157	169	182	191	199	207	222	232	248
55–59	128	162	173	183	191	198	203	213	228	263

ZUTPHEN, THE NETHERLANDS

Height (cm)

Age	N	1	2	3	4	5	6	7	8	9
40–44	181	165	168	171	174	175	177	179	180	183
45–49	237	166	169	172	174	175	176	178	180	183
50–54	235	166	168	170	172	174	175	177	180	182
55–59	225	163	167	169	171	172	174	176	178	182

Relative body weight (%)

Age	N	1	2	3	4	5	6	7	8	9
40–44	181	85	91	93	96	99	102	105	108	111
45–49	236	85	89	92	95	97	100	103	106	111
50–54	234	82	88	91	95	97	100	102	105	113
55–59	224	82	87	91	94	97	99	101	106	110

Sum of skinfolds (mm)

Age	N	1	2	3	4	5	6	7	8	9
40–44	181	14	16	20	22	24	27	29	32	38
45–49	236	13	16	20	22	23	26	28	32	37
50–54	234	13	16	20	22	24	26	30	32	37
55–59	225	14	16	18	21	22	26	28	32	38

Systolic blood pressure (mm Hg)

Age	N	1	2	3	4	5	6	7	8	9
40–44	181	125	130	130	136	140	145	150	153	160
45–49	236	120	129	130	135	140	145	150	156	165
50–54	233	120	128	132	138	140	146	155	163	175
55–59	225	122	130	135	140	145	150	158	168	176

Diastolic blood pressure (5th phase, mm Hg)

Age	N	1	2	3	4	5	6	7	8	9
40–44	180	75	80	80	85	90	90	94	98	100
45–49	236	73	80	80	85	90	90	93	98	104
50–54	233	75	80	80	85	90	90	95	100	108
55–59	225	75	80	82	85	88	90	95	100	106

Serum cholesterol (mg per 100 ml)

Age	N	1	2	3	4	5	6	7	8	9
40–44	174	177	198	209	224	233	244	253	268	285
45–49	219	186	201	215	226	235	247	257	272	298
50–54	224	187	200	209	219	227	239	252	265	289
55–59	214	177	197	206	217	226	238	252	264	292

Table A.1. (continued)

		\multicolumn{9}{c}{Decile}								
Age	N	1	2	3	4	5	6	7	8	9
CRETE, GREECE										
					Height (cm)					
40–44	158	159	162	163	165	166	168	170	172	174
45–49	199	158	161	163	165	166	168	169	171	174
50–54	172	159	161	164	165	166	168	170	171	174
55–59	146	158	160	162	164	165	167	168	170	173
					Relative body weight (%)					
40–44	157	82	86	88	92	94	96	100	104	112
45–49	200	79	82	85	88	91	94	97	103	111
50–54	172	75	81	84	88	92	94	98	102	112
55–59	146	77	81	84	86	88	90	94	97	103
					Sum of skinfolds (mm)					
40–44	160	10	10	12	13	14	17	20	24	30
45–49	202	10	10	11	12	14	15	18	22	28
50–54	175	9	10	12	13	15	17	20	23	27
55–59	148	10	10	11	13	14	15	17	19	23
					Systolic blood pressure (mm Hg)					
40–44	158	112	118	122	128	131	136	142	150	155
45–49	201	116	120	123	130	132	136	140	145	155
50–54	173	115	122	127	130	135	139	145	152	164
55–59	146	119	125	130	134	138	145	152	160	174
					Diastolic blood pressure (5th phase, mm Hg)					
40–44	158	68	72	75	76	80	82	87	90	96
45–49	201	70	72	75	78	80	82	85	89	97
50–54	173	70	72	75	80	81	85	89	90	95
55–59	146	70	73	75	80	83	85	89	90	94
					Serum cholesterol (mg per 100 ml)					
40–44	152	156	169	177	186	198	206	217	233	260
45–49	190	154	169	178	188	199	206	219	235	251
50–54	167	158	176	183	195	210	218	232	250	270
55–59	143	163	172	193	199	208	226	235	245	257
CORFU, GREECE										
					Height (cm)					
40–44	120	159	162	164	166	167	169	172	174	176
45–49	114	158	161	162	164	166	167	170	172	177

		Decile								
Age	N	1	2	3	4	5	6	7	8	9
50–54	169	159	160	162	164	166	167	169	170	172
55–59	126	158	160	161	162	164	165	166	168	172
		Relative body weight (%)								
40–44	120	80	84	88	92	94	100	102	106	114
45–49	114	79	83	87	89	93	100	104	110	115
50–54	168	77	82	85	88	92	95	98	103	110
55–59	126	77	80	83	87	90	94	97	103	111
		Sum of skinfolds (mm)								
40–44	120	10	11	12	14	16	19	20	24	30
45–49	114	10	11	12	14	15	18	20	26	31
50–54	169	10	11	12	13	14	16	19	23	31
55–59	126	10	10	11	12	14	16	19	24	30
		Systolic blood pressure (mm Hg)								
40–44	120	109	115	121	128	130	134	138	140	154
45–49	114	110	119	121	125	130	134	139	146	160
50–54	169	111	120	125	130	134	138	140	151	164
55–59	126	111	120	125	130	135	140	150	158	167
		Diastolic blood pressure (5th phase, mm Hg)								
40–44	120	70	72	76	80	81	82	85	89	92
45–49	114	70	72	75	79	80	82	86	90	98
50–54	169	71	75	78	80	81	85	89	90	97
55–59	126	70	74	76	80	81	85	88	90	95
		Serum cholesterol (mg per 100 ml)								
40–44	120	146	158	172	185	193	203	220	232	262
45–49	111	147	163	176	193	203	209	222	233	259
50–54	165	162	174	186	194	202	216	232	246	258
55–59	125	154	171	180	186	194	201	212	227	251

ROME RAILROAD

		Height (cm)								
40–44	197	160	162	163	165	166	167	169	172	175
45–49	215	159	162	164	165	166	168	169	170	172
50–54	231	158	161	163	164	165	166	168	170	172
55–59	124	157	159	161	163	164	166	168	170	173
		Relative body weight (%)								
40–44	197	90	95	100	104	108	113	117	121	127
45–49	215	90	96	100	104	108	112	116	122	129
50–54	231	87	95	99	103	106	110	113	118	125
55–59	124	82	93	100	104	108	112	114	121	126

Table A.1. (continued)

Age	N	Decile								
		1	2	3	4	5	6	7	8	9
		Sum of skinfolds (mm)								
40–44	197	14	17	20	22	26	30	34	38	44
45–49	215	15	19	21	23	27	30	33	38	45
50–54	231	13	16	20	23	25	28	32	36	40
55–59	124	13	17	20	23	26	29	30	34	39
		Systolic blood pressure (mm Hg)								
40–44	197	119	123	129	131	135	138	140	147	158
45–49	215	118	128	133	136	138	141	145	151	160
50–54	232	118	126	130	135	138	141	148	152	162
55–59	124	122	129	135	140	142	150	155	166	174
		Diastolic blood pressure (5th phase, mm Hg)								
40–44	197	70	76	80	83	86	89	91	96	102
45–49	215	72	79	80	84	89	90	95	100	106
50–54	232	72	80	82	86	89	90	93	98	105
54–59	124	78	80	85	88	90	91	97	100	103
		Serum cholesterol (mg per 100 ml)								
40–44	195	154	168	182	196	207	216	225	234	252
45–49	214	159	173	185	197	206	218	229	240	260
50–54	231	159	173	186	198	209	219	231	242	267
55–59	124	158	170	183	193	204	212	225	239	261

VELIKA KRSNA, YUGOSLAVIA

Age	N	1	2	3	4	5	6	7	8	9
		Height (cm)								
40–44	136	163	164	167	169	171	172	173	175	178
45–49	81	163	164	166	168	170	171	173	174	178
50–54	135	160	163	165	167	168	170	172	174	176
55–59	158	161	164	166	167	168	170	172	174	177
		Relative body weight (%)								
40–44	136	81	85	86	88	89	92	95	99	109
45–49	81	78	81	84	87	88	91	94	100	109
50–54	135	78	81	83	85	88	90	93	96	103
55–59	158	76	78	80	83	86	89	92	95	101
		Sum of skinfolds (mm)								
40–44	136	10	10	11	12	13	14	16	18	23
45–49	81	9	10	11	12	13	14	15	18	25

						Decile				
Age	N	1	2	3	4	5	6	7	8	9
50–54	135	9	10	11	12	13	14	15	18	22
55–59	158	9	10	11	11	12	14	15	19	24
Systolic blood pressure (mm Hg)											
40–44	136	109	112	120	120	124	127	130	130	141
45–49	82	110	117	120	121	128	130	132	140	148
50–54	135	110	119	124	128	130	133	139	144	157
55–59	158	115	120	128	130	130	140	143	150	160
Diastolic blood pressure (5th phase, mm Hg)											
40–44	136	69	70	76	77	78	80	81	87	90
45–49	81	70	76	77	78	80	81	84	88	93
50–54	135	70	76	78	80	80	84	86	88	96
55–59	158	70	76	79	80	80	85	88	90	98
Serum cholesterol (mg per 100 ml)											
40–44	136	121	133	141	149	154	162	168	179	191
45–49	82	120	132	143	151	157	168	178	194	201
50–54	135	116	133	144	152	159	168	179	186	204
55–59	158	126	134	139	149	155	164	179	190	207

ZRENJANIN, YUGOSLAVIA

					Height (cm)					
30–39	111	163	164	167	168	170	171	172	174	177
40–44	148	161	164	165	167	168	170	171	173	175
45–49	100	160	162	164	166	167	168	170	173	176
50–54	169	157	160	162	164	165	167	168	170	173
55–59	99	159	161	164	164	166	168	170	171	174
Relative body weight (%)											
30–39	113	84	88	92	94	97	102	105	112	120
40–44	148	85	91	95	99	103	107	112	118	125
45–49	100	83	89	93	97	100	105	111	114	122
50–54	169	85	89	92	95	100	103	105	110	119
55–59	99	84	87	90	93	97	102	106	112	124
Sum of skinfolds (mm)											
30–39	113	11	12	13	15	17	20	26	32	41
40–44	148	11	13	16	19	23	30	37	40	48
45–49	100	10	13	14	18	23	27	30	37	42
50–54	169	11	13	16	18	22	27	30	35	44
55–59	99	12	13	16	19	22	27	34	39	46

Table A.1. (continued)

Age	N	\multicolumn{9}{c}{Decile}

Age	N	1	2	3	4	5	6	7	8	9
\multicolumn{11}{c}{Systolic blood pressure (mm Hg)}
30–39	110	109	114	119	121	123	127	131	136	140
40–44	148	110	116	120	120	126	130	132	138	142
45–49	100	110	116	120	124	126	130	130	135	142
50–54	169	112	120	124	126	130	138	144	150	160
55–59	99	120	128	130	132	138	144	150	163	177
\multicolumn{11}{c}{Diastolic blood pressure (5th phase, mm Hg)}
30–39	110	69	70	73	75	77	79	84	87	88
40–44	148	70	72	78	80	80	84	88	90	90
45–49	100	70	76	78	80	80	83	86	90	92
50–54	169	72	78	80	82	86	88	90	96	100
55–59	99	74	79	80	84	88	90	90	98	102
\multicolumn{11}{c}{Serum cholesterol (mg per 100 ml)}
40–44	148	126	140	150	158	162	169	175	185	204
45–49	100	134	144	150	160	170	176	181	190	211
50–54	169	133	143	150	160	170	178	187	196	211
55–59	98	131	142	148	155	166	175	182	191	200

UNIVERSITY OF BELGRADE FACULTY, YUGOSLAVIA

Age	N	1	2	3	4	5	6	7	8	9
\multicolumn{11}{c}{Height (cm)}
30–39	77	170	173	175	177	178	179	180	182	184
40–44	239	169	171	173	174	175	177	178	180	183
45–49	69	168	171	172	174	176	177	179	182	184
50–54	142	167	170	172	173	175	177	180	182	184
55–59	88	167	170	171	172	174	175	177	179	182
\multicolumn{11}{c}{Relative body weight (%)}
30–39	77	89	99	100	101	103	105	108	113	119
40–44	239	94	98	102	106	109	111	113	116	119
45–49	70	91	97	100	103	106	109	112	115	121
50–54	142	90	95	100	102	106	108	113	117	125
55–59	87	91	95	100	102	108	111	113	115	122
\multicolumn{11}{c}{Sum of skinfolds (mm)}
30–39	76	18	21	28	31	34	36	40	43	47
40–44	239	23	30	33	36	39	41	46	49	54
45–49	70	26	30	34	36	38	42	45	50	54

						Decile				
Age	N	1	2	3	4	5	6	7	8	9
50–54	142	21	30	34	37	40	42	44	48	54
55–59	87	21	27	32	35	38	41	44	47	55
Systolic blood pressure (mm Hg)											
30–39	76	115	120	120	124	127	129	130	131	137
40–44	238	112	118	120	120	126	128	130	136	149
45–49	69	118	120	126	130	130	136	140	148	156
50–54	142	117	122	126	130	132	136	140	146	155
55–59	88	120	126	130	134	140	141	148	158	164
Diastolic blood pressure (5th phase, mm Hg)											
30–39	76	73	75	77	79	79	81	83	87	90
40–44	238	72	76	80	80	80	84	86	90	93
45–49	69	74	79	80	84	88	90	90	98	106
50–54	142	77	80	82	86	86	88	90	92	100
55–59	88	78	80	80	86	88	90	94	100	103
Serum cholesterol (mg per 100 ml)											
30–39	76	146	163	172	178	190	110	212	218	238
40–44	235	160	174	185	193	200	210	220	230	255
45–49	69	167	182	195	200	206	211	224	235	246
50–54	141	167	183	193	202	212	225	237	256	272
55–59	88	165	186	190	200	212	219	226	242	258

Table A.2. Percentage distribution of body mass index (kilograms per meter height) in men 40–59 years old (weight in underclothes, height without shoes; in all cohorts no significant relationship between body mass index and age).

Body mass index	U.S. RR (N = 2,558)	Rome RR (N = 767)	Dalmatia (N = 668)	Slavonia (N = 683)
<20.0	3.60	2.48	16.77	15.52
20.0–20.9	3.17	3.65	12.57	12.01
21.0–21.9	6.29	5.48	15.57	13.03
22.0–22.9	8.99	5.35	12.28	12.45
23.0–23.9	9.50	7.04	11.68	11.13
24.0–24.9	12.00	8.87	8.68	7.91
25.0–25.9	13.02	10.56	7.19	8.05
26.0–26.9	12.43	10.69	5.09	5.27
27.0–27.9	10.48	11.86	3.89	3.51
28.0–28.9	7.35	8.87	2.25	3.37
29.0–29.9	4.85	7.43	2.10	2.49
≥30.0	8.33	17.73	1.95	5.27

Table A.2. (continued)

Body mass index	E. Finland (N=797)	W. Finland (N=836)	Crevalcore (N=978)	Montegiorgio (N=715)
<20.0	11.17	7.66	3.27	8.25
20.0–20.9	11.04	9.21	3.48	6.43
21.0–21.9	13.68	11.48	7.16	11.33
22.0–22.9	14.18	12.44	9.00	12.17
23.0–23.9	14.30	12.44	11.96	12.73
24.0–24.9	10.54	11.48	11.25	9.65
25.0–25.9	6.78	10.41	10.33	9.79
26.0–26.9	7.03	8.25	9.30	8.11
27.0–27.9	4.14	4.31	9.20	5.87
28.0–28.9	2.26	4.67	6.03	4.48
29.0–29.9	1.88	2.51	5.01	3.64
≥30.0	3.01	5.14	14.01	7.55

Body mass index	Zutphen (N=876)	Crete (N=674)	Corfu (N=529)	Tanushimaru (N=507)
<20.0	5.14	15.13	15.88	18.74
20.0–20.9	8.68	13.06	9.45	18.54
21.0–21.9	8.11	14.69	15.31	20.32
22.0–22.9	12.44	14.54	11.15	14.99
23.0–23.9	14.73	12.17	9.07	12.43
24.0–24.9	15.64	8.46	11.72	5.92
25.0–25.9	12.56	6.68	7.18	3.75
26.0–26.9	9.70	5.04	4.91	2.76
27.0–27.9	5.14	3.12	6.43	1.38
28.0–28.9	4.45	3.56	2.65	0.20
29.0–29.9	1.48	1.63	1.13	0.59
≥30.0	1.94	1.93	5.10	0.39

Body mass index	Ushibuka (N=454)	Velika Krsna (N=510)	Zrenjanin (N=516)	Belgrade (N=538)
<20.0	14.98	21.96	4.46	1.30
20.0–20.9	16.52	15.69	5.62	2.42
21.0–21.9	18.06	17.65	8.91	3.53
22.0–22.9	18.94	15.69	12.60	5.58
23.0–23.9	13.22	10.00	10.08	8.55
24.0–24.9	7.71	6.47	10.66	12.27
25.0–25.9	3.96	2.94	10.47	10.22
26.0–26.9	2.64	2.94	8.91	15.43

Body mass index	Ushibuka (N=454)	Velika Krsna (N=510)	Zrenjanin (N=516)	Belgrade (N=538)
27.0–27.9	1.76	2.55	8.53	14.68
28.0–28.9	1.32	2.35	4.46	11.71
29.0–29.9	0.22	0.59	5.62	5.95
⩾30.0	0.66	1.18	9.69	8.36

References

Acheson, R. M., and Baird, J. T. 1973. Serum cholesterol in a national sample of U.S. adults. A study from prevalence data of its relationship to physique, blood pressure, blood glucose and other variables. *Internat. J. Epidem.* 2:283–292.

Adelson, S. F., and Keys, A. 1962. Diet and some health characteristics of 123 business and professional men. Agricultural Research Service. ARS 62–11. Washington, D.C.: U.S. Department of Agriculture.

Anderson, J. T., and Keys, A. 1956. Cholesterol in serum and lipoprotein fractions: Its measurement and stability. *Clin. Chem.* 2:145–159.

Antonis, A.; Bersohn, I.; Plotkin, R.; Easty, D. L.; and Lewis, H. E. 1965. Influence of seasonal variation: Diet and physical activity on serum lipids in young men in Antarctica. *Am. J. Clin. Nutr.* 16:428–435.

Berkson, D. M.; Stamler, J.; Lindberg, H. A.; Miller, W. A.; Stevens, E. L.; Soyugenc, R.; Tokich, T.; and Stamler, R. 1970. Heart rate: An important risk factor for coronary mortality—ten-year experience of the Peoples Gas Company Epidemiological Study, 1958–68. In *Proceedings of the Second International Symposium on Atherosclerosis*, pp. 383–389, R. J. Jones, ed. New York: Springer-Verlag.

Billings, F. T.; Kalstone, B. M.; Spencer, J. L.; Ball, C. O. T.; and Meneely, G. R. 1949. Prognosis of acute myocardial infarction. *Am. J. Med.* 7:356–370.

Blackburn, H.; Brozek, J.; and Taylor, H. L. 1959. Lung volume in smokers and nonsmokers. *Ann. Int. Med.* 51:68–77.

Blackburn, H.; Parlin, R. W.; and Keys, A. 1967. The inter-relations of electrocardiographic findings and physical characteristics of middle-aged men. *Acta Med. Scand.* suppl. 460, pp. 316–341.

Blackburn, H.; Taylor, H. L.; Parlin, R. W.; Kihlberg, J.; and Keys, A. 1965. Physical activity of occupation and cigarette smoking. *Arch. Environ. Health* 10:312–322.

Borhani, N. O.; Hechter, H. H.; and Breslow, L. 1963. Report of a ten-year follow-up of the San Francisco longshoremen. Mortality from coronary heart disease and from all causes. *J. Chron. Dis.* 16:1251–1266.

Böttiger, L. E., and Carlson, L. A. 1973. The Stockholm Prospective Study 2. New events of coronary heart disease in men in relation to findings at initial examination, 9 year follow-up. In *Early phases of coronary heart disease: The possibility of prediction*, pp. 158–181, J. Waldenstrom, T. Larsson, and N. Ljungstedt, eds. Stockholm: Nordiska Bokhandelns Forlag.

Bronte-Stewart, B.; Keys, A.; and Brock, J. F. 1955. Serum-cholesterol, diet and coronary heart disease. *Lancet* 2:1103–8.

Brownlee, K. A. 1965. *Statistical theory and methodology in science and engineering.* 2d ed. New York: Wiley.

Buzina, R.; Ferber, E.; Keys, A.; Brodarec, A.; Agneletto, B.; and Horvat, A. 1964. Diets of rural families and heads of families in two regions of Yugoslavia. *Voeding* 25:629–640.

Buzina, R.; Keys, A.; Brodarec, A.; Anderson, J. T.; and Fidanza, F. 1966. Dietary surveys in rural Yugoslavia: II, Chemical analyses of diets in Dalmatia and Slavonia. *Voeding* 27:31–36.

Buzina, R.; Keys, A.; Brodarec, A.; and Fidanza, F. 1966. Dietary surveys in rural Yugoslavia. III, Comparison of three methods. *Voeding* 27:99–105.

Carlson, L. A., and Böttiger, L. E. 1972. Ischemic heart disease in relation to fasting values of plasma triglycerides and cholesterol. *Lancet* 1:865–868.

Chapman, J. M.; Coulson, A. H.; Clark, V. A.; and Borun, E. R. 1971. The differential effect of serum cholesterol, blood pressure and weight on the incidence of myocardial infarction and angina pectoris. *J. Chron. Dis.* 23:631–645.

Chapman, J. M.; Goerke, L. S.; Dixon, W.; Loveland, D. B.; and Phillips, E. 1957. The clinical status of a population group under observation for two to three years. *Am. J. Publ. Health* 47(Suppl. 4):33–72.

Chapman, J. M., and Massey, F. J. 1964. The interrelationship of serum cholesterol, hypertension, body weight and risk of coronary disease: Results of the first ten years follow-up in the Los Angeles heart study. *J. Chron. Dis.* 17:933–949.

Comstock, G. W.; Kendrick, M. A.; and Livesay, V. 1966. Subcutaneous fatness and mortality. *Am. J. Epidem.* 83:548–563.

Connor, W. D.; Cerqueira, M. T.; Connor, R. W.; Wallace, R. B.; Malinow, M. R.; and Casdorph, H. R. 1978. The plasma lipids, lipoproteins and diet of the Tarahumara Indians of Mexico. *Am. J. Clin. Nutr.* 31:1131–42.

Cooper, C.; Stamler, J.; Dyer, A.; and Garside, D. 1979. The decline in mortality from coronary heart disease, U.S.A., 1968–1975. *J. Chron. Dis.* 31:709–720.

Dawber, T. R.; Kannel, W. B.; and Friedman, G. D. 1966. Vital capacity, physical activity and coronary heart disease. In *Prevention of ischemic heart disease: Principles and practice*, pp. 254–265, W. Raab, ed. Springfield, Ill.: Charles C Thomas.

Dawber, T. R.; Kannel, W. B.; and Lyell, L. P. 1963. An approach of longitudinal studies in a community: The Framingham Study. *Ann. N.Y. Acad. Sci.* 107:539–556.

Dawber, T. R., and McNamara, P. M. 1967. Coronary heart disease: Identification of susceptible individual. In *Atherosclerotic vascular disease*, pp. 130–146, A. N. Brest and J. H. Moyer, eds. New York: Appleton-Century-Crofts.

Dawber, T. R.; Moore, F. E.; and Mann, G. V. 1957. Coronary heart disease in the Framingham Study. *Am. J. Publ. Health* 47(Suppl. 4):4–24.

Dawber, T. R.; Pearson, G.; Anderson, P.; Mann, G. V.; Kannel, W. B.; Shurtleff, D.; and McNamara, P. 1962. Diet and cardiovascular disease in the Framingham Study. II, Reliability of measurement. *Am. J. Clin. Nutr.* 11:226–234.

Dimond, G. E. 1963. Hypertension, body weight, and coronary heart disease. *Arch. Int. Med.* 112:550–554.

Doyle, J. T.; Heslin, A. S.; Hilleboe, H. E.; Formel, P. F.; and Korns, R. F. 1957. A prospective study of degenerative cardiovascular disease in Albany: Report of three years experience. I. Ischemic heart disease. *Am. J. Publ. Health* 47(Suppl. 4):25–32.

Doyle, J. T.; Kannel, W. B.; McNamara, P. M.; Quickenton, P.; and Gordon, T. 1976. Factors related to suddenness of death from coronary disease: Combined Albany-Framingham studies. *Am. J. Cardiol.* 37:1073–78.

Dublin, L. I., and Marks, H. H. 1958. Mortality among insured overweights in recent years. In *Life insurance and medicine*, pp. 436–462, H. E. Ungerleider and R. Gubner, eds. Springfield, Ill.: Charles C Thomas.

Dyer, A. R.; Stamler, J.; Berkson, D. M.; and Lindberg, H. A. 1975. Relationship of relative weight and body mass index to 14-year mortality in the Chicago Peoples Gas Company Study. *J. Chron. Dis.* 28:109–123.

Easty, D. L. 1970. The relationship of diet to serum cholesterol levels in young men in Antarctica. *Br. J. Nutr.* 24:307–312.

Epstein, F. H. 1975. The epidemiology of coronary artery disease: A review from the epidemiologic standpoint. *J. Chron. Dis.* 18:735–774.

Fidanza, F. 1979. Changing patterns of food consumption in Italy (to be published).

Fidanza, F., and Fidanza-Alberti, A. 1967. Dietary surveys in connection with the epidemiology of heart disease: Reliability, sources of variation, and other data from nine surveys in Italy. *Voeding* 28:244–252.

―――― 1975. Food and nutrient consumption of two rural population groups of Italy followed for ten years. *Nutr. Metab.* 18:176–189.

Fidanza, F.; Fidanza-Alberti, A.; Ferro-Luzzi, G.; and Proja, M. 1964. Dietary surveys in connection with the epidemiology of heart disease: Results in Italy. *Voeding* 25:502–509.

Finegan, A.; Hickey, N.; Maurer, B.; and Mulcahy, R. 1968. Diet and coronary heart disease: Dietary analysis on 100 male patients. *Am. J. Clin. Nutr.* 21:143–148.

Fraser, G. E., and Swannell, R. J. 1979. Diet and serum cholesterol in Seventh Day Adventists: A cross-sectional study showing significant relationships. *Am. J. Clin. Nutr.* (in press).

French, A. J., and Dock, W. 1944. Fatal coronary arteriosclerosis in young soldiers. *J. Am. Med. Assoc.* 124:1233–37.

Friedman, G. D.; Klatsky, A. L.; and Sieglaub, A. B. 1976. Lung function and risk of myocardial infarction and sudden cardiac death. *New Engl. J. Med.* 294:1071–1075.

Geizerova, H.; Hejl, Z.; and Santucek, M. 1975. Angina pectoris and risk factors in the urban male population in the sixth decade. *Rev. Czech. Med.* 21:17–25.

Gordon, T.; Garcia-Palmieri, M. R.; Kagan, A.; Kannel, W. B.; and Schiffman, J. 1974. Differences in coronary heart disease in Framingham, Honolulu and Puerto Rico. *J. Chron. Dis.* 27:329–344.

Gordon, T.; Kagan, A.; and Rhoads, C. G. 1975. Relative weights in different populations. Letter to the editor. *Am. J. Clin. Nutr.* 28:304–305.

Gordon, T., and Kannel, W. B. 1973. The effects of overweight on cardiovascular diseases. *Geriatrics* 28:80–88.

Gordon, T., and Kannel, W. B. 1976. Obesity and cardiovascular disease: The Framingham Study. *Clin. Endocrin. Metabol.* 5:367–375.

Hartog, C. den; Buzina, R.; Fidanza, F.; Keys, A.; and Roine, P., ed. 1968. *Dietary studies and epidemiology of heart diseases.* The Hague: Stichting tot wetenschappelijke Voorlichting op Voedingsgebied.

Hartog, C. den; Van Schaik, T. F. S. M.; Dalerup, L. M.; Drion, E. F.; and Mulder, T. 1965. The diet of volunteers participating in a long term epidemiological field survey on coronary heart disease at Zutphen, Netherlands. *Voeding* 26:184–208.

Hegsted, D. M.; McGandy, R. B.; Myers, M. L.; and Stare, F. J. 1965. Quantitative effects of dietary fat on serum cholesterol in man. *Am. J. Clin. Nutr.* 17:281–295.

Hensler, N. M., and Giron, D. J. 1963. Pulmonary physiological measurements in smokers and non-smokers. *J. Am. Med. Assoc.* 186:885–889.

Heyden, S. 1975. Risk factors of ischemic heart disease. Study monograph. Mannheim, Germany: Boerhringer-Mannheim.

Hilleboe, H. E. 1967. Geographic distribution of arteriosclerotic heart disease. In *Cowdry's arteriosclerosis: A survey of the problem*, 2d ed., pp. 623–678, H. T. Blumenthal, ed. Springfield, Ill.: Charles C Thomas.

Hutchinson, J. J. 1961. Clinical implications of extensive actuarial study of build and blood pressure. *Ann. Int. Med.* 54:90–96.

Jacobs, D. R.; Anderson, J. T.; and Blackburn, H. 1979. Diet and serum cholesterol: Do zero correlations negate the relationship? *Am. J. Epidem.* (in press).

Johnson, B. C.; Epstein, F. H.; and Kjelsberg, M. O. 1965. Distributions and familial studies of blood pressure and serum cholesterol in a total community: Tecumseh, Michigan. *J. Chron. Dis.* 18:147–160.

Jolliffe, N., and Archer, M. 1959. Statistical association between international coronary heart disease death rates and certain environmental factors. *J. Chron. Dis.* 9:636–652.

Kagan, A. 1960. Atherosclerosis of the coronary arteries: Epidemiological considerations. *Proc. Roy. Soc. Med.* 53:18–22.

Kahn, H. A. 1963. The relationship of reported coronary heart disease to physical activity of work. *Am. J. Publ. Health* 53:1058–67.

Kahn, H. A.; Medalie, J. H.; Neufeld, H. N.; Riss, E.; Balogh, M.; and Groen, J. J. 1969. Serum cholesterol: Its distribution and association with dietary and other variables in a survey of 10,000 men. *Israel J. Med. Sci.* 5:1117–27.

Kannel, W. B.; Dawber, T. R.; Kagan, A.; Revotskie, N.; and Stokes, J., III. 1961. Factors of risk in the development of coronary heart disease, six-year follow-up experience: The Framingham study. *Ann. Int. Med.* 55:33–50.

Kannel, W. B., and Gordon, T. 1974. Obesity and cardiovascular disease. The Framingham study. In *Obesity*, W. L. Burland, P. D. Samuel, and J. Yudkin, eds. London: Churchill-Livingston.

―――, eds. 1968. *The Framingham study: An epidemiological investigation of cardiovascular disease*. Sections 1, 2, 6. Washington, D.C.: Superintendent of Documents, U.S. Government Printing Office.

Kannel, W. B.; Gordon, T.; and Schwartz, M. S. 1971. Systolic and diastolic blood pressure and risk of coronary heart disease: The Framingham study. *Am. J. Cardiol.* 27:335–356.

Kannel, W. B.; LeBauer, E. J.; Dawber, T. R.; and McNamara, P. M. 1967. Relation of body weight to development of coronary heart disease: The Framingham study. *Circulation* 35:734–744.

Kemsley, W. F. F.; Billewicz, W. Z.; and Thomson, A. M.; 1962. A new weight-for-height standard based on British anthropometric data. *Br. J. Prev. Soc. Med.* 16:189–195.

Keys, A. 1949. The physiology of the individual as an approach to a more quantitative biology of man. *Fed. Proc.* 8:523–529.

―――. 1952. The cholesterol problem. *Voeding* 13:539–555.

―――. 1953a. Atherosclerosis: A problem in newer public health. *J. Mt. Sinai Hosp.* 20:118–139.

―――. 1953b. Prediction and possible prevention of coronary heart disease. *Am. J. Publ. Health* 43:1399–1407.

―――. 1954. Obesity and degenerative heart disease. *Am. J. Publ. Health* 44:864–871.

―――. 1955a. Obesity and heart disease. J. Chron. Dis. 1:456–461.

―――. 1955b. Weight changes and health of men. In *Weight Control*, pp. 18–28, E. S. Eppright, P. Swanson, and C. A. Iverson, eds. Ames: Iowa State College Press.

―――. 1956. Field studies in Italy, 1954. In *World trends in cardiology: I, Cardiovascular epidemiology*, pp. 50–61, A. Keys and P. D. White, eds. New York: Hoeber-Harper.

―――. 1957a. Diet and the epidemiology of coronary heart disease. *J. Am. Med. Assoc.* 164:1912–19.

―――. 1957b. Epidemiological aspects of coronary artery disease. J. Chron. Dis. 6:552–559.

———. 1965. Dietary survey methods in studies on cardiovascular epidemiology. *Voeding* 26:464–483.
———. 1967. Diet effects on the blood lipids of man. *Med. Prisma*, no. 3. Ingelheim on Rhein: C. H. Boeringer Sohn.
———. 1971. Sucrose in the diet and coronary heart disease. *Atherosclerosis* 14:193–202.
———. 1975. Coronary heart disease: The global picture. *Atherosclerosis* 22:149–192.
———. 1978. Die Angina Pectoris in der Seven Countries Study. In *Angina pectoris*, pp. 275–290, E. Gill, ed. Stuttgart: Gustave Fischer Verlag.
———. 1979. Dietary survey methods. In *Nutrition, lipids, and coronary heart disease*, pp. 1–23, R. I. Levy, B. M. Rifkind, B. H. Dennis, N. D. Ernst, eds. New York: Raven Press.
———, ed. 1970. Coronary heart disease in seven countries. *Am. Heart Assoc.* Monograph number 29. *Circulation*, Suppl. I, vols. 41, 42, I-1–I-211.
Keys, A.; Anderson, J. T.; and Grande, F. 1957. Prediction of serum-cholesterol responses of man to changes in fats in the diet. *Lancet* 2:959–966.
Keys, A.; Anderson, J. T.; and Grande, F. 1965a. Serum cholesterol response to changes in the diet. I, Iodine value of dietary fat versus 2S–P. *Metabolism* 14:747–758.
———. 1965b. Serum cholesterol response to changes in the diet. II, The effect of cholesterol in the diet. *Metabolism* 14:759–765.
———. 1965c. Serum cholesterol response to changes in the diet. III, Differences among individuals. *Metabolism* 14:766–775.
———. 1965d. Serum cholesterol response to changes in the diet. IV, Particular fatty acids in the diet. *Metabolism* 14:776–787.
Keys, A.; Aravanis, C.; Blackburn, H.; Djordjevic, B. S.; Dontas, A. S.; Fidanza, F.; Karvonen, M. J.; Menotti, A.; and Taylor, H. L. 1972a. Lung function as a risk factor for coronary heart disease. *Am. J. Publ. Health* 62:1506–11.
Keys, A.; Aravanis, C.; Blackburn, H.; van Buchem, F. S. P.; Buzina, R.; Djordjevic, B. S.; Fidanza, F.; Karvonen, M. J.; Menotti, A.; Puddu, V.; Taylor, H. L. 1972b. Probability of middle-aged men developing coronary heart disease in five years. *Circulation* 45:815–828.
Keys, A.; Aravanis, C.; Blackburn, H.; van Buchem, F. S. P.; Buzina, R.; Djordjevic, B. S.; Dontas, A. S.; Fidanza, F.; Karvonen, M. J.; Kimura, N.; Lekos, D.; Monti, M.; Puddu, V.; and Taylor, H. L. 1967. Epidemiological studies related to coronary heart disease: Characteristics of men aged 40–59 in seven countries. *Acta Med. Scand.* Suppl. 460, 392 pp.
Keys, A.; Aravanis C.; and Sdrin, H. 1966. The diets of middle-aged men in two rural areas of Greece. *Voeding* 27:575–586.
Keys, A.; and Blackburn, H. 1963. Background of the patient with coronary heart disease. *Prog. Cardiovasc. Dis.* 6:14–44.

Keys, A.; Fidanza, F.; Karvonen, M. J.; Kimura, N.; and Taylor, H. L. 1972c. Indices of relative weight and obesity. *J. Chron. Dis.* 25:329–343.

Keys, A.; Karvonen, M. J.; and Fidanza, F. 1958. Serum-cholesterol studies in Finland. *Lancet* 26 (July):175–178.

Keys, A.; Kimura, N.; Kusukawa, A., Bronte-Stewart, B.; Larsen, N.; and Keys, M. H. 1958. Lessons from serum cholesterol studies in Japan, Hawaii and Los Angeles. *Ann. Int. Med.* 48:83–94.

Keys, A.; Mickelsen, O.; Miller, E. v. O.; Hayes, E. R.; and Todd, R. L. 1950. The concentration of cholesterol in the blood serum of normal man and its relation to age. *J. Clin. Invest.* 29:1347–53.

Keys, A.; and Parlin, R. W. 1966. Serum cholesterol response to changes in dietary lipids. *Am. J. Clin. Nutr.* 19:175–181.

Keys, A.; Taylor, H. L.; Blackburn, H.; Brozek, J.; Anderson, J. J.; and Simonson, E. 1963. Coronary heart disease among Minnesota business and professional men followed fifteen years. *Circulation* 28:381–395.

Klinebaum, D. G.; Kupper, L. L.; and Cassel, J. C. 1971. Multivariate analysis of the risk of coronary heart disease in Evans County, Georgia. *Arch. Int. Med.* 128:943–948.

Kozarevič, D.; Pirc, B.; Dawber, T. R.; Gordon, T.; Zukel, W. J.; and Vojvodič, N. 1976. The Yugoslavia cardiovascular disease survey. I, The incidence of coronary heart disease by area. *J. Chron. Dis.* 29:405–414.

Larsson, B. 1978. Obesity: A population study of men with special reference to development and consequences for health, 146 pp. Göteborg.; Gotab, Kungälv,

Leon, A. S., and Blackburn, H. 1977. The relationship of physical activity to coronary heart disease and life expectancy. *Ann. N.Y. Acad. Sci.* 301:561–578.

Liu, K.; Stamler, J.; Dyer, A.; McKeever, J.; McKeever, P. 1978. Statistical methods to assess and minimize the role of intra-individual variability in obscuring the relationship between dietary lipids and serum cholesterol. *J. Chron: Dis.* 31:399–418.

McDonough, J. R.; Hames, C. G.; Stulb, S. C.; and Garrison, G. E. 1965. Coronary heart disease among Negroes and Whites in Evans County, Georgia. *J. Chron. Dis.* 18:443–468.

Mancini, M., and diMarino, L. 1973. Alimentazione e aterosclerosé. *L'Ospedale Maggiore* 68(5):304–313.

Mann, G. V. 1974. The influence of obesity on health. *New Eng. J. Med.* 291:178–195, 226–232.

———1977. Current concepts, diet-heart: End of an era. *New Eng. J. Med.* 297:644–680.

Mann, G. V.; Pearson, G.; and Gordon, T.; and Dawber, T. R. 1962. Diet and cardiovascular disease in the Framingham Study: I, measurement of dietary intake. *Am. J. Clin. Nutr.* 11:200–225.

Mantel, N., and Haenszel, W. 1959. Statistical aspects of the analysis of data from retrospective studies of disease. *J. Nat. Cancer Inst.* 22:719.

Masironi, F. 1970. Dietary factors and coronary heart disease. *Bull. WHO* 42:103–114.

Medallie, J. H.; Neufeld, H. N.; Riss, E.; Groen, J. J.; Kahn, H. A.; and Bachrach, G. H. 1968. Variations in prevalence of ischemic heart disease in defined segments of the male population of Israel. *Israel J. Med. Sci.* 4:755–788.

Menotti, A. 1973. Epidemiologia delle complicazioni dell'arteriosclerosi. *Minerva Med.* 64:1233–41.

Menotti, A.; Capocacia, R.; Conti, S.; Farchi, G.; Mariotti, S.; Verdecchia, A.; Keys, A.; Karvonen, M.; and Punsar S. 1977. Identifying subsets of major risk factors in multivariate estimation of coronary risk. *J. Chron. Dis.* 30:557–565.

Menotti; A., Puddu; V.; Monti, M.; and Fidanza, F. 1969. Habitual physical activity and myocardial infarction. *Cardiologia* 54:119–128.

Montoye, H. J. 1975. *Physical activity and health: An epidemiologic study of an entire community.* Englewood Cliffs, N.J.: Prentice-Hall.

Montoye, H. J.; Block, W. D.; Metzner, H. L.; and Keller, J. B. 1976. Habitual physical activity and serum lipids: Males 16–64 in a total community. *J. Chron. Dis.* 29:697–709.

Morris, J. N.; Chave, S. W. P.; Adam, C.; Sirey, C.; Epstein, L.; and Sheehan, D. J. 1973. Vigorous exercise in leisure time and the incidence of coronary heart disease. *Lancet* 1:333–339.

Morris, J. N.; Heady, J. A.; and Raffle, P. A. B. 1956. Physique of London busmen: Epidemiology of uniforms. *Lancet* 2:569–570.

Morris, J. N.; Heady, J. A.; Raffle, P. A. B.; Roberts, C. G.; and Parks, J. N. 1953. Coronary heart disease and physical activity of work. *Lancet* 2:1053–7, 1111–20.

Paul, O. 1971. Risks of mild hypertension: A ten year report. *Br. Heart J.* 33(Suppl. 6): 116–121.

Paul, O.; Lepper, M. H.; Phelan, W. H.; Dupertuis, G. W.; McMillan, A.; McKean, H.; and Park, H. 1963. A longitudinal study of coronary heart disease. *Circulation* 28:20–31.

Pekkarinen, M. 1967. Chemical analysis in connection with dietary surveys in Finland. *Voeding* 28:609–616.

Pekkarinen, M.; Kivioja, S.; and Jortikka, A. 1967. A comparison of the food intake of rural families estimated by one-day recall and precise weighing methods. *Voeding* 28:470–476.

Pooling Project Research Group. 1978. Relationship of blood pressure, serum cholesterol, smoking habit, relative weight and ECG abnormalities to incidence of major coronary events: Final report of the Pooling Project. *J. Chron. Dis.* 31:201–306.

Punsar, S., and Karvonen, M. J. 1976. Physical activity and coronary heart disease in populations from East and West Finland. *Adv. Cardiol.* 18:196–207.

Robertson, T. L.; Kato, H.; Gordon, T.; Kagan, A.; Rhoads, G. C.; Land, C. E.; Worth, R. M.; Belsky, J. L.; Dock, D. S.; Miyanishi, M.; and Kawamoto, S.

1977. Epidemiologic studies of coronary heart disease and stroke in Japanese men living in Japan, Hawaii, and California. *Am. J. Cardiol.* 39:244–249.

Roine, P.; Pekkarinen, M.; and Karvonen, M. J. 1964. Dietary studies in connection with epidemiology of heart diseases: Results in Finland. *Voeding* 25:384–393.

Roine, P.; Pekkarinen, M.; Karvonen, M. J.; and Kihlberg, J. 1958. Diet and cardiovascular disease in Finland. *Lancet* 26 (July):173–175.

Rose, G. A. 1962. The diagnosis of ischaemic heart pain and intermittent claudication in field surveys. *Bull. WHO* 27:645–658.

Rose, G. A., and Blackburn, H. 1968. *Cardiovascular survey methods.* Geneva: World Health Organization mono. no. 56.

Rosenman, R. H.; Brand, R. J.; Jenkins, C. D.; Friedman, M.; Straus, R.; and Wurm, M. 1975. Coronary heart disease in Western Collaborative Group Study: Final follow-up experience in 8½ years. *J. Am. Med. Assoc.* 233:872–877.

Seltzer, C. C. 1966. Some re-evaluations of the build and blood pressure study, 1959, as related to ponderal index, somatotype and mortality. *New Eng. J. Med.* 274:254–259.

Seltzer, C. C., and Mayer, J. 1965. Simple criterion of obesity. *Postgrad. Med.* 38:A101–A107.

Seltzer, C. C.; Siegelaub, A. B.; Friedman, G. D.; and Collen, M. F. 1974. Differences in pulmonary function related to smoking habits and race. *Am. Rev. Resp. Dis.* 110:598–608.

Shurtleff, D. 1974. Some characteristics related to the incidence of cardiovascular disease and death: The Framingham Study, 16-year follow-up (section 30). W. B. Kannel and T. Gordon, eds., Washington, D.C.: DHEW publ. no. (HIH) 74–599.

Sokolow, M. and Perloff, D. 1961. The prognosis of essential hypertension treated conservatively. *Circulation* 23:697–713.

Stamler, J. 1973. Primary prevention in mass community efforts to control the major coronary risk factors: The challenges and possibilities—critical issues and outlook for the future. *J. Occup. Med.* 15:54–59.

Stamler, J. 1978. Lifestyles, major risk factors, proof and public policy. George Lyman Duff Memorial Lecture. *Circulation.* 58:3–19.

Stamler, J.; Berkson, D. M.; Mojonnier, L.; Lindberg, H. A.; Hall, Y.; Levinson, M.; M.; Burkey, F.; Miller, W.; Epstein, M. B.; and Andelman, S. L. 1968. Epidemiological studies on atherosclerotic coronary heart disease: Causative factors and consequent preventive approaches. *Progr. Biochem. Pharmacol.* 4:30–49.

Stamler, J.; Lindberg, H. A.; Berkson, D. M.; Shaffer, A.; Miller, W.; Poindexter, A. 1960. Prevalence and incidence of coronary heart disease in strata of the labor force of a Chicago industrial corporation. *J. Chron. Dis.* 11:405–420.

Stamler, J.; Stamler, R.; and Shekelle, R. B. 1970. Regional differences in prevalence, incidence and mortality from atherosclerotic coronary heart disease. In

Ischaemic heart disease, J. H. deHaas, H. C. Hemker, and H. A. Snellen, eds. Leiden, Netherlands: Leiden University Press.
Taylor, H. L. 1978. Personal communication and unpublished data.
Taylor, H. L.; Blackburn, H.; Brozek, J.; Parlin, R. W.; and Puchner, T. 1967. Railroad employees in the United States. *Acta Med. Scand.* Suppl. 460, pp. 55–115.
Taylor, H. L.; Blackburn, H.; and Keys, A. 1970. Five-year follow-up of employees of selected U.S. railroad companies. *Am. Heart Assoc.* Mono. 29, pp. 120–139.
Taylor, H. L.; Buskirk, E. R.; and Remington, R. D. 1973. Problems in temperature regulation and exercise. *Fed. Proc.* 32:1623–27.
Taylor, H. L.; Parlin, R. W.; Blackburn, H.; and Keys, 1966. Problems in the analysis of the relationship of coronary heart disease to physical activity or its lack with special reference to sample size and occupation withdrawal. In *Physical activity in health and disease*, pp. 242–261, K. Evang and K. Lange Andersen, eds. Oslo: Oslo Universitetsborlaget.
Tibblin, G.; Wilhelmsen, L.; and Werkö, L. 1975. Risk factors for myocardial infarction and death due to ischemic heart disease and other causes. *Am. J. Cardiol.* 35:514–528.
Truett, J.; Cornfield, J.; and Kannel, W. 1967. Multivariate analysis of the risk of coronary heart disease. *J. Chron. Dis.* 20:511–524.
Walker, S. H., and Duncan, D. B. 1967. Estimation of the probability of an event as a function of several independent variables. *Biometrika* 54:167–179.
West, R. O.; and Hayes, O. B. 1968. Diet and serum cholesterol levels. A comparison between vegetarians and non-vegetarians in a Seventh Day Adventist group. *Am. J. Clin. Nutr.* 21:853–862.
Westlund, K., and Nicolaysen, R. 1972. Ten-year mortality related to serum cholesterol. *Scand. J. Clin. Lab. Invest.* 30:Suppl. 127.
White, P. D. 1956. Clinical studies in Italy, 1954. In *World trends on Cardiology*, pp. 62–68, A. Keys and P. D. White, eds. New York: Heober-Harper.
Wilhelmsen, L.; and Tibblin, G. 1966. Tobacco smoking in fifty-year old men: I, Respiratory symptoms and ventilatory function tests. *Scand. J. Resp. Dis.* 47:121–130.
Wilhelmsen, L.; Wedel, H.; and Tibblin, G. 1973. Multivariate analyses of risk factors for coronary heart disease. *Circulation* 48:950–958.
Wilson, A. C. 1958. Biological and social factors which influence life insurance selection. In *Life insurance and medicine: The prognosis and underwriting of disease*, pp. 379–419, H. E. Ungerleider, and R. S. Gubner, eds. Springfield, Ill.: C. C. Thomas.
Yater, W. M.; Traum, A. H.; Brown, W. G.; Fitzgerald, R. P.; Geisler, M. A.; and Wilson, B. B. 1948. Coronary artery disease in men 18–39 years of age: Report of 866 cases, 450 with necropsy examination. *Am. Heart J.* 36:344, 683.
Yerushalmy, J., and Hilleboe, H. E. 1957. Fat in the diet and mortality from heart disease. *NY J. Med.* 57:2343–54.

Index

Accidents, deaths due to, 68–69
Acheson, R. M., 132
Adelson, S. F., 254
Age: of cohorts, 3, 15; as risk factor, 14, 96–97, 100, 101–102, 320, 321, 341; distribution and standardization, 22–24; of prevalence men, 43–45, 51–53; and incidence of CHD, 94–95, 100–101; and ten-year death rate, 97–98; correlated with other variables, 98–99; and comparability of cohorts, 99–100; and blood pressure, 105, 106, 119, 321, 322; and cholesterol, 132; and weight, 163, 168, 186, 190; and physical activity, 198; and pulse rate, 220, 221, 233; and respiratory function, 236–239, 246, 332; and vital capacity, 239–241, 243
Aging, normal response to, 338
Albany, N.Y., 1, 2, 191, 315; follow-up studies in, 11; prevalence of CVD at entry, 39; studies on blood pressure, 105
Anaerobic exercise, 213–214, 217, 330
Anderson, J. T., 249, 250, 255, 258, 340
Angina pectoris: definition of, 13, 14, 18–19; in Framingham, 39; comparability of data on, 40; prevalence of, at entry, 44; deaths from, 48–53; incidence and ten-year coronary death rate, 91; and relative body weight, 180–181, 184, 192
Antarctica, 255
Antonis, A., 255
Aravanis, Christ, 7, 248, 249
Archer, M., 259
Areas represented in study, 6–7. *See also* Cohorts
Arrhythmias, 91–92

Atherosclerosis: and blood pressure, 119; and smoking habits, 152

Baird, J. T., 132
Bantu, 316
Belgrade, cohort from University of, 6, 9, 15; incidence among, 10; ten-year deaths, 65, 67, 69; ten-year incidence, 86, 88; age correlated with other variables, 98; age of men at entry, 100; blood pressure, 104; cholesterol, 122, 133; smoking habits, 136, 137, 138, 139; relative weight and fatness, 164–166, 168, 175, 185–186; physical activity, 198, 200, 201; resting pulse rate, 220, 221, 222; respiratory function, 237; vital capacity, 245; diet, 250–253; multivariate analyses of, 266, 268. *See also* Yugoslavia
Berkson, D. M., 190, 218
Billewicz, W. Z., 163
Billings, F. T., 191
Blackburn, Henry, 18, 19, 161, 203, 212, 213, 244, 258
Blood pressure, 1; measurement of, 17–18; of prevalence men, 44–45; and age, 98, 119, 321, 322; as risk factor, 100, 109–114, 293, 294, 315, 319–320, 321–323, 341; and ten-year death rates, 104, 106–109; correlated with other variables, 105–106; systolic vs. diastolic, 105, 118, 282–283, 299–301, 321; and incidence, 114–115; validity of multivariate model, 115–117; population comparisons, 117–118; cause and effect in, 118–119; summary of, 119–120; and BMI, 168, 187; and physical activity, 199; and pulse rate, 220, 221; and vital capacity, 243,

Blood pressure (*Continued*)
246; and respiratory function, 244; multivariate analyses of, 278–283; changes in, 299–302, 314
Body mass index (BMI): and CHD, 45; and blood pressure, 105–106; and relative weight, 162–163, 186–187; and other characteristics, 168; in multivariate analyses, 265–271; other studies of, 271–274; as risk factor, 274
Bologna, 1, 256–257
Borhani, N. O., 189
Böttiger, L. E., 189, 193
Breslow, L., 189
Brock, J. F., 1, 152
Bronte-Stewart, B., 1, 152
Brownlee, K. A., 25
Brozek, J., 244
Buzina, Ratko, 6, 72, 248, 249, 257

Cagliari, 1, 256–257
California, 14, 249, 316; follow-up studies in, 11, 13. *See also* Los Angeles
Cancer: in ten-year study, 79–80; and smoking habits, 146–148, 327
Cardiovascular disease (CVD): categories of, 18–20; men free of, 19; prevalence of, at entry, 24
Carlson, L. A., 189, 193
Changes over time, 338–339
Chapman, J. M., 2, 39, 192
Chicago, study of Peoples Gas Co. in, 2, 11, 335; prevalence of CVD at entry, 39; ten-year deaths, 82–83; blood pressure, 105; relative weight, 189–190, 328, 336; resting pulse rate, 218; multivariate analyses of, 272–273, 294
Cholesterol, dietary, 320, 323–325, 334. *See also* Serum cholesterol
Claudication, 19
Cohorts, in study: definition of, 3, 9; rural men, 3–4; railroad men, 4–5; other, 5–6; enrollment of, 316–317; prior characteristics of, 339–340
Comparability, 2, 10; and the Pooling Project, 12–13; of data from examinations, 17; of cohorts, 99–100
Comstock, G. W., 190
Confidence limits, 30–31
Connor, W. D., 257
Cooper, C., 313
Corfu, 4, 7, 9; incidence, 10, 86; ten-year deaths, 65, 67, 69; vs. Crete, 87–88; age, 98, 100; blood pressure, 104; cholesterol, 122, 133; smoking habits, 136, 137, 138, 139; relative body weight and fatness, 164–166, 168, 174, 184–185; physical activity, 198, 210; pulse rate, 220, 221, 222; respiratory function, 237; vital capacity, 245; diet, 250–253; multivariate analyses of, 266, 268. *See also* Greece
Cornfield, J., 26, 27, 264
Coronary heart disease (CHD): definition of, 13; men free of, 19; "hard," 20, 201; prevalence of, at entry, 24; "disappearance" of, 62; death rate vs. incidence, 89–92; death rates from, vs. noncoronary heart disease, 318, 341; incidence of, 319–320
Crete, 4, 7, 9; incidence, 10, 86, 87–88, 319; ten-year deaths, 65, 67, 69; age correlated with other variables, 98; age of men at entry, 100; blood pressure, 104; cholesterol, 122, 133; smoking habits, 136, 137, 138, 139; relative body weight and fatness, 164–166, 168, 174, 184–185; physical activity, 198, 210; pulse rate, 220, 221, 222; respiratory function, 237; vital capacity, 245; diet, 250–253; multivariate analyses of, 266, 268; field trials in, 315. *See also* Greece
Crevalcore, Italy, 4, 9; incidence, 10, 86; age of men from, 22, 100; ten-year deaths, 65, 67, 73; age correlated with other variables, 98; blood pressure, 104; cholesterol, 132, 133; smoking habits, 136, 137, 138, 139; relative body weight and fatness, 164–166, 168, 173; physical activity, 198; pulse rate, 220–221, 222; respiratory function, 237; vital capacity, 245; diet, 250–253; multivariate analyses of, 266, 268; changes in, 305, 307–309
Croatia (Dalmatia, Slavonia), 8, 15; prevalence of CVD at entry, 34–36; NCHD men in, 57–60; ten-year deaths, 72; ten-year incidence of CHD, 87; hypertension, 117–118; cholesterol, 130–131; relative body weight and fatness, 170–171, 180–181; pulse rate, 229; weight change, 297; blood pressure change, 300–301; cholesterol change, 303, 304; smoking habits, 312
Czechoslovakia, 41

Dalmatia, 3, 6, 9; incidence, 10, 86; ten-year deaths, 65, 67, 69; age, 98, 100; blood pressure, 104, 110–112; cholesterol, 122, 133; smoking habits, 136, 137, 138, 139; relative body weight and fatness, 164–166;

physical activity, 198; pulse rate, 220, 221, 222; respiratory function, 237; diet, 250–253; multivariate analyses of, 266, 268. *See also* Croatia

Dawber, T. R., 2, 38, 82, 192, 235, 254

Deaths: causes of, 20–21; attribution of, 21–22; expected, 29–30; from all causes vs. CHD, 48–53; incidence of diagnostic classes, 89–92; and blood pressure, 106–114; and smoking habits, 137. *See also* Ten-year deaths

Decile classification, 31–32

Diagnoses: comparability of, 13; criteria for, 18

Diet, 248–262; and incidence, 251–254; correlated with serum cholesterol, 254–258, 320; vital statistics, 259–261; summary of, 261–262; changes in, 284, 298, 307–311, 314, 339; and risk, 333–335

Di Marino, L., 259

Dimond, G. E., 191

Djordjevic, B. S., 7

Dock, W., 188

Dols, M. J. L., 7

Dontas, A. S., 7

Doyle, J. T., 2, 39, 105, 191

Dublin, Louis, 163, 188

Duncan, D. B., 26, 33, 109, 264, 293

Dyer, A. R., 190, 272, 273

Easty, D. L., 255

Electrocardiogram (ECG), 17; as criterion for diagnosis, 18–19; abnormalities in, as risk factors, 59–60; resting pulse rate from, 218

Entry examination, 7–8, 317; prevalence of CVD at, 34–38

Eskimos, 316

Europe: south vs. north, 80; rural vs. urban, 80–82

Europe, northern (East and West Finland, Zutphen): death rates and smoking habits in, 140, 143–144, 146–147; incidence and smoking habits, 148, 151, 153, 154–158, 159; pulse rate, 223, 224; multivariate analyses of, 269, 276, 279, 280, 281, 283, 290–291; prediction of deaths in, 285–290

Europe, southern (Italy, Greece, Yugoslavia): death rates and smoking habits in, 146–147; incidence and smoking habits, 151, 153, 154–158; pulse rate, 227, 228; multivariate analyses of, 268, 276, 279–280, 283, 290–291; prediction of deaths in, 285–290, 342

Evans County, Ga., 11, 39–40, 193

Fats: saturated, 259, 261, 334; in diet, 316; and serum cholesterol, 320

Fiber, dietary, 334

Fidanza, Flaminio, 6, 248, 249, 307, 308, 309, 340

Fidanza-Alberti, A., 248, 249, 307, 308

Finegan, A., 255

Finland (East and West), 1, 14–15, 316; cohorts in, 3–4, 7, 9, 15; incidence, 10, 86, 319; prevalence of CVD at entry, 34–36; NCHD men in, 57–60; ten-year deaths, 65, 67, 72–73; incidence and age, 94, 100–101; age correlated with other variables, 98; age of men at entry, 100; blood pressure, 104, 109–111, 117–118; cholesterol, 122, 124–125, 128–129, 133, 134; smoking habits, 136, 137, 138, 139, 158, 312, 326; relative body weight and fatness, 164–166, 168, 171–172, 179, 180–181; physical activity, 198, 200, 201, 203–205, 216, 331; pulse rate, 220, 221, 222, 227, 229; respiratory function, 237, 240–243; vital capacity, 237, 238, 244–245; diet, 250–253; multivariate analyses of, 266, 268, 275; weight change, 297; blood pressure change, 300–301; cholesterol change, 303, 304, 305

Follow-up, 8–9; plans for, 3; studies of, 9, 11

Forced expiratory volume (FEV): as risk factor, 242–243, 247, 332–333

Framingham, Mass., studies in, 1, 2, 11, 12, 315; prevalence of CVD at entry, 38–39; deaths, 82–83; blood pressure, 105, 118, 278; obesity, 189, 191, 192; pulse rate, 230–231, 233; vital capacity, 235–236; diet, 254, 335; BMI, 271–272

Fraser, G. E., 256, 258

French, A. J., 188

Friedman, G. D., 235

Geizerova, H., 41

Giron, D. J., 244

Glucose tolerance test, 341

Gordon, T., 40, 118, 189, 192, 193, 284

Gothenburg, Sweden, 11; prevalence of CVD at entry, 40; and relative weight, 189, 193

Grande, F., 249, 250, 255

Greece (Crete, Corfu), 7; trials in, 15; prevalence of CVD at entry, 34–36; ten-year deaths, 76; ten-year incidence, 87; blood pressure, 110–112, 117–118; cholesterol, 124–125, 130–131, 132, 134; smoking habits, 141–142, 143–144, 149–150, 157, 158, 326; relative body weight and fatness,

Greece (*Continued*)
173–174, 184–185; physical activity, 200, 201, 210, 211, 216; pulse rate, 223–224, 229; vital capacity, 237–239, 244; respiratory function, 240–243; weight change, 297; blood pressure change, 300–301; cholesterol change, 303, 306; smoking-habit change, 312. *See also* Corfu; Crete

Green Bay, Wisc., 4
Gyarfas, Ivan, 8

Haenszel, W., 25, 33
Hartog, C. den, 248, 254
Hawaii, 14, 249, 284, 316; prevalence of CVD at entry, 40; relative body weight, 193
Hayes, O. B., 256
Heart disease, *see* Cardiovascular disease; Coronary heart disease; Noncoronary heart disease
Hechter, H. H., 189
Hegsted, D. M., 249
Height and respiratory function, 236–239, 246, 332
Hejl, Z., 41
Hensler, N. M., 244
Heyden, S., 193
Hilleboe, H. F., 259
Honolulu, 284
Hungary, 8
Hutchinson, J. J., 161
Hypertension: degrees of, 103, 323; and CHD death rates, 117; and body weight, 191. *See also* Blood pressure
Hypertensive vascular disease, 61

Incidence of heart disease: crude data on, 10; follow-up studies, 11; comparability of rates, 12–13; age-standardized, 24–25, 100–101; and blood pressure, 114–115; and cholesterol, 128–132; and smoking habits, 148–152; and obesity, 180–186; and pulse rate, 227–230; and diet, 251–254; variations in, 319–320. *See also* Ten-year incidence
Infarcts, *see* Myocardial infarction
Infectious diseases: deaths due to, 68–69; and body weight, 179
Intermittent claudication, 61–62
International Classification of Diseases (ICDA), 20–21, 29
Ireland, 255
Israel: follow-up studies in, 11, 13; prevalence of CVD at entry, 40; diet in, 255
Italy, 1, 5, 9; choice of, 6, 15; prevalence of CVD at entry, 34–36; NCHD men in, 57–60; ten-year deaths, 71–72, 73; blood pressure, 104, 117–118; cholesterol, 122, 124–125, 130, 134; smoking habits, 141–142, 143–144, 149–150, 157, 158–159, 326; relative body weight and fatness, 164–166, 168, 173, 182–183; pulse rate, 223–224, 229; diet, 259–261; multivariate analyses of, 266, 268; weight change, 297; blood pressure change, 300–301; cholesterol change, 303, 305; smoking-habit change, 312; field trials in, 315. *See also* Crevalcore; Montegiorgio; Rome

Italy, rural: incidence of CHD, 87; age and incidence, 100–101; blood pressure, 110, 112; BMI, 179; physical activity, 200, 201, 205–207, 216, 331; respiratory function, 240–243; vital capacity, 244; multivariate analyses of, 275; dietary change, 307–309

Jacobs, D. R., 258
Japan, 1, 14, 316; cohorts from, 3–4, 15; choice of, 6–7; follow-up studies, 11; prevalence of CVD at entry, 34–36, 53–54; NCHD men in, 57–60; blood pressure, 117–118; cholesterol, 126–127, 135, 292; smoking habits, 144, 147, 154, 157, 159, 292, 312, 326; relative body weight and fatness, 177, 292; physical activity, 200, 201, 210–211, 216, 331; pulse rate, 229–230; multivariate analyses, 269–270, 292; deaths from all causes, 292; dietary change, 309–310
Jolliffe, N., 259
Jortikka, A., 248

Kagan, A., 193
Kahn, H. A., 213, 255
Kaiser-Permanente Hospitals, 235–236
Kannel, W. B., 26, 27, 105, 118, 189, 192, 235, 264
Karvonen, Martti J., 7, 248, 340
Kemsley, W. F. F., 163
Kendrick, M. A., 190
Keys, A.: (1949), 1; (1950), 132, 304; (1952), 1, 259; (1953a), 1, 14, 259; (1953b), 1; (1954), 161; (1956), 1, 14; (1957), 1, 259; (1958), 284, 340; (1965), 249, 254, 257; (1967), 3, 17, 31, 32, 161, 164, 255; (1970), 3, 17, 18, 22, 25, 31, 32, 179, 192, 248, 251, 265; (1972a), 17, 118, 235, 284; (1972b), 26; (1972c), 163; (1975), 118; (1979), 248, 254

Kimura, Noboru, 7, 53
Kivioja, S., 248
Klatsky, A. L., 235
Klinebaum, D. G., 284
Kupper, L. L., 284
Kyushu Island, 74–75, 316

Laboratory for Physiological Hygiene (LPH), University of Minnesota, 2, 15, 19–20
Lamm, George, 8
Lard, 72
Larsson, B., 193
Laterality/linearity, 162, 168, 187
Leon, A. S., 213
Life insurance companies: and body weight, 187–189
Likelihood ratio statistic (LRS), 28
Lipoprotein fractionation of blood serum, 340–341
Liu, K., 258
Livesay, V., 190
Lombardy, 259
London, 213
London School of Hygiene Cardiovascular Questionnaire, 19
Longshoremen, studies of, 9–10
Los Angeles, 1, 2, 11, 315; prevalence of CVD at entry, 39; and relative body weight, 192–193
Lung cancer, 73
Lyell, L. P., 192

McDonough, J. R., 39
McNamara, P. M., 192
Madrid, 14
Mancini, M., 259
Mann, G. V., 2, 38, 82, 192, 193, 212, 254
Mantel, N., 25, 33
Mariani, A., 308
Marks, H. H., 188
Masironi, F., 259
Massey, F. J., 192
Mathematical models, 335–338
Maximum likelihood statistics (MLS), 28
Mayer, J., 161
Medallie, J. H., 40
Mediterranean groups: ten-year deaths, 82; incidence and age, 94; blood pressure, 110, 112, 322
Menotti, Alessandro, 18, 28, 205, 208, 259, 265
Metchnikoff, Élie, 76
Methods, 17–33; blood pressure measurement, 17–18; diagnosis and disease classification, 18–22; age distribution and standardization, 22–24; incidence, 24–25; multivariate analysis, 25–32; summary of, 32–33
Metropolitan Life Insurance Co., 161, 187–188
Minneapolis, 335
Minnesota, 1, 2, 315; follow-up studies in, 11
Minnesota, University of. *See* Laboratory for Physiological Hygiene
Montegiorgio, Italy, 4, 9; incidence, 10, 86; age, 22, 98, 100; ten-year deaths, 65, 67, 73; blood pressure, 104; cholesterol, 122, 133; smoking habits, 136, 137, 138, 139; relative body weight and fatness, 164–166, 168, 173; physical activity, 198; pulse rate, 220, 221, 222; respiratory function, 237; vital capacity, 245; diet, 250–253; multivariate analyses of, 266, 268; changes in, 304–305, 307–309. *See also* Italy
Moore, F. E., 2, 38, 82, 192
Morris, J. N., 213
Multiple Risk Factor Intervention Trial (MRFIT) program, 118
Multivariate analyses of Seven Countries data, 263–295; methods compared, 263–265; relative body weight, 265–271; other studies, 271–274; obesity, 275–276; physical activity, 276–277; resting pulse rate, 277–278; blood pressure, 278–283; predictive value of, 284–290, 335–338; coefficients, 290–293; summary of, 293–295
Multivariate analysis, 25–32; multiple linear equation, 26; multiple logistic equation, 26; expected deaths, 29–30; measures of variation and significance, 30–31; decile classes, 31–32
Multivariate model, validity of, 115–117
Myocardial infarction: definition of, 19–21; prevalence of, at entry, 44; deaths from, in ten-year follow-up, 48–50; classes of, 50–51; and age, 51–53; vs. ten-year deaths from CHD, 90

Naples, 1, 14
Nashville, Tenn., 191
Navajo Indians, 316
Neoplasms: and smoking habits, 146–148, 157, 159, 327
Netherlands, 7, 15, 319, 326. *See also* Zutphen
New Zealand, 256
Nicotera, Italy, 7

Noncoronary heart disease (NCHD): prevalence of, at entry, 54–57; follow-up, 57–60; hypertensive vascular disease, 61; intermittent claudication, 61–62; death rates of, vs. coronary heart disease, 318

Obesity, and overweight, 161–195; as risk factor, 161–162, 187–193, 320, 327–329, 341–342; measures of relative weight, 162–164, 275; differences among cohorts, 164–169; ten-year death rate, 169–179; and incidence, 180–186; correlated with other variables, 186–187; other studies of, 187–193; summary of, 193–195. *See also* Body mass index; Relative body weight; Weight

Olive oil, 72, 80, 87
Oslo, 11, 13
Overweight. *See* Obesity

Parlin, R. W., 212, 249
Paul, Oglesby, 39, 105, 163
Pekkarinen, M., 248
Perloff, D., 191
Physical activity, 196–217; and prevalence of CHD, 46–48; of NCHD men, 54–56; and ten-year deaths, 69–71, 200–212; classes of, 196–198; as risk factor, 198, 206, 215–216, 294, 320, 329–332, 341; correlated with other variables, 198–200; and prevalence vs. incidence rates, 212; other studies of, 212–215; summary of, 215–217; and pulse rate, 220, 222, 233; and vital capacity, 243; multivariate analyses of, 276–277; changes in, 298
Poisonings, deaths due to, 68–69
Polyunsaturated fatty acids, 253
Ponderal index, 132, 163
Pooling Project Research Group, 2, 12; incidence and age in, 94–95; multivariate analyses, 273–274
Prevalence of CHD: at time of entry, 34–38; in other studies, 38–41; characteristics of prevalence men, 41–46; and physical activity, 46–48; at ten-year follow-up, 48–53; of heart disease other than CHD, 54–62; "disappearance" of CHD, 62; summary of, 62–63
Prognosis, data for, 19
Puerto Rico, 11, 40
Pulse rate. *See* Resting pulse rate

Railroad men, United States, 4–5, 15; prevalence of CVD at entry, 34–36; ten-year deaths among, 64–65. *See also* Rome; United States
Reexaminations, 15. *See also* Ten-year follow-up
Relative body weight: measures of, 162–164; multivariate analyses of, 265–274; as risk factor, 274, 293–294, 320, 327–329; changes in, 297–299, 313. *See also* Body mass index; Obesity
Respiratory function, 235–247; measurement of, 236; relation of, to height and age, 236–239; and ten-year death rate, 239–243; as risk factor, 239, 242, 332–333; correlated with other variables, 243–246; summary of, 246–247
Resting pulse rate, 218–234; and BMI, 168, 187; and physical activity, 199; differences in, among cohorts, 219–220; as risk factor, 219, 220, 223, 227, 233, 294, 332; correlated with other variables, 220–223; and ten-year death rate, 223–227; and incidence of CHD, 227–230; other studies of, 230–233; summary of, 233–234; and vital capacity, 243; multivariate analyses of, 277–278
Rhoads, C. G., 193
Risk factors, 1; blood pressure, 1, 17–18, 100, 109–114, 293, 294; serum cholesterol, 1–2, 133–135, 293, 323–325; age, 14, 96–97, 100, 101–102; smoking habits, 145, 152; obesity, 161–162, 270, 274, 275–276, 327–329; physical activity, 198, 206, 294, 329–331; resting pulse rate, 219, 220, 223, 227, 294, 332; respiratory function, 239, 242, 332–333; vital capacity, 239, 294; forced expiratory volume, 242–243; diet, 259–261; relative body weight, 293–294; early choices of, 315–316; mathematical analysis of, 335–338; conclusions concerning, 341–342
Robertson, T. L., 193, 284
Roentgenograms, 340
Rohrer index, 163
Roine, P., 1, 248
Rome, railroad men in, 5, 9; incidence, 10, 86, 318; ten-year deaths, 65, 67, 71–72, 318; age, 98, 100; cholesterol concentration, 133; smoking habits, 136, 137, 138, 139; relative body weight, 173; physical activity, 198, 200, 201, 207–208, 216; pulse rate, 220, 221, 222; diet, 250–253
Rose, G. A., 19

Rosenman, R. H., 193
Rural areas: advantages of study in, 3; vs. urban, 80–81; changes in, 296–297. *See also* Italy, rural

Saint Louis, 4
San Francisco, longshoremen in, 4, 11, 189
Santucek, M., 41
Sardinia, 259
Schwartz, M. S., 118
Sdrin, H., 248, 249
Seattle, 4
Seltzer, C. C., 161, 244
Serbia (Belgrade, Velika Krsna, Zrenjanin), 4, 6, 7, 15; prevalence of CVD at entry, 34–36; NCHD men in, 57–60; ten-year deaths, 76–77; ten-year incidence, 87; blood pressure, 117–118; cholesterol, 129; relative body weight and fatness, 168, 175, 185–186; pulse rate, 229; respiratory function, 240–243; vital capacity, 244; weight change, 297; blood pressure change, 300–301; cholesterol change, 303, 306; smoking-habit change, 312. *See also* Belgrade; Velika Krsna; Zrenjanin
Serum cholesterol, 121–135; as risk factor, 1, 14, 121, 293, 315, 319–320, 323–325, 341; in prevalence men, 44–45; and age, 99, 339; and blood pressure, 105; figures for cohorts, 121–123; ten-year death rate, 123–128; and incidence, 128–132; correlated with other variables, 132–133; summary of, 133–135; and smoking habits, 152–153; and BMI, 168, 187; and physical activity, 199; and pulse rate, 220, 221; and vital capacity, 243; and diet, 249, 254–258; changes in, 302–307, 314. *See also* Cholesterol, dietary
Seventh-Day Adventists, 256
Shekelle, R. B., 259
Shurtleff, D., 231, 233, 236, 271–272
Siegelaub, A. B., 235
Skinfold thickness: as measure of obesity, 164, 165; and heart-disease death rate, 166; and BMI, 168, 193; in multivariate analyses, 275, 294
Slavonia, 6, 9; ten-year deaths, 65, 67, 69; ten-year incidence of CHD, 86; age, 98, 100; blood pressure, 104; cholesterol, 122, 133; smoking habits, 136, 137, 138, 139; relative body weight and fatness, 164–166; physical activity, 198; pulse rate, 220, 221, 222; respiratory function, 237; diet, 250–253; multivariate analyses of, 266, 268; changes in, 304
Smoking habits, 136–160; of men with and without CHD at entry, 41–43, 136; of NCHD men, 56–57; and blood pressure, 105; and ten-year death rate, 140–146; as risk factor, 145, 152, 154, 315, 320, 325–327, 341; and death from neoplasms, 146–148; and incidence, 148–152; regional differences in, 152–154; and probability of death, 154–158; summary of, 158–159; and BMI, 168, 187; and pulse rate, 220, 221; and vital capacity, 244, 246; changes in, 311–313
Sokolow, M., 191
South Africa, 1, 14, 316
Spain, 1, 316
Stamler, Jeremiah, 39, 82–83, 105, 249, 258
Stamler, R., 259
Standard errors of means, 30–31
Stockholm, 193
Stroke (cerebrovascular disease), 19, 75
Sucrose: as risk factor, 252–253, 262, 320, 334
Swanell, R. J., 256, 258
Sweden, 193. *See also* Gothenburg; Stockholm

Tanushimaru, Japan, 4, 9; incidence, 10, 86; ten-year deaths, 65, 67, 74–75; age, 98, 100; blood pressure, 104; cholesterol, 122, 133; smoking habits, 136, 137, 138, 139, 144; relative body weight and fatness, 164–166, 168, 177–178; physical activity, 198; pulse rate, 218, 220, 221, 222; diet, 250–253; multivariate analyses, 266, 268, 269–270. *See also* Japan
Tarahumara Indians, 257
Taylor, H. L., 4, 46, 203, 213, 244
Tecumseh, Mich., 2, 11, 12
Ten-year deaths, 317–318; from all-causes vs. CHD, 64–67; of NCVD men at entry, 67–68; from causes other than heart disease, 68–69; by cohorts, 69–77; by national groups, 77–79; from cancer and other neoplasms, 79–80; comparison of cohort groupings, 80–82; other studies, 82–83; summary of, 83–84; and age, 97–98; and cholesterol, 123–128; and smoking habits, 137, 140–146; and BMI, 169–179, 194, 267; and physical activity, 200–212; and pulse rate, 223–227; and respiratory function, 239–243; multivariate analyses of, 290–293
Ten-year follow-up, changes at, 296–314; body weight, 297–299; blood pressure,

Ten-year follow-up (*Continued*)
299–302; cholesterol, 302–307; diet, 307–311; smoking habits, 311–313; summary of, 313–314
Ten-year incidence, of CHD, 85–95; comparisons of cohorts within regions, 85–89; incidence of diagnostic classes vs. CHD death rate, 89–92; summary of, 93–94; and age, 94–95; and body weight, 180–186, 194
Thomson, A. M., 163
Tibblin, G., 40, 189, 244
Tobacco, 327
Truett, J., 26, 27, 263, 264
Twin City, 254
Tuberculosis: deaths due to, 69; and body weight, 179

Underweight, as hazard, 328, 342
United States, railroad men in study, 4–5, 9, 15; incidence, 10; NCHD men in, 57–60; ten-year deaths, 65, 67, 69–71, 318; age, 98, 100; blood pressure, 104, 109–110, 117–118; cholesterol, 122, 124, 133, 134; smoking habits, 136, 137, 138, 139, 141–143, 150–151, 156–157, 158; relative body weight and fatness, 164–166, 168, 169–170; physical activity, 198, 200, 201–203, 216, 330–331; pulse rate, 220, 221, 222; respiratory function, 237, 240; vital capacity, 239–243, 244–245; diet, 250–253; multivariate analyses of, 266, 268, 270–271, 275, 276, 279, 281, 283, 291; changes in, 298–299, 302, 305–307, 314; dietary change, 310–311; smoking-habit change, 311–313
United States, vital statistics on age in, 22–23
Urban areas, vs. rural, 80–81
Ushibuka, Japan, 3, 4, 9; incidence, 10, 86; ten-year deaths, 65, 67, 74–75; age, 98, 100; blood pressure, 104; cholesterol, 122, 133; smoking habits, 136, 137, 138, 139, 144; relative body weight and fatness, 164–166, 168, 177–178; physical activity, 198; pulse rate, 218, 220, 221, 222; diet, 250–253; multivariate analyses of, 269–270, 292. *See also* Japan

Velika Krsna (Serbia), 4, 9; incidence, 10, 86; ten-year deaths, 65, 67, 76–77; age, 98, 100; blood pressure, 104; cholesterol, 122, 133; smoking habits, 136, 137, 138, 139; relative body weight and fatness, 164–166, 168, 175, 185–186; physical activity, 198; pulse rate, 220, 221, 222; respiratory function, 237; vital capacity, 245; diet, 250–253; multivariate analyses of, 266, 268
Violence, deaths due to, 68–69
Vital capacity: and physical activity, 199–200; pulse rate, 220, 221; respiratory function, 237; and age, 246; as risk, 295, 333
Vital Statistics of the United States, 22, 29, 83, 97, 318

Walker, S. H., 26, 33, 109, 264, 293
Washington, D.C., 213
Wedel, H., 40
Weight (obesity; skinfolds): of prevalence men, 46; and age, 99, 339; and blood pressure, 105; and fatness, 162; under- vs. over-, 274. *See also* Body mass index; Obesity; Relative body weight
Werkö, L., 189
West, R. O., 256
Western Collaborative Group Study, 193
White, P. D., 1
Wilhelmsen, L., 40, 189, 244
Wilson, A. C., 188
World Health Organization, 318

Yater, W. M., 188
Yerushalmy, J., 259
Yugoslavia (Dalmatia, Slavonia, Velika Krsna, Zrenjanin, Belgrade), 9, 11, 15; cholesterol levels, 126, 134; smoking habits, 140–141, 143–144, 148–149, 159, 326; relative body weight and fatness, 168, 175; physical activity, 200, 201, 209–210, 216, 331; pulse rate, 225

Zrenjanin (Serbia), 6, 9, 15; ten-year deaths, 65, 67, 76–77; incidence, 86; age, 98, 100; blood pressure, 104; cholesterol, 122, 133; smoking habits, 136, 137, 138, 139; relative body weight and fatness, 164–166, 168, 175, 185–186; physical activity, 198; respiratory function, 237; vital capacity, 245; diet, 250–253; multivariate analyses of, 266, 268. *See also* Serbia
Zutphen (Netherlands), 5–6, 9, 15; incidence, 10, 86, 88–89; age, 22, 98, 100; prevalence of CVD at entry, 34–36; NCHD men in, 57–60; ten-year deaths, 65, 67, 74; blood pressure, 104, 117–118; cholesterol, 122, 126–127, 128–130, 133, 134; smoking habits, 136, 137, 138, 139, 158; relative

body weight and fatness, 164–166, 168, 175–177, 179, 183–184; physical activity, 198, 200, 201, 208–209, 216, 331; pulse rate, 220, 221, 222, 227, 228, 229; diet, 250–253; multivariate analyses of, 266, 268, 275; weight change, 297; blood pressure change, 300–301; cholesterol change, 303, 305, 307; smoking-habit change, 312

Bei Fragen zur Produktsicherheit wenden Sie sich bitte an:
If you have any questions regarding product safety,
please contact:

Walter de Gruyter GmbH
Genthiner Straße 13
10785 Berlin
productsafety@degruyterbrill.com